Strabismus Symposium

Documenta Ophthalmologica Proceedings Series volume 32

Editor H.E. Henkes

Dr W. Junk Publishers   The Hague–Boston–London   1982

Strabismus Symposium
Amsterdam, September 3–4, 1981

Edited by A.Th.M. van Balen
and W.A. Houtman

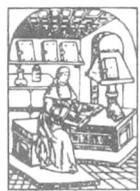

Dr W. Junk Publishers   The Hague–Boston–London   1982

Distributors:

for the United States and Canada

Kluwer Boston Inc.
190 Old Derby Street
Hingham, MA 02043
USA

for all other countries

Kluwer Academic Publishers Group
Distribution Center
P.O. Box 322
3300 AH Dordrecht
The Netherlands

Library of Congress Cataloging in Publication Data

Strabismus Symposium (1981 : Amsterdam, Netherlands)
    Strabismus Symposium, Amsterdam, September 3-4, 1981.

    (Documenta ophthalmologica. Proceedings series ;
v. 32)
    1. Strabismus--Congresses. I. Balen, A. Th. M. van.
II. Houtman, W. A. III. Series. [DNLM: 1. Strabismus--
Congresses. W3 DO637 v. 32 1981 / WW 415 S896s 1981]
RE771.S85 1981   617.7'62   82-16
                                                 AACR2

ISBN-13: 978-94-009-7999-4   e-ISBN-13: 978-94-009-7997-0
DOI: 10.1007/978-94-009-7997-0

Cover design: Max Velthuijs

Dr W. Junk Publishers, P.O. Box. 13713, 2501 ES The Hague, The Netherlands.

CONTENTS

OPENING ADDRESS

Ladies and Gentlemen, my dear colleagues:

The meeting of the CESSD in Amsterdam has been opened. Maybe this will be the last meeting in its present form. A transformation is taken into consideration. Well, it is an astonishing coincidence that this event is to take place in this year and in this country. As regards the time, it is now exactly twenty years ago since the CESSD was founded in Paris, namely in the autumn of 1961. As regards the place, the Netherlands, a decisive impetus to the foundation of the CESSD was given by a Dutchman, namely by our colleague Mr. Jonkers.

I suppose that a vast majority of the participants in this meeting do not know, be it for reasons of age, the way that led to the foundation of the CESSD. In order to prevent this fact from leading to false ideas concerning the original meaning and purpose of the organization (which, in my view, too, needs reforms) I am going to take the liberty of taking a short look back at the history of the association.

After the last world war, the ophthalmologists on the European continent who were particularly interested in the problems of strabismus formed an infinitely small group. Switzerland was, to a certain degree, an exception, not the least thanks to the work of Bangerter, and it was, therefore, not a matter of pure chance that owing to an initiative taken by Streiff, stabismus was the main subject of the 1955 meeting of the Schweizer Ophthalmologische Gesellschaft. The meeting was a fruitful one, in all respects, and offered the first opportunity for an exchange of ideas on the continental level.

On the other hand, the 1958 international congress of ophthalmologists in Brussels, from which quite a number of people had expected much, was, to a large extent, as regards strabology, a failure, although strabismus was one of its main subjects. There were numerous reasons for that failure, let me just point out one of them, namely the fact, clearly recognized at the time by Jonkers, that a decisive impediment to productive cooperation, in particular with Anglo-Saxon colleagues, had resulted from the fact that we had neither a uniform terminology nor uniform diagnostic methods with common fundamental principles. To put it exaggeratedly: We were discussing with one another without being sure that we understood one another.

Through the endeavours of several years, Jonkers succeeded in getting

Docum. Ophthal. Proc. Series, Vol. 32, ed. by A.Th.M. van Balen & W.A. Houtman
© *1982, Dr W. Junk Publishers, The Hague. ISBN 90 6193 728 0*

colleagues who were interested in the problems to join up and form a group. Later on, the members of that group were appointed official representatives by their respective national ophthalmological societies. The CESSD was thus officially founded in the autumn of 1961, under the direction of Jules François. Its task consisted in co-ordinating, within a small group on a European level, problems of strabology and in passing the results on to national working parties, which were taking shape more and more everywhere. Those activities were completed by regular meetings on the European level, partly held, intentionally, without dependence on general ophthalmological congresses, somewhat in the style of today's meeting.

From the very beginning, the CESSD called itself a European organization, but that was not true, it being, in the first stage, limited to Western Europe. The credit goes to Thomas, who thanks to his personal contacts with the World Health Organization, created the possibility of the CESSD being joined by representatives of the so-called socialist countries in 1964. Our colleague, Avetisov, of the Moscow Helmholtz Institute became one of our vice-presidents. The sole exception has been up to now, as far as I know, Albania.

This all-European union has been not only a theoretical construction but has withstood many a strain in spite of the political situation that was difficult at that time, too. Numerous colleagues from the other side of the 'Iron Curtain' were in this way offered the possibility of taking part in meetings held in the West for the first time, for example in the 1966 symposium at Giessen.

Vice versa, it was also possible to hold a symposium in 1968 in Leipzig that was harmonious in all respects under the direction of Sachsenweger, despite the entry of troops into Czechoslovakia.

Ladies and Gentlemen,

When presenting you with the historic evolution of the CESSD, I was induced to do so for several reasons. First, because I felt bound to give, here and now, our colleague Mr. Jonkers, our thanks for his contributions. Secondly, I did it for the sake of rectifying false notions. The CESSD has never been a Strabological Society in the usual meaning. I for my part, at least, have always, since its foundation, seen it as an all-European committee charged with the task of creating contacts for mutual understanding and endeavouring to achieve harmony. The fact that, in addition, symposiums with general admission have been organized by the respective national representatives does, in my view, not change the fundamental structure. If we want to keep to that task, we have to question ourselves as to what is the most suitable reform of the CESSD for pursuing that aim. With good will on all sides, we shall certainly find a solution.

Irrespective of the said problem, I wish you full success for your work within the framework of this meeting. I thank you very much for your attention.

C. Cüppers (President)

PHYSIOLOGICAL FIXATION DISPARITY

C. RASHBASS

(Groningen, The Netherlands)

INTRODUCTION

Any dialogue between physiologist and clinician introduces the risk of language difficulties, and these are somewhat different from the language difficulties at any European meeting. The latter arise from a desire to use different words to express the same ideas, but the problem when physiologist confronts clinician is the wish to use the same words for different concepts. In order to try to avoid such misunderstandings some clear definitions are needed at the outset.

The fundamental concepts that are used in talking about the eyes' vergence control system are 'vergence', 'target vergence' and 'disparity'. These are defined in Fig. 1. 'Fixation disparity' is a disparity present during the steady binocular fixation of a target. The question of physiological interest is whether fixation disparity needs to be non-zero in order to maintain the state of vergence of a person with a well-developed, healthy vergence system, when viewing a target situated at any distance within the range of distances at which binocular viewing is unstrained. The most complete studies of the vergence control system fail to answer this question satisfactorily. Westheimer & Mitchell (1956) reported a substantial fixation disparity but Rashbass &

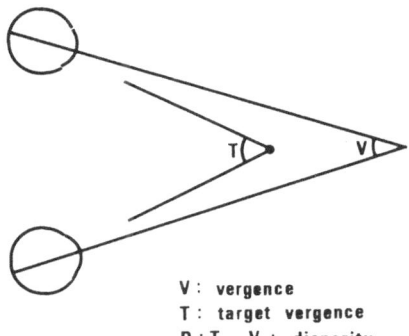

V : vergence
T : target vergence
D : T − V : disparity

Fig. 1. Illustrates the definition of the primary terms: vergence (v): the angle of intersection of the lines of sight; target vergence (t): the vergence that would obtain were the lines of sight directed through the target; disparity (d): the difference between vergence and target vergence.

Docum. Ophthal. Proc. Series, Vol. 32, ed. by A.Th.M. van Balen & W.A. Houtman   3
© *1982, Dr W. Junk Publishers, The Hague. ISBN 90 6193 728 0*

Westheimer (1961) considered this probably to be a recording artifact. Riggs & Niehl (1960), using a contact-lens recording method, considered that any fixation disparity was less than 2'. Rashbass & Westheimer (1961) calibrated their recording system on the assumption of zero fixation disparity. Zuber & Stark (1968) show results implying a large fixation disparity but themselves raise the possibility that it is of instrumental origin.

Does it matter?

There is little doubt that if fixation disparity is non-zero during normal binocular viewing, it is certainly rather small. If our concern were with the question of how well the vergence system functions then such a small error in vergence would not constitute an important deficiency of function. If, on the other hand, our concern is with the question of how the vergence system functions, then the presence or absence of fixation disparity becomes crucial. In the jargon of control-systems theory the presence of a positional error in the stationary steady state implies a zero-order system; if steady-state control is achieved without error then the system is first order or higher and contains at least one non-leaky integrator (Fig. 2). In every-day terms, if vergence requires disparity in order to maintain it, then at any moment during steady binocular fixation the disparity that is present is sufficient incoming information to specify what the level of the vergence should be. By contrast, if different vergence levels can be maintained all with zero disparity then a very different neural process, one involving some form of storage or memory, is required to achieve this.

The argument is sometimes advanced that, in general, a non-zero binocular disparity must be present during fixation because, if one or both eyes are covered the state of vergence will change. When one or both eyes are covered there is no disparity. Whence it follows that during steady binocular fixation there must be a disparity. This argument is fallacious and results from the confusion of two different concepts. When one eye only is fixating there is indeed no disparity, but this is very different from the situation where both eyes are open, where the visual system is being informed that the value of the disparity is zero. An analogous difference exists in comparing the behaviour of an amplifier whose input is taken to zero by grounding it, with the behaviour

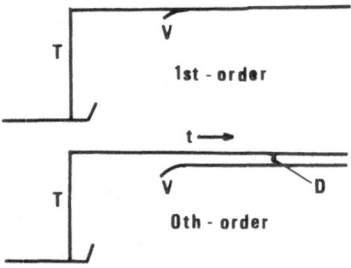

Fig. 2. A diagrammatic illustration of the difference between 1st order systems and zero-order systems. The time course of the change in vergence is omitted as it is irrelevant here. In the state of steady fixation, only zero-order systems have a maintained disparity.

4

of the same amplifier when it has no input, that is its input terminal is not connected to anything, in which situation the amplifier output is generally undefined.

METHODS

What methods are available to discover whether there is a fixation disparity?

Broadly they can be classified into two classes: subjective and objective. The objective methods involve recording eye position and to be suitable for detecting a small fixation disparity require to satisfy two conditions. The first condition is that the method be absolutely callibrated without reference to fixation positions of the eyes, for it is the precision of these that is in question. If that condition is satisfied then it is further required that the method be able to record eye position with a precision of about 1'. In general, existing methods do not satisfy these conditions. Subjective methods are variants of the method described by Ogle; two vertical nonius lines of which each eye sees only one, are surrounded by a binocularly viewed fixation target. This method suffers from two defects. Firstly, it is not possible to fixate the binocular surround and, at the same time, retain an adequate vernier acuity at the position of the nonius lines. Secondly, it is assumed that the subjectively perceived position of the lines accurately reflects the retinal position of their images. Since it is known that within Panum's fusional area, binocularly viewed lines can retain a fair amount of variation in their disparity, and yet still be perceived by both eyes as being in the same place, it is difficult to be convinced that the link between retinal and perceived position is not equally flexible in the monocular situation.

An attempt to resolve the question of whether fixation disparity is zero under physiological condition has been made by G. Bijl and myself by using afterimages. The method relies on the ability to make stereoscopic judgements about binocular afterimages. It is not obvious, a priori, that this is possible, although some confidence that it is can be drawn from the observations of Shortess & Krauskopf (1961) that the stereoacuity of stabilized images is unimpaired.

The apparatus we used is shown in Fig. 3. The subject views binocularly the virtual image of a fixation target seen by reflection in a thin sheet of glass angled at 45°. The fixation target is adequately illuminated for easy fixation, the rest of the room being in darkness. The reflected image is 90 cm distant from the subject (vergence 4°). Lurking in the darkness on the far side of the sheet of glass is a photographic flash gun, masked down to a vertical slit about 0.5 mm wide and 2 cm high. The distance of the flash gun from the subject can be adjusted by the experimenter. The subject fixates the reflected target, and when he is satisfied that binocular fixation is as accurate as possible he releases a flash. After a few moments a fused binocular afterimage develops, which has a disparity that is determined by the position at which the experimenter has fixed the flash gun. We have used afterimages of this sort for three experiments.

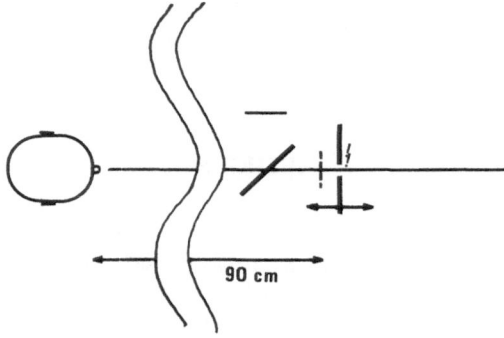

Fig. 3. A diagram of the apparatus. A plate of glass, angled at 45°, allows the subject to see the virtual image (dashed line) of a fixation target at a distance of 90 cm. A flash gun, masked to a vertical slit, can be positioned at distances somewhat less than or greater than 90 cm.

Experiment 1

The purpose of this experiment is to confirm that the disparity of a binocular afterimage can provide stereoscopic information. The subject is instructed to continue fixating the target at 90 cm and to report whether the afterimage is seen in front or behind the fixation target, the choice being forced. After-images will usually be considered to be in front of any opaque surface onto which they are projected because it is not usual to be able to see anything behind such a surface. In order to avoid this misleading occlusal clue we provide a slit in the fixation screen. The subject can easily project the afterimage into this space and an unprejudiced stereoscopic judgement can be made.

If the disparity of the afterimage is available for stereoscopic vision then we should expect that those afterimages formed with +ve (crossed) disparity will be seen in front of the fixation target, and vice versa. We generated after-images with +ve and —ve disparities of $0'$, $3'$ and $6'$ in random order, and in all cases the answers that the subjects gave were correct (Fig. 4). When the disparity was zero the subjects were aware of the uncertainty and arbitrarily

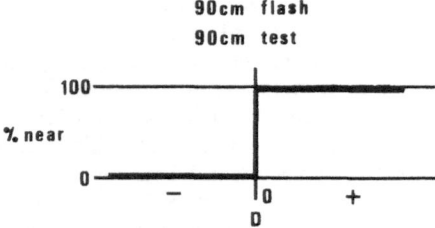

Fig. 4. The result of experiment 1. The disparity imposed on the afterimage is plotted horizontally, and the percentage of such presentations that are reported as appearing nearer to the subject than the fixation target plotted vertically. The thick black line indicates that subjects always saw afterimages with +ve disparity as closer than the fixation target and vice versa.

6

chose to report the afterimage 'nearer' of 'further' in order to co-operate in the forced-choice design of the experiment. We conclude from this experiment that afterimages are valid objects for stereoscopic judgements and proceed to experiment 2.

Experiment 2

This experiment is in all essentials the same as experiment 1 except that immediately after the flash has been released the light illuminating the fixation target at 90 cm is extinguished and a similar fixation target 30 cm from the subject is illuminated. As in experiment 1 the experimenter randomly selects the position of the flashgun to produce a range of +ve and −ve disparities and the subject is again required to report whether the afterimage is seen nearer or further than the fixation target, now at 30 cm.

The result to be expected from this experiment will depend on whether or not the disparity is different when fixating binocularly at 30 cm from what it was when fixating at 90 cm. If the disparity is the same, and in that case, by definition, zero, then flashes with +ve disparity will be seen nearer than the fixation target, and those with −ve disparity, further. If, on the other hand, the disparity at 30 cm is different (probably more +ve) than it was when the flash was released while fixating at 90 cm, then the afterimage having the same disparity as is present while fixating at 30 cm will be seen in the plane of the target. Disparities smaller than that, although they may be positive, will be seen behind the fixation target. These two possible outcomes are illustrated diagrammatically in Fig. 5. In the event, subjects had no difficulty in assigning all the afterimages produced with +ve disparity to the front of the fixation target, and all those with −ve disparity, behind. Of course all the afterimages appeared to be very close to the target. An afterimage produced by a flash 1 cm in front of the 90 cm target is seen only about 1 mm in front of the target at 30 cm. This is the result of the non-linear relation between distance and vergence. Despite this contraction of distance, disparities as small as 3′ were confidently correctly judged. This suggests that if any disparity is required to hold vergence to a distance of 30 cm, it is not greater than 1.5′.

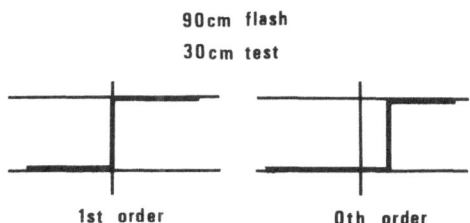

Fig. 5. The two possible results of experiment 2. The ordinate and abscissa are the same as in Fig. 4. If a disparity is present when fixating at 30 cm then afterimages with that disparity will be seen in the place of the target. In the event the results indicated a 1st-order system.

Finally we attempted to confirm this result by carrying out a further experiment. We formed afterimages with disparities selected from the range $3'$, $6'$, $9'$ and $12'$. In this case they were always +ve. As soon as the flash had been released all lights were extinguished and the subject instructed to fixate the afterimage. The vergence loop is now open – vergence movements do nothing to change the disparity. This experiment also is expected to discriminate between a control system that requires error (i.e. disparity) to maintain its output and one that does not. The possible results are shown diagrammatically in Fig. 6.

If no disparity is required in order to maintain binocular fixation, then any attempt to look directly at an afterimage formed with +ve disparity will cause the eyes to converge. Owing the perfectly open feedback loop, this movement will not reduce the disparity. The movement will therefore continue until the eyes can converge no further. Different disparities will cause similar effects. The rate of convergence may depend on the size of the disparity, and the limiting convergence may also depend on the disparity (in the figure it is shown as constant). The crucial expectation is that, as experiment 2 has shown that maintained fixation at 30 cm requires a disparity less than $1.5'$, then in experiment 3 any disparity equal to or greater than that should reach a limiting convergence closer than 30 cm. If, on the other hand, the vergence control system does require disparity to maintain vergence, then looking at an afterimage which has +ve disparity will not drive convergence to a limit, but only to that value which requires the existing disparity to maintain it.

After the subject has released the flash and formed a binocular afterimage with +ve disparity, all lights are extinguished and the subject is required to fixate the afterimage. The afterimage is seen by the subject to move towards him and, after several seconds, to come to rest. The subject now has to esti-

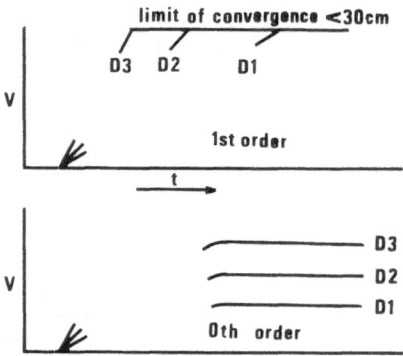

Fig. 6. A diagrammatic representation of the vergence response to fixed disparities (D1, D2, D3). As in Fig. 2 the course of the movement is omitted. First-order systems are expected to generate extreme vergence for all disparities. In zero-order systems the steady state vergence will be strongly dependent on disparity. In the event the system behaves as zero-order.

is provided with a small light, that can be momentarily lit by his pressing a button. He can also adjust the distance that this light is from him. The subject continues to fixate the afterimage carefully and occasionally causes the small light to come on briefly. Usually he can judge whether this brief appearance is seen closer or further than the floating afterimage. He then adjusts the position of the light to bring it closer to the afterimage and tests again. In this way he can rather rapidly find the apparent distance of the afterimage. Precision need be no better than a few centimeters. It soon became very clear that subjects who, in experiment 2, could converge on to a real target at 30 cm with a disparity less than 1.5′, would view an afterimage with a disparity as large as 12′ at a distance much greater than 30 cm, suggesting that the vergence control system does require a disparity in order to maintain vergence.

We conclude from these experiments that binocular fixation of a real target is disparity-free. Fixation of an afterimage, on the other hand, does require disparity. The most likely properties of afterimages to account for this behaviour are that they are stable in retinal position and that they are not affected by accommodation. A better understanding of the behaviour of afterimages as fixation targets requires further study.

REFERENCES

Westheimer, G. & A.M. Mitchell. Eye movement responses to convergence stimuli. Arch. Ophthal., N.Y., 55: 858–856 (1956).
Rashbass, C. & G. Westheimer. Disjunctive eye movements. J. Physiol., 159: 339–360 (1961).
Riggs, L.A. & E.W. Niehl. Eye movements recorded during convergence and divergence. J. opt. Soc. Amer. 50: 913–920 (1960).
Zuber, B.L. & L. Stark. Dynamical characteristics of the fusional vergence eye movement system. IEEE Trans. Sys. Sci. Cyber., SCC4, 72–79 (1968).
Shortess, G.K. & J. Krauskopf. Role of involuntary eye movements in stereoscopic activity. J. opt. Soc. Amer. 51: 555–559 (1961).

Author's address:
Lab. Animale Fysiologie
Rijksuniversiteit
Groningen, The Netherlands

FIXATION DISPARITY AND THE INTERACTION
OF FOVEAL AND NON-FOVEAL FUSION

W. RÜSSMAN & C. VOM EYSER
(Cologne, F.R.G.)

INTRODUCTION

The objective misalignment of haploscopic vernier lines induced by some oculomotor imbalance (e.g. prism strain, heterophoria) is called fixation disparity (Fig. 1; Ogle et al. 1967). As a matter of fact fixation disparity is to correspond to some mismatch of the fusion pattern in the test person's subjective space. How can this mismatch be processed in the test person's visual system? Can this be done by straightforward sensory fusion or is it achieved by partial suppression of bifoveal vision? The interactions between fixation disparity and foveal suppression have been discussed in the literature (Ogle et al. 1967) but — to our best knowledge — nobody really tried to show them.

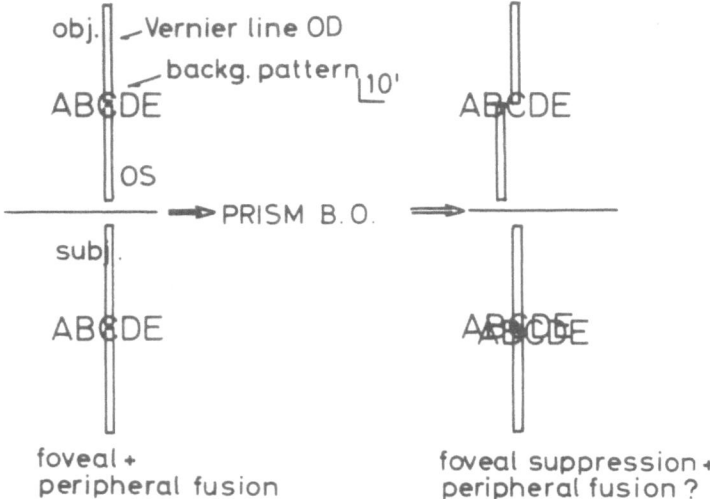

Fig. 1. Schematic representation of fixation disparity settings of a normal test person. Test person's view is shown in the lower part, observer's view in the upper. The prism induced misalignment of vernier lines seen by the observer (upper right = fixation disparity) is to correspond to fusion mismatch in the test person's subjective space.

METHODS

We designed two experimental set-ups to show the presence of suppression with fixation disparity.

In the first set-up (Fig. 2) we projected a rectangle consisting of two triangles visible to each eye separately. This rectangle was at a distance of 20 to 30 min of arc from the stationary vernier line seen by the right eye only. The test person had to realign the vernier first. He was then asked if he could see the both triangles simultaneously or in rapid alternation at least. If not so the test person's statements were interpreted as suppression.

It is obvious from the test design that it indicates the processing of retinal rivalry rather than proving straightforward foveal suppression. For this reason the rectangle was replaced by a small circular mark visible to the right eye only in the second set-up (Fig. 2). The luminance of this mark could be modified by a let of neutral density filters (Table 1). Thus the contrast of the mark could be set to five different levels. Again the test person had to adjust the vernier first. Now the circular mark was presented at increasing contrasts to the level the test person could detect. The respective thresholds were recorded. Measurements were repeated three to five times each in both set-ups.

We used the phase difference haploscope of Aulhorn for the vernier in both set-ups. In the first set-up the haploscope was fitted with additional polarizing foils for the triangular controls. The circular mark used in the second set-up was projected by the third projector of the haploscope.

Figs. 3 and 4 show fixation disparity curves obtained from two normal test persons, Fig. 3 with first set-up, Fig. 4 with second. As usual prism vergence is shown on the abscissa in prism diopters, base out prisms to right, base in prisms to the left. The ordinate gives fixation disparities in min of arc, eso-disparity above, exo-disparity below. Full circles in Fig. 3 indicate disparity settings with simultaneous perception of triangular controls while suppression is shown by empty circles. The latter is found only in the end portion of normal curves with increasing fixation disparities. In Fig. 4, black bars on inset scales indicate threshold contrasts in the second set-up, ranging from 0.13 to 0.25. The total length of black bars on a single

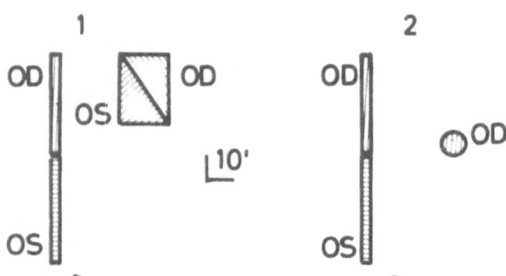

Fig. 2. Modified set-ups to measure fixation disparities. First set-up (left) uses triangular controls to detect foveal fusion failure. Second set-up (right) works with a small circular mark.

Table 1. Background and target (vernier, control) luminance and target contrast in experimental set-up 1 and 2.

	luminance (cd/m²)	contrast
Experiment 1		
background	2	
vernier	8	3.00
control	8	3.00
Experiment 2		
background	4	
vernier	18	3.50
control	4.5	0.13
	5.0	0.25
	6.5	0.63
	9.0	1.25
	12.0	2.00

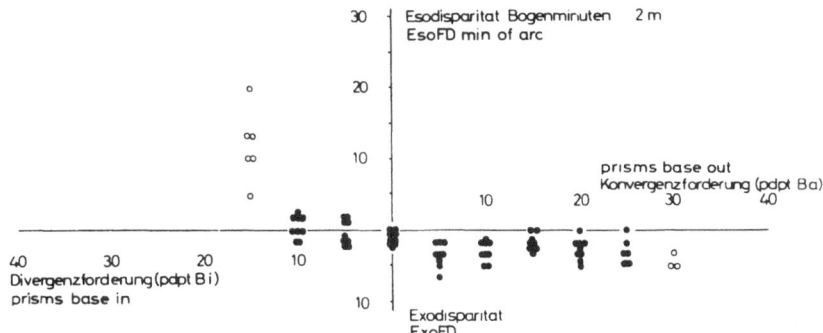

Fig. 3. Fixation disparity curve of a normal test person (first set-up). Full circles indicate simultaneous perception of triangular controls, empty circles suppression.

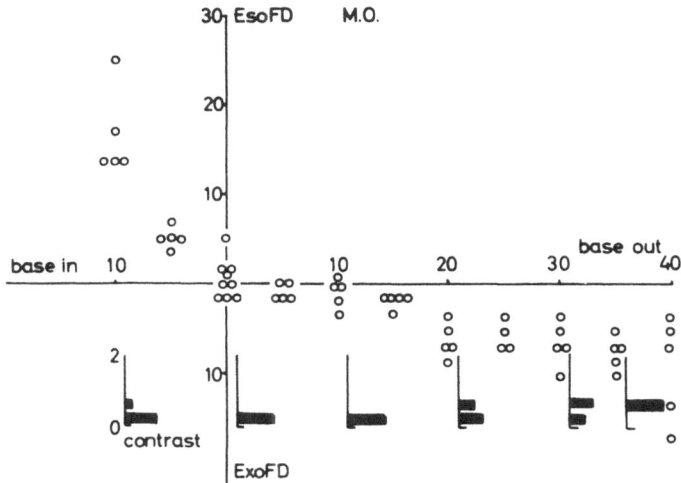

Fig. 4. Fixation disparity curve of a normal test person (second set-up). Black bars on inset scales indicate contrast thresholds. Sum of bar length = 5 single settings.

13

inset scale corresponds to the number of five different settings. There is a slight but definite increase of thresholds in forced convergence only whilst fixation disparities keep growing on both directions. We suppose this might result from the test character favouring the detection of temporal suppression in exo-disparity.

Such signs of foveal suppression have been found in most normal subjects and in a number of all patients with intermittent divergent squint or convergent microtropia. Figs. 5 and 6 have been obtained from two patients with

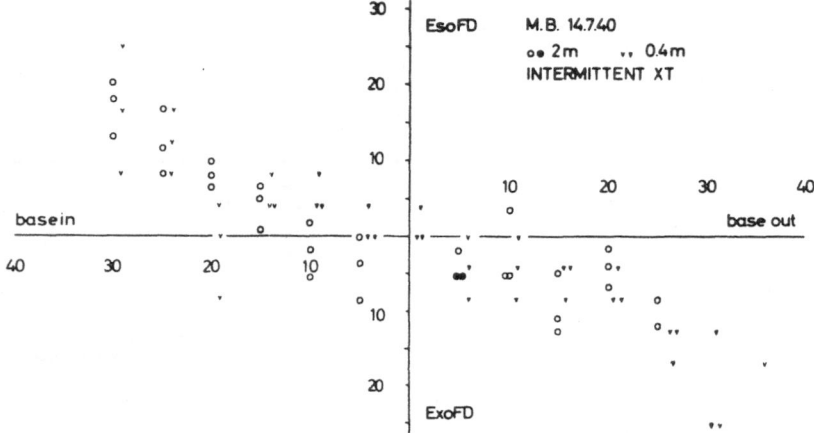

Fig. 5. First set-up diagram of a patient with intermittent divergent squint. Note prevailing suppression (empty circles).

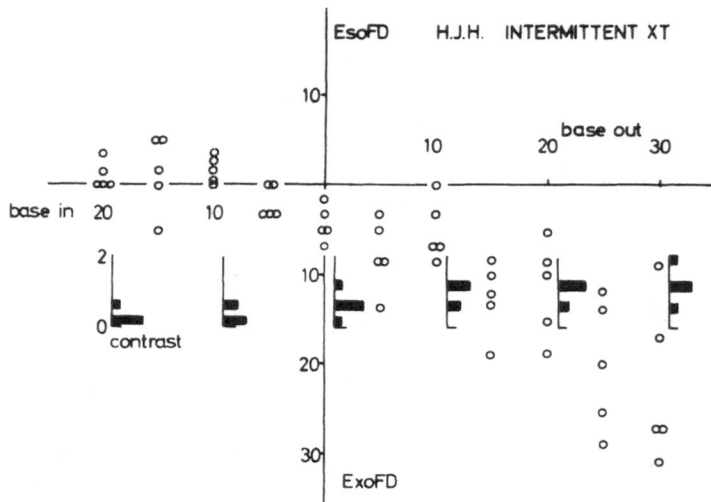

Fig. 6. Second set-up data in a patient with intermittent divergent squint. Note threshold shift with base out prisms increasing.

intermittent divergent squint. First set-up data in Fig. 5 show that empty circles indicating suppression of triangular controls are prevailing. From Fig. 6 a definite increase of contrast thresholds is obvious with prisms base out. Large fixation disparities parallel these signs of suppression in both diagrams.

In the patient of Fig. 5 a simple recess resect procedure preceded by some prism treatment reduced fixation disparities to normal values. In the postoperative fixation disparity curve (Fig. 7) full circles are predominant indicating the simultaneous decrease of suppression achieved by the surgical relief of the oculomotor imbalance.

Certainly these findings need further support from additional measurements with refined controls in the first set-up and with moving the circular mark next to the vernier in the second. Thus we might overcome the obvious drawbacks of our present procedures. With these limitations in mind it may be allowed to rise two questions: (1) How can we explain the suppression joint with fixation disparity? (2) What may this suppression mean to our understanding of fixation disparity?

To answer the first question we may recall the well accepted fact (Bishop 1975) that binocular vision depends on cortical neurones tuned to both eyes. Most of their binocular receptive fields are found at corresponding retinal sites. Any disparate stimulation of these corresponding retinal fields will decrease the activity to those cortical neurones they are connected to. Certainly this should especially afflict bifoveal vision because of the tiny receptive fields mediating it. Thus some suppression of bifoveal vision seems to be rather natural adjunct to fixation disparity.

This concept may provide an answer to the second question as well. We feel the idea might prove quite consistent with the views of Ogle et al. (1967), Jampolsky et al. (1957), Crone (1973), and Dedecker et al. (1976) concerning fixation disparity curves in normal, heterophoric, and microtropic sub-

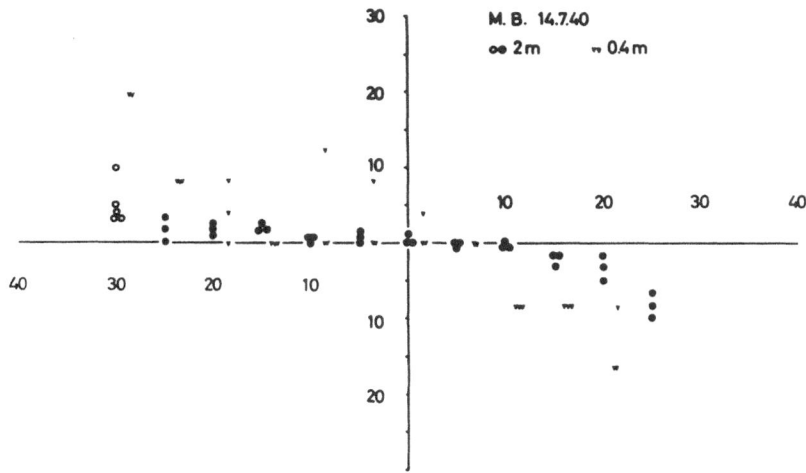

Fig. 7. Same patient as Fig. 5 – first set-up diagram changed after recess resect procedure.

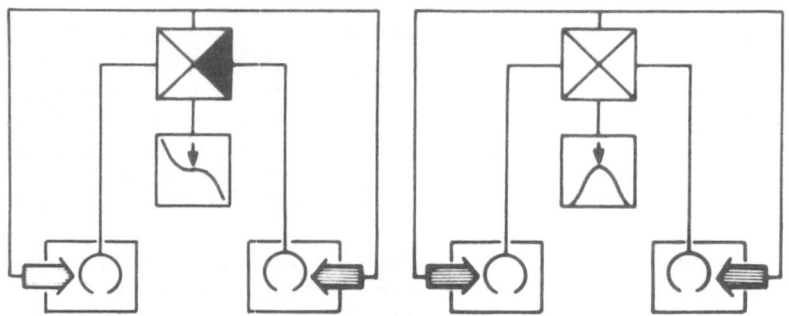

Fig. 8. Block diagram illustrating vergence control models. Left model uses fixation disparity to set motor fusion at zero disparity if possible. Right model sums monocular inputs and sets motor fusion at maximum gain of sensory fusion.

jects. But we find some difficulties from our point of view with the suggestion of Crone (1978) that fixation disparity represents a retinal error signal needed to control motor fusion efforts. Instead of subtracting binocular inputs to compute the error signal the system might rather add them up and set motor fusion at maximum gain of sensory fusion (Fig. 8; Friedburg 1978). In this context it would be quite natural to say: fixation disparity is indicating some depression of bifoveal sensory fusion that results in a shift of motor fusion control to the non-foveal subsystem.

REFERENCES

Bishop, P.O. Binocular vision. In: Moses, R.A., ed.: Adler's physiology of the eye. 6th ed. The C.V. Mosby Co. St. Louis 1975, p. 558 ff.

Crone, R.A. Diplopia. Excepta Medica Amsterdam 1973.

Crone, R.A., J.L. Vrooland & S. Hardjowijoto. Proportionalregelung der Fusion, Integralregelung der willkuerlichen Konvergenz. In: Kommerell, G., Hrsg.: Augenbewegungsstoerungen. J.F. Bergmann Verlag Muenchen 1978, p. 323.

Dedecker, W., Th. Scheffel & J. Baenge. Fixation disparity and the origin of microstrabismus. In: Moore, S., J. Mein, L. Stockbridge. Orthoptics – past, present, future. Symposia specialists Miami 1976, p. 155.

Friedburg, D. Ist Fixationsdisparitaet der Motor der Fusion? Ber. Dtsch. Ophthal. Ges. 75: 473 (1978).

Jampolsky, A., B.C. Flom & A.N. Freid. Fixation disparity in relation to heterophoria. Amer. J. Ophthal. 43: 97 (1957).

Ogle, K.N., T.G. Martens & J.A. Dyer: Oculomotor imbalance in binocular vision and fixation disparity. Lea & Febiger Philadelphia 1967.

Authors' address:
Universitäts-Augenklinik
Joseph-Stelzmann-Str. 9
D-5000 Köln 41, F.R.G.

FIXATION DISPARITY IN VERTICAL VERGENCE MOVEMENTS

W.A. HOUTMAN & B.A.E. VAN DER POL

(*Groningen, The Netherlands*)

ABSTRACT

The vertical vergence response generally is smaller than the presented disparity. Yet fixation disparity seems not obligatory for the vertical fusional response. Fixation disparity is modeled as a phenomenon due to interaction of a fast and a slow vergence system.

INTRODUCTION

When the vergence response is unequal to the magnitude of the stimulus, a binocular fixation error exists, which is called 'fixation disparity'. Fixation disparity can be plotted as a function of the magnitude of the stimulus. The stimulus can be either versional or accommodative (Ogle et al. 1967).

As long as fixation disparity is within Panum's area, the images will be perceptually fused. Panum's area is strongly dependent on the configuration of the binocular targets (Julesz & Fender, cit. Julesz 1971).

No agreement exists about the clinical significance of the phenomenon of fixation disparity. Carter (1980) considered (spontaneous) fixation disparity to be an 'ultra' microstrabismus in the presence of normal retinal correspondence and normal single binocular vision. The magnitude of the fixation disparity within the limits imposed by Panum's area, is considered to be a function of the difficulty of maintaining precise motor function.

The term 'associated phoria' is used (against dissociated heterophoria) for the amount of prisms necessary to reduce fixation disparity to zero. Palmer & Von Noorden (1978) rejected a causal relationship between fixation disparity and the heterophoria, because a lack of correlation exists between the magnitude and direction of fixation disparity and the heterophoria.

The interpretation of the subjective measurements of fixation disparity is based on the assumption that the perceived direction of the reference or nonius lines (Fig. 1) represent the position of the lines of sight. Hebbard's (1962) data showed close agreement between objective and subjective measurements.

Fixation disparity and the shape of the response curves are influenced by the following factors: 1. The size of the dichoptically presented targets has

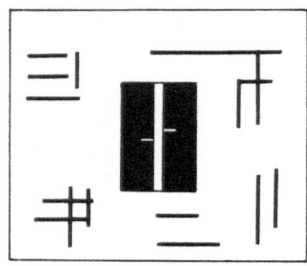

Fig. 1. Target for measurement of fixation disparity. The left nonius (or reference) line is seen by one of the eyes, the right by the other eye only. The lines are situated in a central field without cues for fusion. The magnitude of the fixation disparity (in min. arc) can be estimated from the amount of displacement which is necessary to align the reference lines.

hardly any influence. Nonius lines allow the most precise measurements (Ogle et al. 1967). 2. Diminution of contrast and luminance do increase fixation disparity (Herzau 1975). 3. Increasing size of the central field lacking cues for fusion, does increase fixation disparity (Hebbard 1960; Ogle et al. 1967; Herzau 1975). 4. On the contrary, when one adds more central contours, the shape of the response curves will be more flat, and fixation disparity decreases. Mitchell & Ellerbrock (1955), Hebbard (1960), Monjé et al. (1975) concluded that fixation disparity does not disappear completely when one stimulates as centrally as possible. However, Riggs & Niehl (1960) concluded from objective recordings that the vergence response was equal to the stimulus amplitude within moderate amplitudes of the stimulus. 5. Fixation disparity decreases with prolonged exposure (Ogle et al. 1967; Schubert 1943; Ellerbrock 1950; Carter 1965). The largest part of compensation for the prism induced vergence takes place within three to ten minutes, but can go on for hours. Adaptation in convergent direction was not constantly found by all authors.

Perceptual as well as motor functions are attributed to the residual disparity. In projection fusion theories disparity and residual disparities (eventually after setting the interocular position) create forces in a network which were called 'synchisis' (Von Kries) 'allelotropie' (Von Tschermak) and 'Attraktion' (Van Linschoten). These 'forces' underlie binocular perceptual processes. In the local sign fusion theory a motor function could be attributed to a residual disparity, the images being fused within Panum's area. It is not fully clear when disparate images should have either a perceptual (sensory) or a motor function. Alpern (1969) made a distinction between oculocentric disparity as the stimulus for sensory function, and egocentric disparity as the stimulus for motor fusion.

Ogle (Ogle et al. 1967) was probably the first who attributed a motor function to fixation disparity. He considered the residual error to be 'the stimulus for the direction and magnitude of the innervations that provide the fusional movements, and for the maintenance of the tensions to the convergence divergence muscle synergies to prevent diplopia. If a disparity between

18

all images of the object does not exist, there is no stimulus to the fusional processes at all; this could occur only when there is no oculomotor imbalance' (pg. 329).

Crone et al. (1978) meant that fixation disparity is a property of the fusional system; the (voluntary) convergence fully compensates an error (fusion being a proportional, the voluntary vergence an integral control system).

Schor (1979) modeled fixation disparity as a steady state error of the fast fusional vergence system, being necessary to maintain alignment because of the 'leaky' integrator character of the system. Fixation disparity was found inversely related to prism adaptation.

Semmlow & Hung (1979) found that a high level of overconvergence at least half of fixation disparity can be attributed to accommodative interaction. Fixation disparity response curves are shaped by the combined influence of accommodative and fusional vergence.

Because of the absence of voluntary and accommodative input fixation disparity in vertical vergence can be studied as a function of fusional vergence.

In earlier studies (Houtman et al. 1981) it was found that the dynamic vertical motor response generally is smaller than the magnitude of the stimulus. However, the inequality between the magnitude of the response and of the stimulus is dependent on the size and composition of the binocular targets, and dependent on the stimulus amplitude. The same is true for the horizontal fusional vergence at the limits of the fusional range (Houtman 1981). The influence of target size and target composition decreases for lower stimulus amplitudes, creating the possibility that within very narrow limits the vertical system may be independent of the target characteristics, as in horizontal vergence (Rashbass & Westheimer 1961). To prove that fixation disparity is obligatory for the vertical response, it should be excluded that fixation disparity is absent for very small disparities, when binocular targets are used as large and complex as possible (Houtman 1979).

METHODS

Eye movement recordings were possible by an electro-magnetic coil method. For a full description of the methods, see Houtman et al. 1981.

Binocular targets, subtending a visual angle of 10.9 dg. arc, were composed of high and low frequency contours. The size of the targets was limited by technical reasons. Disparities were presented as step functions. To avoid adaptation the targets were viewed in the rest position during at least 20 seconds, before the next disparity was presented. Only in the experiments in which the target moved from a +7.5 to a −7.5 min. arc disparity, the position of the targets was altered every 15 sec. Except for the targets, the room was dark.

In another series of experiments the subjective and objective responses were compared. With the aid of a Riley prism (total amount 4 diopters) disparities of 17, 34, 51 and 68 min. arc were presented, while the subject was viewing the center of the target for measuring fixation disparity. The width of the polarized nonius lines subtended a visual angle of two min. arc; the central field 2°33 × 3°66 dg. arc. The room was moderately illuminated.

The magnitude of the motor response from the recordings was measured from the eye position at the beginning of the response and the position of the eye at the moment the nonius lines were horizontally aligned. The nonius lines were continuously illuminated. Drifts during viewing the device through the polaroid filters were within 10–12 min. arc, within periods of 20–30 seconds. In experiments determining the subjective fixation disparity, the residual disparity was measured after the subjectively observed displacement of one of the nonius lines stopped.

EXPERIMENTS AND RESULTS

In a number of experiments with a 10.9 dg. arc complex target never an average response was found that equalled the stimulus amplitude, even in the case when the targets were driven from a positive to negative disparity of 7.5 min. arc (total disparity 15 min. arc). In the graph (Fig. 2) an evident relationship between response and stimulus amplitude cannot be recognized. The findings possibly could be interpreted as a proportional relationship as suggested by Crone (1978) for the fusional control system. This is contrary to our findings in the case of stimulation as a sinusoidal function of time. These responses are more stable than step responses (Houtman et al. 1981). The ratio response/stimulus amplitude less than 1.0 for very small amplitudes of the stimulus may be also caused by a small dead zone, or due to prediction.

The use of prisms afforded the possibility to enlarge the size of the stimulated retinal area. Generally in that case the response was also lower than the stimulus amplitude (Fig. 4).

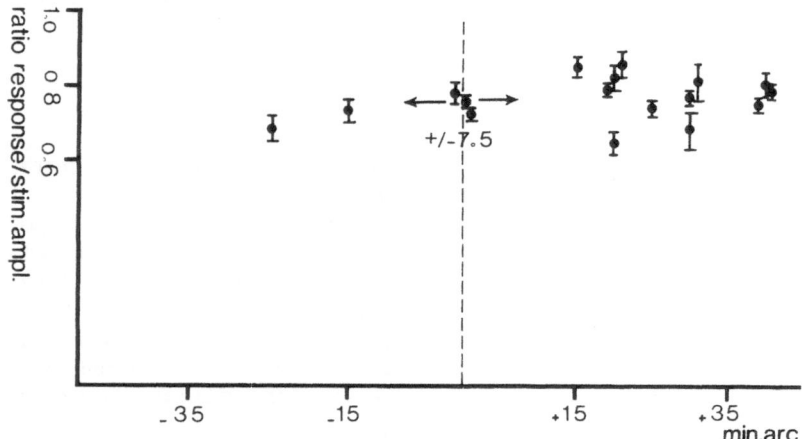

Fig. 2. *Vertical vergence*, subj. H. Motorresponses on suddenly imposed disparities (closed-loop). Complex target. Left neg., right pos. disparities, centre responses on +/−7.5 min. arc disparities. Average values of 5–10 responses with standard error of the mean; four sessions of experiments.

20

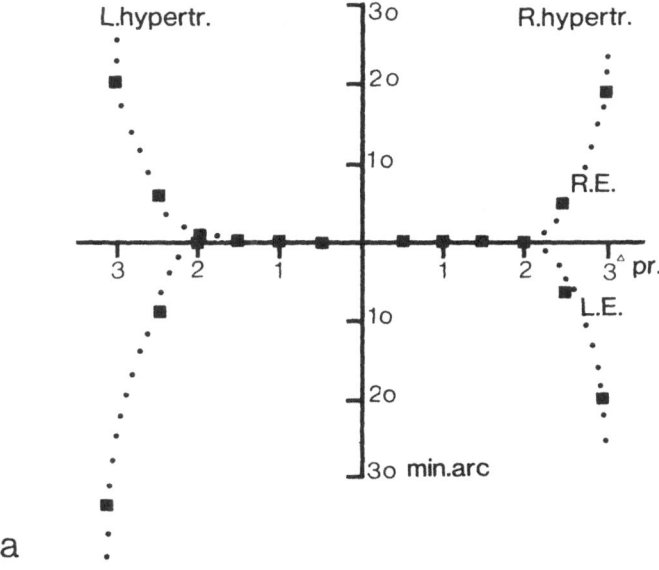

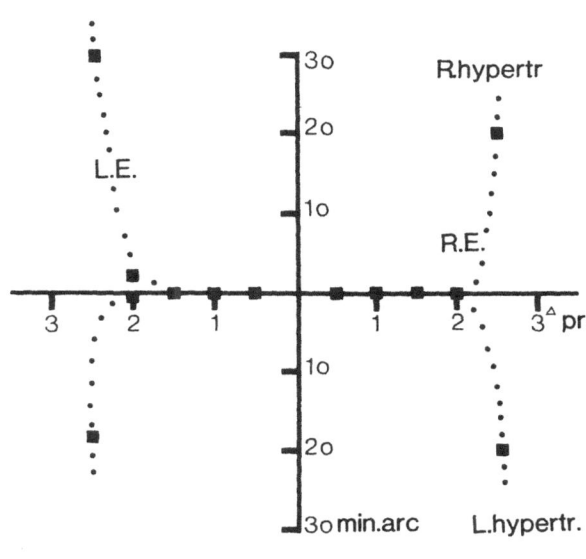

Fig. 3. *Vertical Fusion*, a (subj. P), b (subj. H). Fixation disparity response curves, subj. measured. RE, LE: prisms before right, left eye respect.

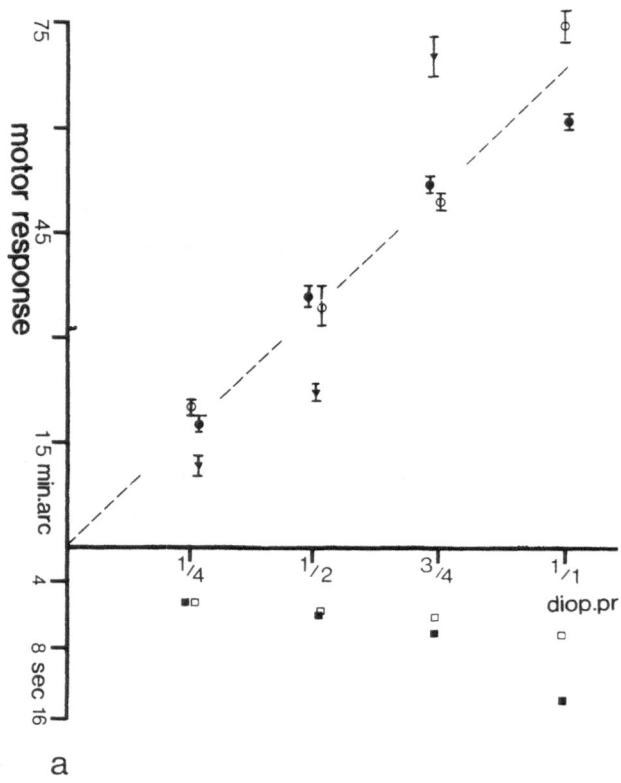

Fig. 4a.

However, both subjects showed a subjective fixation disparity response curve with a large flat zone along the abscis (Fig. 3). Average values from recordings of the objective responses appeared to be in good agreement with the stimulus amplitude (Fig. 4).

The time course of the larger responses from the initial eye position (the rest position) exceeds that of the response in the reverse direction. Smaller responses have a symmetrical shape in both directions (Fig. 5). The same non-linearity is known from the divergent response at the limits of the fusional range (Houtman 1981). The finding of the asymmetrical responses suggests the possibility that is dealt with two mechanisms in the fusional response.

Other findings may also support the idea that a second, slowly acting system is operative within the vertical fusional response. When one eye is occluded after a response, the movement in the direction of the rest position is slower than the normal vergence response. This phenomenon seems to be influenced by exposure time (Fig. 6). When a response to a disparity of 40 min. arc is immediately followed by an additive disparity of 30 m. arc, a further response is impossible. If this disparity is added after prolonged viewing time one can respond again (Fig. 7).

22

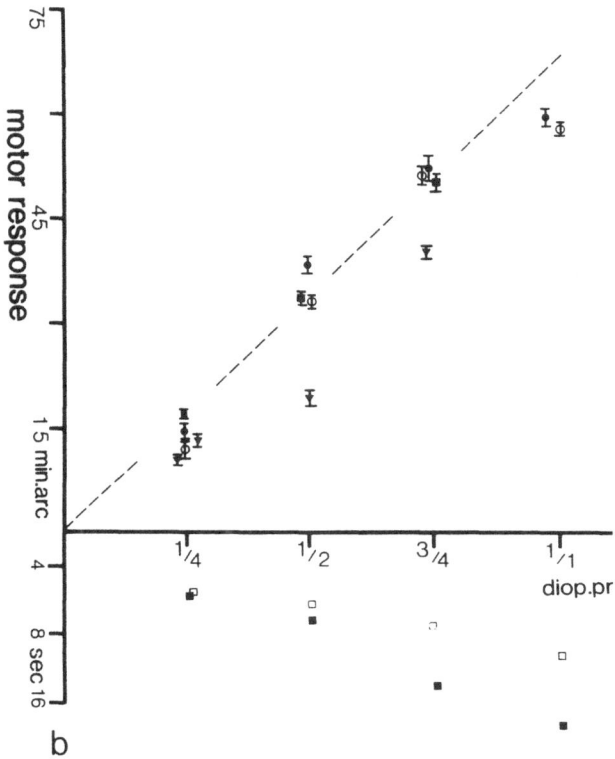

b

Fig. 4. Vertical Vergence, a (subj. P), b (subj. H). Magnitude of the objective responses versus stimulus amplitude. Responses measured at the time when horizontal alignment of the nonius lines of the fixation disparity target is observed. Average values of 18–20 responses with standard error of the mean.

●, ○, ■   various sessions of experiments,

▼   responses in experiments viewing the fix. disp. target without polaroid filters.

(below) time course of responses, from the position of rest (■), and (□) and the reverse direction.

DISCUSSION

Contrary to our findings Ogle's vertical fixation disparity response curves show a more linear relationship between the residual disparity and the amount of prisms. More sigmoid-like curves than Ogle's ones were found by Carter (1980) for horizontal vergence in normal subjects. The magnitude of the objectively measured responses at the moment of perceptual alignment of the horizontal lines correspond rather well with the stimulus amplitude, i.e. the amount of prism value by which the motor response was evoked. Apparently, the possibility to control the alignment and/or the tendency to align the horizontal lines adds something to the motor response,

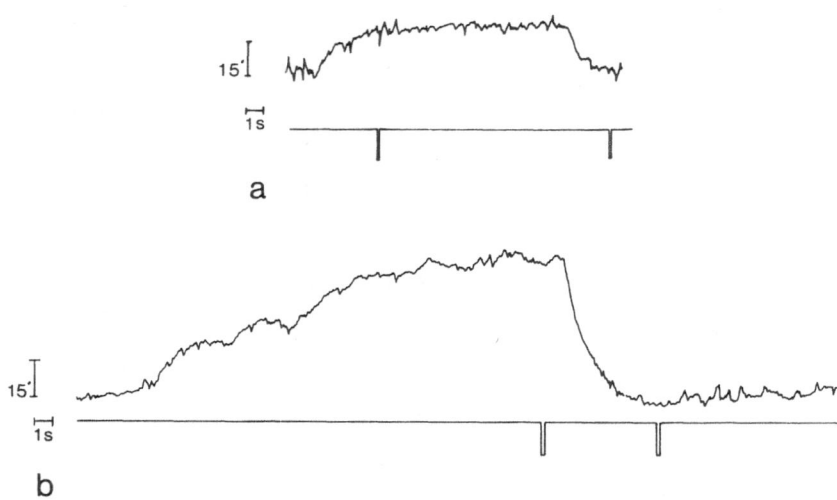

Fig. 5. Vertical Vergence. Objective responses from the experiments of Fig. 3. Stimulus-amplitude 17 (a, subj. H), 68 (b, subj. H) min. arc ⊔ indicates alignment of the nonius lines.

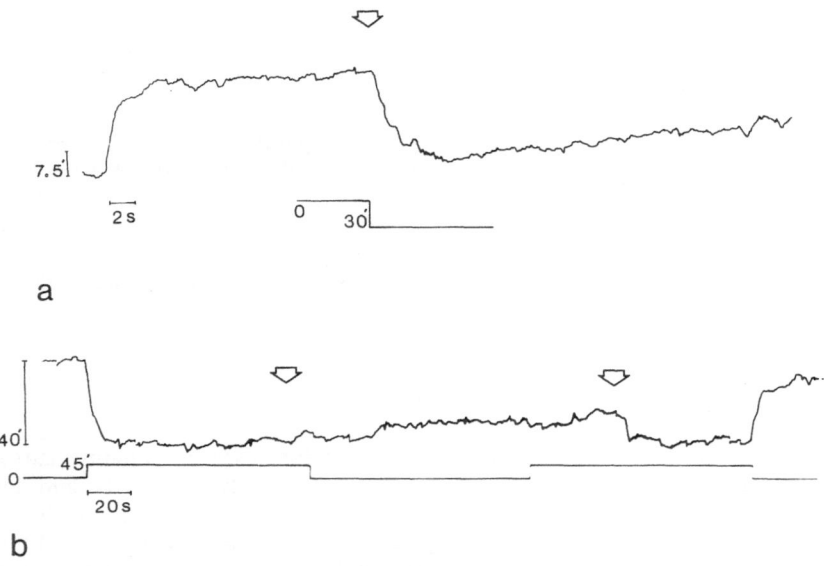

Fig. 6. Autonomous behavior. The eye occluded after having made a fusional movement slowly runs back to the rest position. a. Vertical vergence (subj. H). Occlusion just after a response is finished. The eye slowly runs back to the rest position. b. Vertical vergence (subj. P). After prolonged viewing the measurement is slower. At second arrow response after uncover.

24

when one considers the inequality between response and stimulus amplitude in the other experiments. This can mean either that the procedure to measure fixation disparity does not afford a suitable parameter for the fusional response, or that fixation disparity is not obligatory for the vertical motor response. But above all that fixation disparity is dependent on the target composition and the amplitude of the stimulus.

However, there is another finding which is not consistent with a residual error (Rashbass & Westheimer 1961; Toates 1974). When a disparity is suddenly imposed and maintained at a constant level, subsequently it evokes a uniform movement (up to the saturation level). This is also the case in vertical vergence (Houtman 1981).

An alternative possibility might be that fixation disparity is either the result of interactive processes, such as between a relative fast (which is actually very slow; initial velocities of suddenly imposed disparities are between 15–35 min. arc/s) and slow fusional vergence system, or is caused by the latter system.

The findings from the experiments of Fig. 7, suggest that there is indeed a slowly operating mechanism that gradually relieves the fusional movement to go, farther than the initial fast response, and which for a time limits the amplitude of the response.

Ideas about the existence of two operating systems in vergence are old. By some (Schubert 1943) a distinction is made between a kinetic and static element in the fusional response. The description of the static element appears to be very alike the description of motor fusion by Hofmann & Bielschowsky (1900), a tonic innervation which aim is to keep the alignment of the eyes and to provide an adaptational process in cases of disturbance of the alignment.

This definition in part is synonymous with that of tonic vergence, which is considered to be a long term operative neuronal mechanism which determines the position of rest (Toates 1974; Westheimer 1976). When there are indeed two systems, a relatively fast response and a slowly operating system, the question rises how the systems do interact and what is the input of the slow system? Ogle et al. (1967) meant that the both systems were active together.

Because the amplitude of the vertical response is set dependent on the size and complexity (or contourrichness) of the targets, a releasing interaction of the slow system should be influenced by a visual input. The slow system in that case could be more dependent either on the size of the stimulated retinal area, or on peripheral contours and less on foveal and parafoveal stimulation. This is contrary to the opinion of Schor (1979), who meant that the slow fusional vergence is stimulated by the output or effort of the fast system. He precludes visual input because slow fusional vergence occurs after retinal image disparity is nulled out, and because slow fusional vergence is small or non-existent when the observers are unable to fuse diplopic images.

The fast and slow vertical vergence system can be modeled as a parallel operating 'bang-bang' control system and a parametric adaptive control system respectively. The 'bang-bang' control system (Fig. 8) is consistent

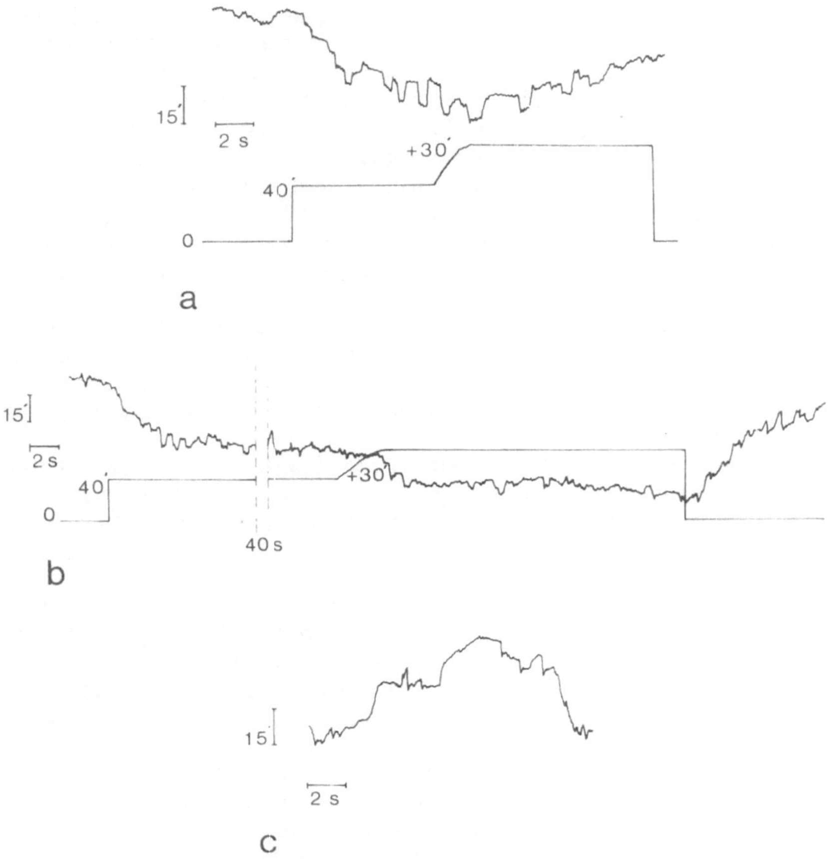

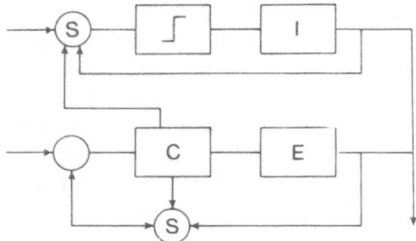

Fig. 7. Vertical Vergence, (subj. H). A superimposed disparity of 30 min. arc to a disparity of 40 min. arc cannot be fused, when this disparity is immediately presented after the response (a), but one can respond after prolonged viewing to the first disparity (b). Initial response to a disparity (85 min. arc) that ultimately cannot be fused (c).

Fig. 8. Model of vertical vergence. Parallel operating 'bang-bang' control model for fast fusional vergence, and a parametric-adaptive control system for slow vergence. S Saturator, I integrator, E effector, S summing junction. For further legend see text.

with much of the dynamic features of the vertical vergence response: the uniform movement to a suddenly imposed disparity (when the feed-back loop is opened) and the constant velocity of the open-loop step response, which is independent of the magnitude of the disparity (15—35 m. arc/s). This control system gives also rise to a reason for the slowness of the vertical movements. The system should be very unstable, if not extremely slow. However, fixation disparity is not consistent with such a system. When one adds yet a parallel operating parametric adaptive controller to the model, it affords the possibility to describe some other characteristics of vertical vergence, included the fixation disparity. In parametric feedback control the error signals, i.e. the disparity error, is averaged over relatively long periods of time (Carpenter 1977).

The model is consistent with an amplitude dependent non-linearity of the ratio between magnitude of the response and the magnitude of the stimulus. And also with the responses to a secondly added disparity and the adaptation of the response, both after prolonged viewing at a fusional stimulus. It is also consistent with an initial response to a disparity which ultimately cannot be fused (Fig. 7).

When a disparity is presented, it evokes a fast fusional response. The output of the parametric adaptive control system will be lower than the value of the presented disparity, at least for the time it averages over a period before and after the presentation. When this value is subtracted from the disparity signal for the fast fusional system, it is understandable that the response (for a time) will be lower than the disparity. The residual disparity will increase when the presented disparity is larger.

In horizontal vergence there must exist a somewhat different situation. In the normal viewing condition (without a preset vergence angle) vergence movements in divergent direction share much of the properties of the vertical vergence (Houtman 1979). Because these findings are independent of the absolute vergence angle, it can be concluded that the horizontal rest position (and event. the phoria position) is set to a reference frame of the particular viewing distance. Factors limiting the range in convergent direction must have been released in the horizontal system.

For strabological practice the fixation disparity method seems of limited value, and restricted to those cases in which one of the nonius lines is not suppressed. Possibly, in the presence of (nearly) foveal stimulation one could determine which cases of dissociated phoria are normal, and which cases are to be considered as an 'ultra' microstrabismus on basis of the occurrence of a spontaneous fixation disparity. The 'ultra' microstrabismus expresses the smooth borders between the straight eye position and squint. The amount of (dissociated) phoria may vary interindividually in these last cases, just as the phoria in microstrabismus.

The value of a fixation disparity plot above the conventional measuring of the fusional range would be confined to a possible indication concerning the relationship between the magnitude of the motor and the sensory fusional response.

REFERENCES

Alpern, M. In: The Eye, vol. III: Muscular Mechanisms (2nd ed.). Ed.: Davson, H. Academic Press, New York (1969).

Carpenter, R.H.S. Movements of the eyes. Pion Limited, London (1977).

Carter, D.B. Fixation disparity and heterophoria following prolonged wearing of prisms. Am. J. Optometry and Arch. Am. Acad. Optometry 42: 141–152 (1965).

Carter, D.B. Parameters of fixation disparity. Am. J. Optometry and Physiol. Optics 57: 610–617 (1980).

Crone, R.A., J.L. Vrooland & S. Hardjowijoto. Proportionalregelung der Fusion, Integralregelung der willkürlichen Konvergenz. In: Augenbewegungsstörungen. Ed: Kommerell, G. 323–328, J.F. Bergmann Verlag, München (1978).

Ellerbrock, V.J. Tonicity induced by fusional movements. Am. J. Optometry and Arch. Am. Acad. Optometry 27: 8–20 (1950).

Hebbard, F.W. Foveal fixation disparity measurements and their use in determining the relationship between accommodative convergence and accommodation. Am. J. Optometry and Arch. Am. Acad. Optometry 37: 3–26 (1960).

Hebbard, F.W. Comparison of subjective and objective measurements of fixation disparity. J. Opt. Soc. Am. 52: 706–712 (1962).

Herzau, V. Fixationsdisparität bei verschiedenen Darbietungsbedingungen. Albrecht v. Graefes. Arch. klin. exp. Ophthalmol. 197: 193–202 (1975).

Hofmann, F.B. & A. Bielschowsky. Ueber die der Willkür entzogenen Fusionsbewegungen der Augen. Pflügers Arch. ges. Physiol. 80: 1–40 (1900).

Houtman, W.A. Verticale Vergentie. Dissertatie. Drukkerij Dijkstra Niemeyer B.V., Groningen (1979).

Houtman, W.A., J.H. Roze & W. Scheper. Vertical vergence movements. Doc. Ophthalmol. 51: 199–207 (1981).

Houtman, W.A. Vertical vergence and fusional movements. In: Orthoptics, Research and Practice. Ed.: Mein, J. & S. Moore, Henry Kimpton Publ., London (1981).

Julesz, B. Foundations of cyclopean perception. The University of Chicago Press, Chicago (1971).

Mitchell, A.M. & V.J. Ellerbrock. Fixation disparity and the maintenance of fusion in the horizontal meridian. Am. J. Optometry and Arch. Am. Acad. Optometry 32: 520–534 (1955).

Monjé, M., H. Stingl & W. de Decker. Fixationsdisparität bei peripherem und zentralem Binokularsehen unter phorischer Belastung. Albrecht v. Graefes Arch. klin. exp. Ophthalmol. 194: 95–107 (1975).

Ogle, K.N., T.G. Martens & J.A. Dyer. Oculomotor imbalance in binocular vision and fixation disparity. Lea and Febiger, Philadelphia (1967).

Palmer, E.A., & G.K. von Noorden. The relationship between fixation disparity and heterophoria. Am. J. Ophthalmol. 86: 172–175 (1978).

Rashbass, C. & G. Westheimer. Disjunctive eye movements. J. Physiol. (Lond.) 159: 339–360 (1961).

Riggs, L.A. & E.W. Niehl. Eye movements recorded during convergence and divergence. J. Opt. Soc. Am. 50: 913–920 (1960).

Semmlow, J.L. & G. Hung. Accommodative and fusional components of fixation disparity. Invest. Ophthalmol. & Vis. Sci., 18: 1082–1086 (1979).

Schor, C.M. The relationship between fusional vergence eye movements and fixation disparity. Vision Res., 19: 1359–1367 (1979).

Schubert, G. Grundlagen der beidäugigen motorischen Koordination. Pflügers Arch. 279–291 (1943).

Toates, F.M. Vergence eye movements. Doc. Ophthalmol., 37: 153–214 (1974).

Westheimer, G. Oculomotor control: The vergence system, 55–64. In: Eye movements and psychological processes. Eds.: Monty, R.A. & J.W. Senders. Lawrence Erlbaum Associates Inc. Publ., New Jersey (1976).

Authors' address:
University Eye Clinic, Oostersingel 59, 9713 EZ Groningen, The Netherlands

VERTICAL FIXATION DISPARITY AND STEREOPSIS

J.B. WEISS

(Paris, France)

SUMMARY

A vertical disparity fixation induces a vertical retinal disparity; for oblique lines this vertical retinal disparity is interpreted as a horizontal retinal disparity. This results in a stereoscopic depthness.

INTRODUCTION

For a figure composed of points, a horizontal fixation disparity (H.F.D.) or a vertical one (V.F.D.) generally does not induce a perception of depthness.

However, for oblique lines, a V.F.D. can produce a perception of depthness. Linksz (1952) reports experiments performed by Ames on a figure with two vertical and one oblique line (Fig. 1).

A similar phenomenon is observed on figures made of oblique and vertical lines. This is especially true when aniseiconia is measured with a device derived from Ames' spatial eiconometer.

Let us take, for example, two identical stereograms made of an oblique cross with its branches 01 and 02 (Fig. 2). If there is no Vertical Fixation Disparity the cross is perceived in a frontal plane. On the other hand, if a V.F.D. is present, as long as the branches of the cross are long enough, the vertical retinal disparity is interpreted as being horizontal.

Indeed, the oblique branch 01 is in crossed and 02 in uncrossed retinal disparity. Both branches 01 and 02 are perceived in different frontal planes.

This is a disturbing phenomenon when one wishes to measure aniseiconia

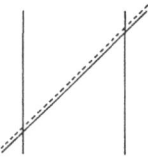

Fig. 1. Ames' phenomenon. A vertical retinal disparity does not modify the perception of the vertical lines. On the contrary, for the oblique line, this vertical retinal disparity acts as a horizontal retinal disparity and so induces stereopsis.

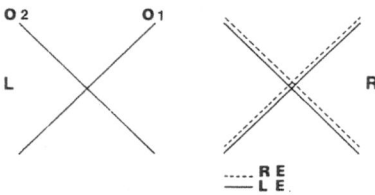

Fig. 2. The test of the oblique cross. A. When there is no vertical disparity, the two branches of the cross seem to lie in the same frontal plane. B. The vertical retinal disparity induces a horizontal disparity, crossed for the oblique 01 and uncrossed for the oblique 02. Hence the two branches of the cross no longer seem to be in the same plane. 01 seems to be nearer than 02.

in a patient with a V.F.D. On the other hand, this phenomenon can be used to detect easily such a Vertical Fixation Disparity.

EXPERIMENTS IN FREE SPACE

Forty patients, seen at the outpatient clinic of the Orthoptic Department were examined. All patients had a stereoacuity of at least 60 seconds of arc with the Wirt test.

Each patient was asked to look at two vertical strings and a third one at an oblique 45 degree angle, all located in the same frontal plane placed at a 40 centimeters distance. The strings were contained in a box, the front of which had two apertures for the eyes. The bottom of the box was translucid. Under these testing conditions when a positive V.F.D. is present in the right eye, the oblique string seems located in back of the two vertical strings. The patient was only asked whether the oblique string was located in the same plane as the vertical ones or whether it was nearer or further away from them.

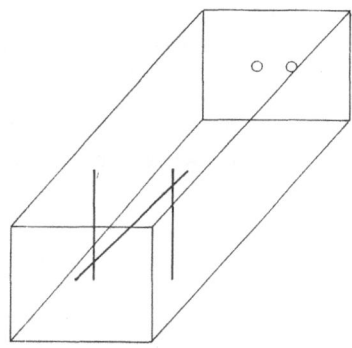

Fig. 3. Free space test. Two vertical lines and an oblique one lie in the same frontal plane, inside a close box. The bottom of the box is translucid. The observer looks inside through two apertures in the front of the box. He is asked if the oblique line is nearer, further or in the plane of the two verticals.

Five patients could not give precise answers. Among the 35 others, 29 perceived the three strings in a same frontal plane. On the other hand 6 patients perceived the oblique string either in front or in back of the two vertical strings.

A definite correlation was found between the V.F.D. and the vertical heterophoria measured with the Maddox wing (Table 1).

In these six patients the determination of the minimal vertical prismatic correction necessary to eliminate the spatial distortion was made and repeated a number of times (Table 2).

Our results show that this minimal correction is as a rule lower than the measured vertical heterophoria.

Table 1. Free space experimentation. Forty subjects from the outpatient clinic of the Orthoptic Department. Vision was 20/20 O.U. and the stereoacuity was at least 60 seconds of arc. The vertical phoria was measured with the Maddox wing.

Number of subjects	Vertical Phoria (Maddox Wing)	Spatial disparity Test
5		Responses too imprecise
29	< 1 prismatic diopter	Obliques in the verticals' plane
4	Hd > 1 Prismatic Diopter	Oblique 01 located farther
2	Hg > 1 Prismatic Diopter	Oblique 01 located nearer

Table 2. Free space experimentation. Six patients presented a Vertical Fixation Disparity. There is a correlation between the vertical phoria, measured with the Maddox wing, and the vertical prismatic correction zeroing the spatial distortion.

Vertical phoria measured with the Maddox wing	Prismatic correction zeroing the spatial distortion
RH 2	1 diopter base down R.E.
RH 2	1 diopter base down R.E.
RH 4	2 diopters base down R.E.
RH 5	2 diopters base down R.E.
LH 2	1 diopter base down L.E.
LH 3	2 diopters base down L.E.

EXPERIMENTS WITH THE SYNOPTOPHORE

Thirty patients seen at the outpatient clinic of the Orthoptic Department were examined. In all patients the stereoacuity measured with Random Dots Stereograms was 200 seconds of arc or better. The vertical heterophoria measured with the Maddox wing was found to be less than 1 prism diopter in 22 patients.

The tests used are reproduced in Fig. 4. The cross is perceived binocularly.

31

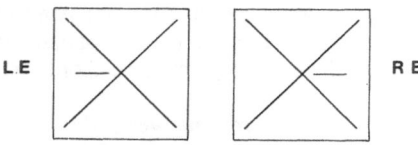

L E   R E

Fig. 4. Test for the synoptophore. With these tests it is possible to detect a vertical fixation disparity upon two different criteria, the spatial distortion of the cross and the nonalignment of the horizontal lines.

Each one of the two horizontal lines is seen monocularly. These seem to be aligned only in the absence of a V.F.D.

The first experiment (E1) consisted of setting the synoptophore so that both arms of the cross were perceived in a same frontal plane. In the second experiment (E2) the setting was modified in such a way that both horizontal lines seemed aligned.

For the 22 patients without a vertical heterophoria a difference of less than 1 prism diopter in the vertical setting of the Synoptophore's arms was found in both experiments.

For the eight patients with a vertical heterophoria greater than 1 prism diopter, the vertical disalignment of the synoptophore's arms was greater than 1 prism diopter (Table 3).

Table 3. Measures obtained with a synoptophore. Thirty patients, with a visual acuity of 20/20 O.U. and a stereoacuity of at least 200 seconds of arc were tested. There is a correlation between the vertical phoria measured with the Maddox wing and the vertical shift of the synoptophore's arms necessary to nullify the spatial distortion (E1) or giving the alignment of the horizontal lines (E2).

Vertical phoria measured with the Maddox wing	Vertical shift used to suppress the distortion	Vertical shift used to obtain the alignment
	Experiment E1	Experiment E2
22 patients < 1 Diopter	< 1 Diopter	< 1 Diopter
HD 2	1 P.D. UP R.E.	1 P.D. UP R.E.
HD 2	2 P.D. UP R.E.	2 P.D. UP R.E.
HD 2	2 P.D. UP R.E.	2 P.D. UP R.E.
HD 4	3 P.D. UP R.E.	3 P.D. UP R.E.
HD 5	3 P.D. UP R.E.	4 P.D. UP R.E.
HG 2	2 P.D. UP L.E.	2 P.D. UP L.E.
HG 3	2 P.D. UP L.E.	2 P.D. UP L.E.
HG 4	3 P.D. UP L.E.	4 P.D. UP L.E.

COMMENTS

The test described above (Cross Test) is simple to use. Detection of a Vertical Fixation Disparity and therefore the associated vertical heterophoria is quick and simple.

32

A determination of the prismatic correction necessary to eliminate the V.F.D. is easily done. This prismatic correction is as a rule lower than what the amount of vertical heterophoria found with the Maddox wing and might give the patient more comfort.

This last point will be discussed in another paper under preparation.

REFERENCES

Linksz, A. Physiology of the eye. Volume 2.835. Grune & Stratton, New York. (1952).
Weiss, J.B. & E. Muller Feuga. Utilisation des stereogrammes a points aleatoires. Jour. Franc. Orthopt. 14. (1982).

Author's address:
Laboratoire Emile Javal
Physiologie de la Vision Binoculaire
Ecole Pratique des Hautes Etudes
39 Avenue Mathurin Moreau
75019 Paris, France

Departement d'Orthoptie
Fondation A. de Rothschild
29 Rue Manin
75019 Paris, France

461 CURVES OF HORIZONTAL PRISM FIXATION DISPARITY IN AN ORTHOPTIC DEPARTMENT

R.A. CRONE & A.M. NOORDENBOS

(*Amsterdam, The Netherlands*)

ABSTRACT

Prism fixation disparity curves have been classified into five types: sigmoid with flat centre, sigmoid, flat, above abscissa, below abscissa. On casuistical and theoretical grounds these curves were considered characteristic for five clinical situations: Normality, convergence defect, fusion defect, esophoria, exophoria, respectively. In a survey of 461 curves from patients with asthenopia and oculomotor imbalance the presumed relation between orthoptic data and type of curve was confirmed.

Prism fixation disparity curves, determined according to Ogle's method, may have various shapes (Crone 1969). In 1969 we distinguished five types which were considered to be characteristic of five different types of oculomotor imbalance (Fig. 1).

I. The normal curve is sigmoid and has a flat central section. Between the primary eye position and a certain degree of convergence there is no fixation disparity. The curve is not so characteristic in all cases, but in normal subjects the exodisparity over a large area of convergence is of small magnitude.

II. A sigmoid curve is characteristic of convergence insufficiency and convergence palsy. Apart from the disturbance of the mechanism of convergence, the binocular vision in such patients is intact, as is shown, inter alia, by an intact vertical vergence.

III. A flat curve is indicative of weak binocular vision: intermittent diplopia, tendency towards suppression, etc. In such patients, the amplitude of convergence can be very great, especially following orthoptic exercises.

IV. A curve with spontaneous esodisparity which is maintained during prismatic convergence is characteristic of esophoria.

V. A curve which reveals spontaneous exodisparity and which is entirely below the abscissa is characteristic of exophoria. The theoretical basis of this classification was discussed again at length in 1979 (Crone & Hardjowijoto 1979). To be brief it comes to this that fixation disparity is an element of the fusion mechanism, while the flat part of the curve, coinciding with the abscissa, points to the integrity of the convergence-accommodation synergy. In curves IV and V binocular vision is only possible in the presence

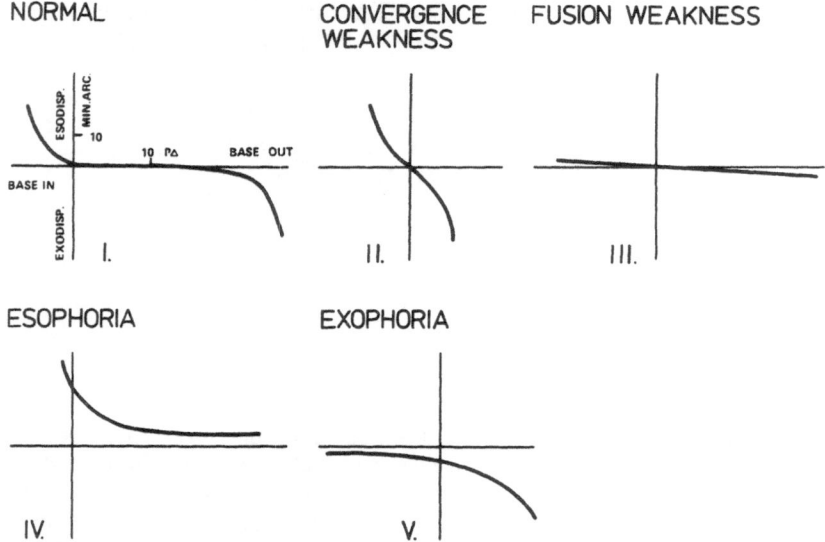

Fig. 1.

of a very small angle of squint. Fusion in such cases is 'micro-anomalous'. Curves of type IV and V that never reach the abscissa are 'obligatory micro-anomalous'. Similar curves that, with strong prisms, eventually do cross the abscissa, are 'facultatively micro-anomalous'.

The above classification has been defended in various papers on the basis of illustrative cases. Up till now there was no statistical survey of cases and prism fixation disparity curves to prove the presumed correlation between the type of curve and the type of oculomotor imbalance.

This study gives an analysis of all prism fixation disparity curves which have been determined in patients with oculomotor imbalance since 1968. We excluded all curves of vertical fixation disparity in patients with vertical imbalance and some 20 cases with paretic strabismus or spasm of convergence. There remained 461 curves of patients which had been referred to the orthoptic department with the following complaints: Asthenopia, intermittent diplopia, intermittent squint, presumed ocular headache which was not caused by errors of refraction. The curves of these 461 patients were classified into type I–V without previous knowledge of the clinical data. Because there are many transitions between 'ideal types', the classification is somewhat arbitrary; it is not, however, biased by the clinical symptomatology (Table 1).

The next step was to classify each patient in one of five groups according to their orthoptic data (Table 2). Patients who had less that 1° of heterophoria, 3° or less convergence 'weakness' at the Maddox Wing and did not have intermittent suppression, were considered normal.

The Figs. 2–8 show which clinical diagnosis was made (1–5 of Table 2) in

Table 1. Classification of cases according to five types of prism fixation disparity curve.

I	('normal')	159 cases	
II	('convergence weakness')	52	
III	('fusion weakness')	54	
IV	('esophoria')	130	
V	('exophoria')	71	

Table 2. Classification of cases into five types according to orthoptic measurements.

1.	normal	97	
2.	convergence weakness $\geqslant 3°$	111	
3.	fusion weakness (intermittent suppression)	77	
4.	esophoria $> 1°$	116	
5.	exophoria $> 1°$	60	

patients with curve I–V. The obligate and facultative micro-anomalous curves of type IV and V have been considered separately.

Curve I (Fig. 2) was seen in all types of oculomotor imbalance, but most in patients which were orthoptically normal or had a (usually slight) weakness of convergence.

Curve II (Fig. 3) was almost pathognomonic of (often severe) convergence weakness. In cases of severe convergence weakness there is very often a superimposed exophoria at distance. The combination of exophoria and convergence weakness was classified as convergence weakness when complaints were predominantly present during near vision.

Curve III (Fig. 4), on theoretical grounds considered to be characteristic of fusion weakness, was seen most frequently in cases of intermittent suppression. The majority of these patients had intermittent exotropia.

Curve IV (Fig. 5) appeared to be highly characteristic of esophoria. The

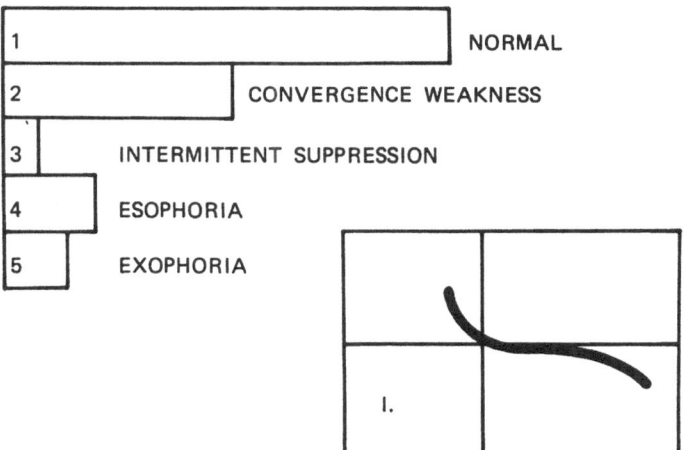

Fig. 2.

37

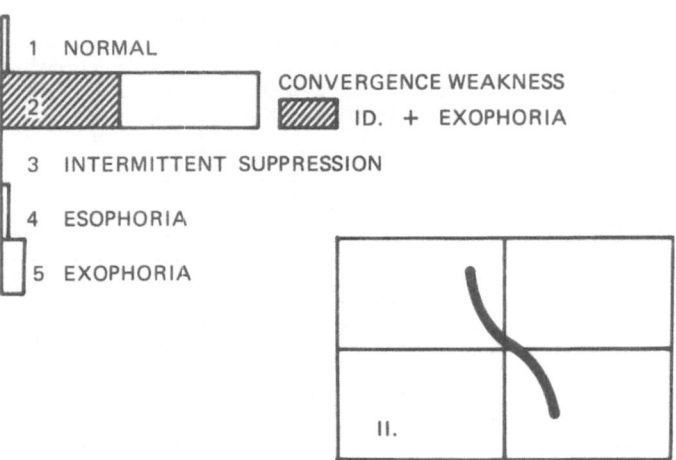

Fig. 3.

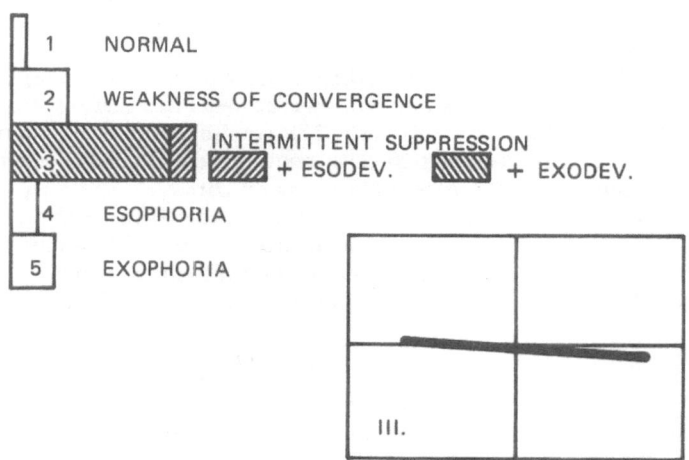

Fig. 4.

patients with 'obligate micro-anomalous vision' (type IVA) had more severe asthenopia. Most of them also had intermittent diplopia (Fig. 6).

Curve V (Fig. 7) proved to be characteristic of exodeviations, pure exophoria as well as intermittent exotropia. The clinical complaints were, again, more severe in the patients with obligate micro-anomalous curves. Intermittent exotropia was more frequent in patients with type A curves than with type B curves (Fig. 8).

Summarizing we can state that in a large group of patients the — theoretically consistent — classification of prism fixation disparity curves into five types correlates well with orthoptical routine findings. It is difficult to say whether the correlation would have been still better if the clinical

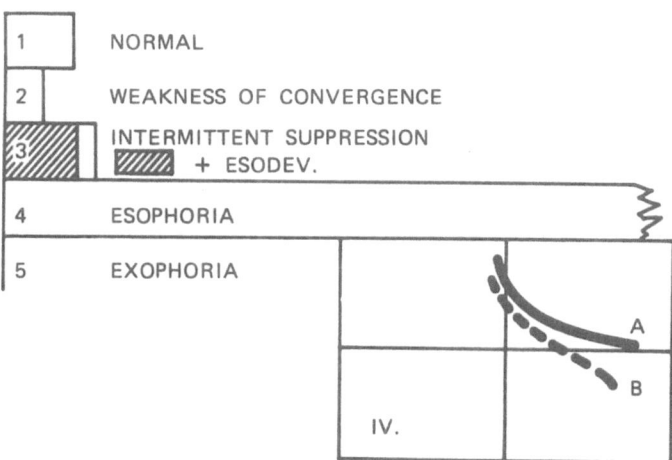

Fig. 5.

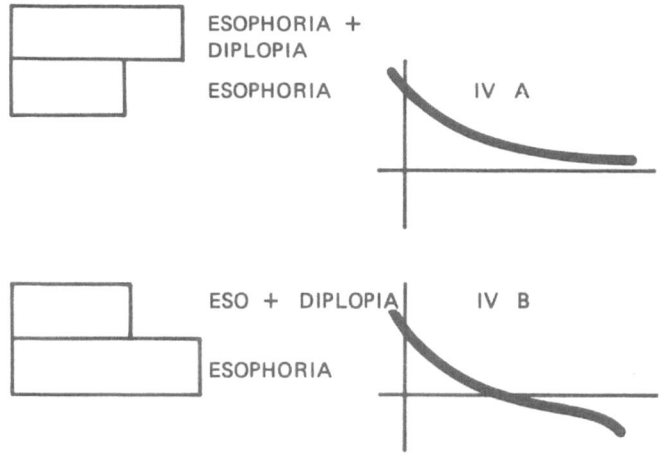

Fig. 6.

criteria had been formulated differently. Probably that is not the case. We published (Crone 1970) cases of severe asthenopia in which the orthoptic routine measurements were almost normal, but the prism fixation disparity curve highly abnormal. Evidently the fixation disparity curve does not merely reflect what could have been found by other means, but adds a new dimension to the study of oculomotor imbalance.

39

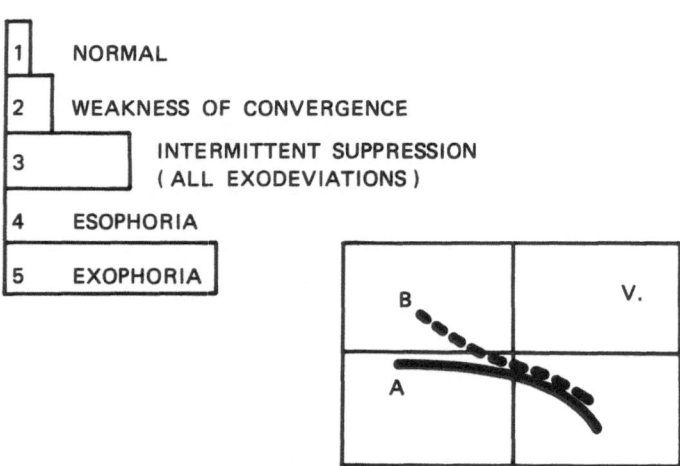

Fig. 7.

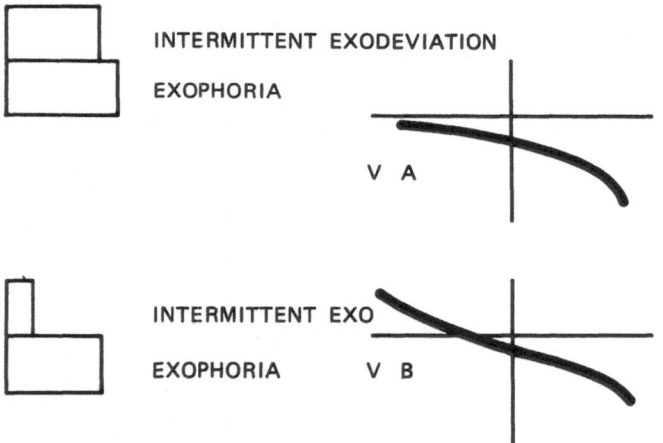

Fig. 8.

REFERENCES

Crone, R.A. Heterophoria. Albrecht v. Graefes Arch. klin. exp. Ophthal. 177: 52–74 (1969).

Crone, R.A. & Sanjoto Hardjowijoto. What is normal binocular vision? Docum. Ophthal. 47: 163–199 (1979).

Crone, R.A. Asthenopia in small angle heterophoria in Strabismus 1969, Transactions C.E.S.S.D., Henry Kimpton, London (1970).

Authors' address:
Eye Clinic of the University of Amsterdam
104 Eerste Helmersstraat
1054 EG Amsterdam, The Netherlands

ANOMALOUS FUSION

B. BAGOLINI

(*Modena, Italy*)

In the classical literature strabismic patients were held to be monocular. The deviated eye was not thought to participate in binocular vision and was thought to be excluded because of scotomatous areas whose purpose was to avoid diplopia and confusion. Anomalous retinal correspondence was thought to be an attempt to reconstruct a type of binocular vision in spite of the deviated eye. This attempt was, however, held to be always abortive and it was never thought that true binocularity could be reached (see for example the classic work of Burian 1945).

Not until the introduction of non-dissociating tests, such as the striated glasses, was it realized that a sort of binocularity could be reached in spite of a deviated eye; this particularly in small angle strabismic patients (Bagolini 1961; 1965; 1967). Dissociation is a word I introduced (see Discussion by Burian of the work of Bagolini 1967), which implies that if we examine a patient in conditions different from those of casual seeing, we may interrupt a weak state of binocularity. The ways in which we can dissociate a binocular state are many: for example if we put a dense red glass in front of one eye we interrupt (or dissociate) a certain binocular adaptation in strabismic patients. This adaptation may be one of suppression of one eye, as occurs in most large angles of strabismus, or it may be a weak state of anomalous binocular vision, as usually occurs in small angles of strabismus. In both cases dissociation with a dense enough red glass leads to diplopia, a condition not normally encountered in an undissociated comitant strabismic patient. Without discussing this phenomenon in detail (for a better explanation see Bagolini 1967), from Fig. 1 we can evaluate the effect of dissociation in 140 strabismic patients tested with various tests of different dissociating power. It is evident that at the striated glasses with patients having an angle of strabismus less than 10 Δ the great majority had a harmonious anomalous correspondence. At the other end, with patients having angles of strabismus above 40 Δ, most of the cases suppressed one eye and were practically monocular. In spite of the fact that the striated glasses have a minimum amount of dissociation, some of the cases were dissociated even by this test and reacted with diplopia. On other tests having a greater dissociating power, the amount of cases showing a harmonious anomalous correspondence were far less than with the striated glasses; according to the test used, they reacted with suppression, diplopia or unharmonious anomalous retinal correspondence.

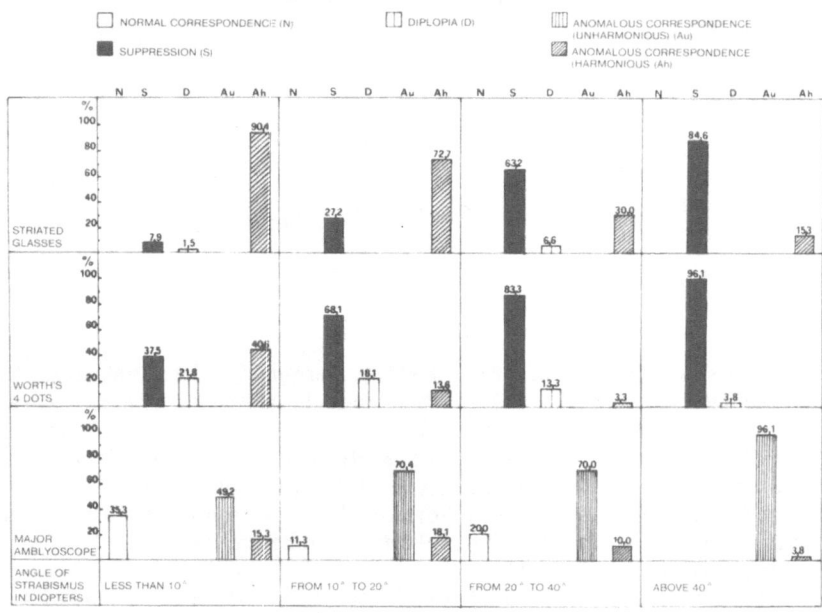

Fig. 1. Clinical findings obtained at the S.G. test, at Worth's 4 dots and Major Amblyo-scope in a group of 165 esotropic patients. The same group has been divided according to the amplitude of the angle of strabismus in prism diopters, into 4 subgroups.

At the S.G. test, it is quite evident that an anomalous binocular vision (anomalous harmonious correspondence) is frequent in small angle strabismus, while in large angle strabismus patients avoid diplopia with suppression. The dissociating effect of the Worth's 4 dot test makes the patient react more easily with suppression even in small angle strabismus. The dissociating effect of the amblyoscope (or Synoptophor) makes the patients react more easily with anomalous retinal correspondence of the unharmonious type. At the major amblyopscope we have considered the correspondence normal or anomalous according to whether there was superimposition, suppression, or crossing at an angle respectively normal or anomalous. The findings at the S.G. test are considered the ones closer to the realm of casual seeing and corresponding to the real sensorial state of the patients.

Cases showing harmonious anomalous retinal correspondence were support-ing a real type of binocular vision. This was proved by studies that examined the subjective space of strabismic patients by means of a horopter apparatus suitably modified. Fig. 2 compares the subjective space of an orthophoric subject (A) with the subjective space of a subjects with small angle strabismus (B). We have inquired if in small angles of strabismus, areas of single binocular vision exist comparable to those of normal subjects. The space was explored by a small light mounted in a horopter apparatus (Bagolini & Tittarelli 1960; Bagolini & Capobianco 1965) and two striated glasses (s.g.) were used in front of each eye, while the patient was looking at a *non*-luminous point P. It was thus possible to detect if the patient was perceiving the light binocularly in a certain region of space around the fixation point P. The result was that in

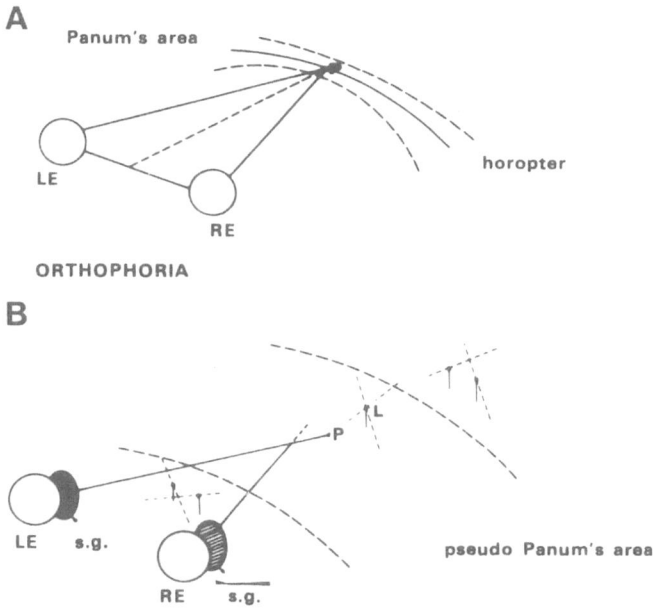

Fig. 2. A. Schematic representation of the Panum's area of binocular single vision in an orthophoric subject. B. Schematic representation of a pseudo-Panum's area supported by anomalous binocular single vision in small angle strabismus. The pseudo-Panum's area is usually larger than the Panum's area in normal subjects. This can be demonstrated by special horopter techniques (Bagolini 1962/1967). It can be easily demonstrated with striated glasses (S.G.) and a pin-point light, when a patient fixes a point *P.* he will see a light (L) crossed by two luminous beams for a certain amount of space in front of and behind of Point P. Outside certain limits (dotted lines) which vary from patient to patient the light L will be perceived double as in physiologic diplopia.

small angles of squint an area similar to the Panum's area of normal subjects could be detected, in which the light was perceived crossed by two luminous beams (each one seen by one eye). This indicates that inside this space, objects were perceived binocularly, while outside this space objects were perceived double, as in the case of physiologic diplopia of normal people. This space of binocular perception (which I call pseudo-Panum's area) has the following characteristics which differentiate it from Panum's area: (1) It is usually larger, indicating that a single retinal point of the fixing eye could correspond in an anomalous way not only to a single point of the deviated eye but also to a retinal area more or less large according to the size of the pseudo-Panum's area. This is geometrically explained in Fig. 3. (2) Owing to the lack of stereo-acuity in squinting subjects, an empirical horopter line can not be found. (3) This state of binocularity is much weaker than normal binocular vision. A suffic-

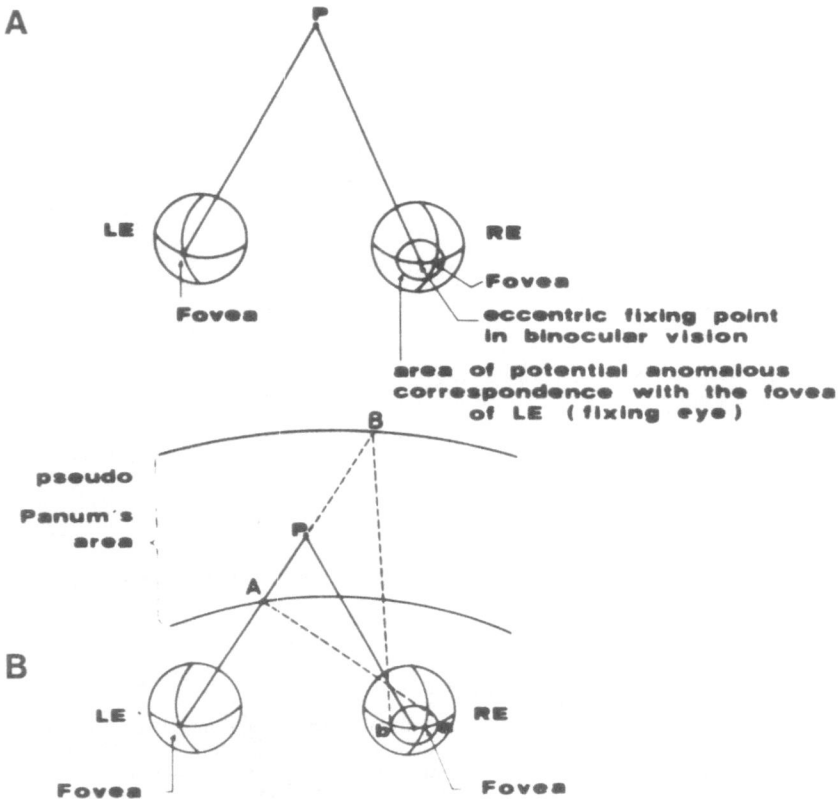

Fig. 3. A. A large pseudo-Panum's area in squinting patients implies that a single retinal point on the fixing eye for example the fovea of the left eye (LE) may correspond to a large retinal area on the deviated eye. This is demonstrated in diagram B. An object P shifting from A to B inside the pseudo-Panum's area is seen singly and binocularly. The image of P is shifting in the deviated eye (RE) on a wide retinal area from *a* to *b* which corresponds in an anomalous way to the fovea of the fixing eye (LE) where the image remains stationary.

iently dense red glass placed in front of one eye can dissociate this binocular state and diplopia appears in the whole subjective space.

Diplopia in squinting subjects appears with filter no denser than number 12 using a red filter ladder with filters numbered according to their density from 1 to 17 (Fig. 4). In normal subjects instead, binocular vision can be interrupted till the point of diplopia only with the denser filters numbers 16 or 17. That binocular vision can be reached in strabismus with small angle deviation has also been demonstrated by my associate Dr. Campos by using campimetric and electrophysiological techniques (Campos & Catellani 1976; Bagolini & Campos 1967; Campos 1980; Campos & Chiesi 1981) He will later demonstrate his findings. Of particular interest is the fact that by campimetric techniques he can demonstrate that in small angles of strabismus with

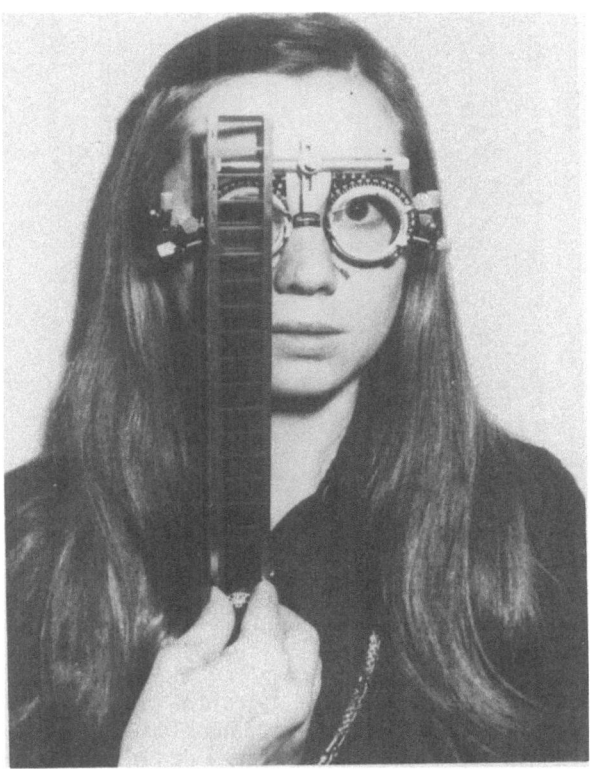

Fig. 4. Filter ladder to measure how deeply rooted the ARC phenomenon and the binocular vision supported by it have become (see text).

anomalous binocular vision the suppression scotomata may completely disappear and confusion and diplopia are avoided by the anomalous correspondence mechanism.

Fig. 5 demonstrates how this is possible. In A a suppression scotoma in the deviated eye is necessary to avoid diplopia. In B where anomalous correspondence has developed, the retinal point X of the deviated eye has acquired the same directional localization of the fovea F of the fixing eye. The image fixed by the fixing eye falls on the fovea of the fixing eye and on the X point of the deviated eye and is perceived binocularly. Suppression is no longer necessary to avoid diplopia since F and X have the same directional localization. This process becomes possible provided that the retinal regions F of the fixing eye and X are stimulated by sufficiently equal retinal images, as occurs in casual seeing. If by haploscopic devices or other tests, we stimulate these two regions with inequal retinal images, we 'dissociate' this sensorial finding and suppression or diplopia is the result. In conclusion we are faced with the following facts: (1) equal retinal images can actually be fused in spite of

45

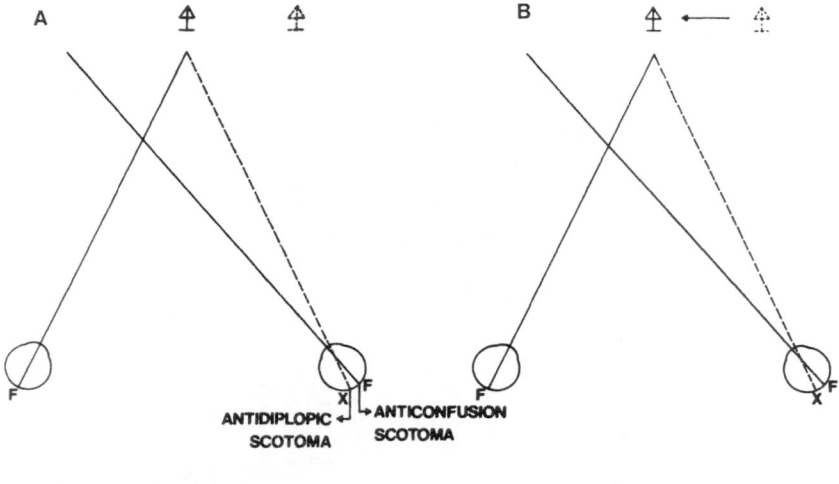

Fig. 5. In A, in which a esotropia of the left eye is supposed, correspondence has remained normal. An antidiplopic scotoma is necessary in X in order for the subject not to perceive double the image of a tree he fixates. In B an harmonious ARC has developed; the retinal point X has acquired the same localization properties of the fovea F of the fixing eye. Suppression scotoma is no longer necessary and the image can be fused in an anomalous way.

a deviated eye, and (2) the subjective space can be divided into regions of binocular vision and regions of diplopia similar to physiological diplopia in normal subjects. These two facts make us believe that in small angles of strabismus a true anomalous sensorial fusion is possible, though much weaker than normal sensorial fusion. In large angles of strabismus, instead, suppression of the deviated eye largely prevails in casual seeing and vision can be considered monocular, as was held in classical literature for all types of squinting subjects. Anomalous sensorial fusion, just like anomalous retinal correspondence, to which it is related, and suppression, can be considered sensorial adaptive phenomena to the angle of strabismus (Burian 1947; Bagolini 1967). These sensorial phenomena in children become more deeply adapted and reinforce themselves with the passing of time.

There is now a sensorio-motorial adaptation to the angle of strabismus which has been only recently studied (Halldén 1952; Maraini & Pasino 1964; Bagolini 1976; Crone 1980). This phenomenon has been highlighted by the widespread use of prisms which has become fashionable in recent years as an attempt at treating sensorial anomalies in comitant strabismus (Bagolini 1961; Berard 1963; Pigassou & Garipuy 1966; Adelstein & Cüppers 1968). If we attempt to correct by prisms the angle of a convergent strabismus, most patients have an increase of the angle of strabismus which may equal the amount of prismatic correction: the prisms 'eating up' as is currently said in orthoptic slang. This phenomenon is almost invariably present and particularly well developed in small angles of strabismus. As has been noted by Adelstein

& Cüppers (1968), a patient may 'eat up' the exact correction but it is almost always possible to find a prismatic overcorrection of such a power that can not be overcome by the patient; sometimes, as first noted by these authors, the hypercorrected angle of strabismus may even decrease. Fig. 6 shows the behaviour of 85 patients with small angle deviation. All of them invariably had an increase of the angle of strabismus when the exact prismatic correction of the deviation was worn. When an overcorrection ranging from 20 to 30 prism diopters equally distributed over the two eyes was given, 56.5% responded with an increase of the angle of strabismus. They are indicated by the arrows pointing up. The lower part of the arrows indicates the original amount of the angle of strabismus in prism diopters. The pointed part of the arrows indicates the variation of the angle of strabismus after an observation of the patient ranging from 10 minutes to 3 hours. 25.5% of this group had total compensation of the prisms. 24.7% of the patients had no increase of the angle of strabismus (represented in the graph by small segments) while 18% showed a decrease of the angle (arrow pointing down). On the whole, observing the prismatic correction of strabismic patients, a few of them do not compensate prism correction, but the majority do. Among a strabismic population that compensates prisms, some of them can only just compensate the prismatic correction of the angle, while others need quite strong prismatic hypercorrection to hamper this peculiar tendency to overconverge. Fig. 7 shows a patient who was able to overcome a prismatic correction of 24 Δ but not overcome a prismatic correction of 40 Δ.

These convergent movements have something in common with normal convergent fusional movements. They are in fact elicited by temporally displacing a retinal image by means of base out prisms, just as occurs for normal converging fusional movements. In a lesser degree, vertical or diverging move-

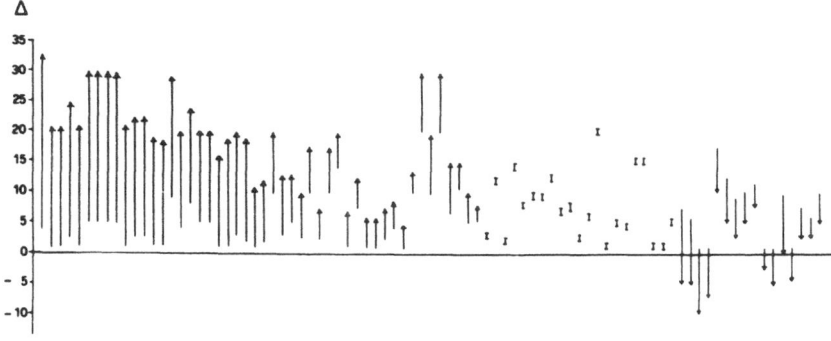

Fig. 6. Behaviour of 85 cases of postoperative esotropias. All the cases invariably increased their angle of deviation when the residual angle of deviation was corrected by prisms. The graph represents their behaviour with a prismatic overcorrection ranging from 20 to 30 diopters. The length of the arrow indicates, in prism diopters (on the ordinate axis) the variation of the angle of deviation. The first cases (arrow pointing up), have completely or partially compensated the prismatic overcorrection by an overconvergence. The cases represented by a small segment did not show any variation of the angle of strabismus, while the last cases (arrow pointing down) have reacted by diverging.

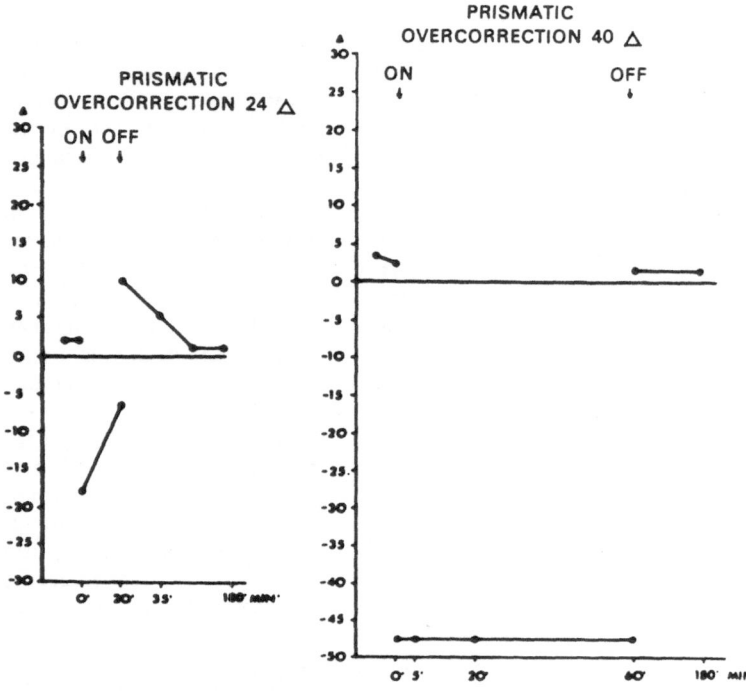

Fig. 7. This diagram shows the behaviour of a patient with small angle of esotropia of 2 diopters. He could compensate an overcorrection of 24 prismatic diopters (diagram to the left) but could not compensate for an overcorrection of 40 prism diopters (diagram to the right). The axis of the abscissa represents, in prismatic diopters, the variations of the angle of strabismus during the time of observation in minutes. Arrow at *on* and *off* represents respectively the moment in which prismatic overcorrections have been applied (on) and removed (off). The various spots represent measurements of the objective deviation (at the cover test) at various lengths of time. The diagram to the left shows that the angle deviation from about 2 diopters eso becomes an artificial exo (negative numbers), after application of base out prisms, of about 17 diopters; after 20 minutes, the artificial exo was only 7 diopters. After removing the prism, the esodeviation was around 11 diopter eso. The esodeviation had therefore increased in 20 minutes by about 9 diopters. The angle of strabismus returned to normal after more than one hour. The diagram on the right shows the behaviour of the same patient after application of 40 diopters. The angle strabismus remained unchanged after an observation of about 1 hour.

ments can be elicited if we displace the retinal image vertically or nasally by vertically placed prims or based in prisms (Campos & Zanasi 1978).

Their similarity with normal fusional movements is then evident. They are elicited by the same type of stimulations, i.e. displacement of retinal images. Like in normal fusional movements convergent movements are strongly developed, but, though less developed, vertical and divergent movements can be elicited in a similar way as for normal fusional movements. They have evidently the aim of bringing equal retinal images over retinal areas which have acquired (in an anomalous way) the same directional localization. That is to say, to bring equal retinal images over areas of anomalous corresponding retinal points; this in a similar way by which normal fusional movements tend to bring equal retinal images over normal corresponding retinal points. They tend to maintain with appropriate ocular movements the anomalous sensorial fusion we have previously described; we therefore believe it can be appropriate to call them anomalous fusional movements (a.f.m.).

They differ, however, from normal fusional movements (n.f.m.) in various features.

a) They are very slow if compared to normal fusional movements. They may take several minutes, hours or even days to reach the final ocular deviation. Unlike n.f.m. they can never be observed by the naked eye because they are too slow. Even in cases of primary microstrabismus, where they may be accomplished rather rapidly, a.f.m. are generally too slow to be detected by observation of the patient's eyes when a base-out prism is placed before one of them. They can only be detected because a variation in the angle of strabismus is observed at the cover test some time after the prisms have been applied.

b) A.f.m. are usually less precise than n.f.m. In fact, while with n.f.m. there is an exact compensation of the prismatic power, in a.f.m. the compensation is frequently only partial.

This last point deserves some comment. We have previously explained that especially in small angle convergent strabismus there is an anomalous sensorial fusion and that this is supported by an anomalous correspondence between a single point of the fixing eye with a large retinal area of the deviated eye (Fig. 3). A.f.m. do not need therefore to compensate completely the prismatic correction, but it is sufficient for them to bring the retinal image inside this area. The larger this area, the smaller need to be the compensatory movements induced by the prism.

If we control the state of binocularity of the patient with striated glasses when we apply prisms, we usually find anomalous binocular vision when the movement has been accomplished. However we find binocular vision even if the movement has compensated only partially the power of the prism. It is evident therefore that the prismatic power is compensated just by that amount which is sufficient to restore an anomalous type of binocular vision. A.f.m. can at times be found even with one eye suppressing or with a certain amount of obstacles artificially created to binocular vision. For explanation of this finding I refer to Bagolini 1976. We have called by the name 'anomalous fusional movements' these sensorio-motorial anomalies that we find in strabismic patients. Similar sensorio-motorial anomalies however have also been found in the past and interpreted in a different way. I am referring to the 'horror fusionis' of Bielschowsky or the 'Widerwillen gegen Einfachsehen' of von Graefe which are different expressions to indicate that a bifoveal fusion is impossible and that ocular movements are accomplished to avoid the bifoveal stimulation. Very probably the movements observed by these Authors are the same as the a.f.m. here described. They were interpreted however as an intolerance (horror) to bifoveal stimulation and the movement had the aim of avoiding a disagreeable situation. We believe that the anomalous movements, here described, cannot be interpreted in this way. In fact if one overcorrects by prisms a convergent strabismus, the image fixed by the dominant eye will be displaced temporally in the deviated eye (Fig. 8); by accomplishing a convergent movement to overcome the prismatic correction, the patient will perform a movement that at least in the first part makes the retinal image shift toward the fovea and not away from it, as is implied in the term 'horror fusionis'. A second interpretation to explain these movements is exemplified by the term 'diplopia phobia' of van der Hoeve. This concept has been recently resumed by Pratt Johnson to explain the ocular movements just described when prisms are applied to correct an angle of strabismus. There is no doubt that in certain cases of strabismus of sudden onset the patient may experience diplopia and may have more or less voluntary movement to increase the angle of deviation. The two equal images will increase their lateral distance and the double image will be less annoying. This explanation can not, however, be applied to the majority of the cases which increase the angle of convergent strabismus by application of base out prisms. We have carefully studied these cases sensorially and the experience of diplopia when prisms are applied is rather the exception than the rule. We believe therefore that particularly in convergent small-angle strabismus a series of adaptational phenomena may take place; these adaptational phenomena leading to anomalous correspondence may support a certain degree of binocularity which reinforces itself in young children with the passing of time. This binocularity consists of an anomalous sensorial fusion and of anomalous fusional movements which tend to stabilize the angle of strabismus.

The knowledge of these sequelae is of practical importance. We do not usually succeed in eliminating a small angle of strabismus by surgery; in fact

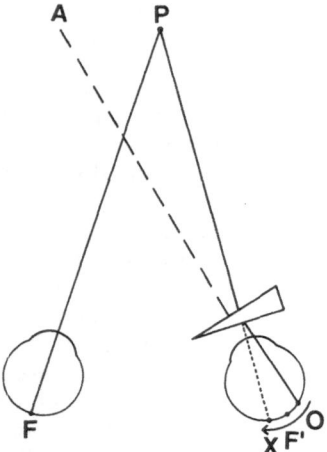

Fig. 8. Shows a patient with small angle of strabismus fixing a point P (the line A–F$_1$ corresponds to the visual axis of the deviated right eye). A prism with a power greater than the prismatic amount of esodeviation will shift the projection of P from a retinal area X to a retinal area O which is situated temporally to the fovea F$_1$. Since the angle of strabismus will increase, the image of P tends to shift (see arrow) from O to X and in the first part of this shifting will go toward the fovea F$_1$ and not away from it as would be implied in the term 'horror fusionis'.

a small amount of surgery is not sufficient to hamper those anomalous fusional movements that tend to restore the previous small-angle deviation. This, particularly if the small angle deviation has been of long standing.

Anomalous sensorial fusion and anomalous fusional movements, however, may have certain advantages. When we obtain postoperatively, from a large angle of esotropia, a small aesthetically disregardable angle of strabismus in sufficiently young children, we may be satisfied with this goal. In fact we usually obtain a type of anomalous binocular vision supported by anomalous sensorial fusion and anomalous fusional movements which may be of some utility in daily life and tends to oppose future variation in the angle of strabismus.

REFERENCES

Adelstein, F. & C. Cüppers. Probleme der operativen Schielbehandlung. Ber. Dtsch. Ophthal. Ges. 69: 580 (1968).

Bagolini, B. Diagnostic et possibilité de traitement de l'état sensoriel du strabisme concomitant avec des instruments peu dissociants (test du verre strié et barre de filtres). Ann. Ocul. 194: 236 (1961).

Bagolini, B. Anomalous correspondence: Definition and diagnostic methods. Doc. Ophthalmol. 23: 346 (1967).

Bagolini, B. Part I – Sensorial anomalies in strabismus (Suppression, anomalas correspondence, amblyopia). Doc. Ophthalmol. 41: 1 (1976).

Bagolini, B. Part II – Sensorio-motorial anomalies in strabismus. (Anomalous movements). Doc. Ophthalmol. 41: 23 (1976).

Bagolini, B. & E.C. Campos. Binocular campimetry in small-angle concomitant esotropia. Doc. Ophthalmol. Proc. Series. Vol. II. Dr W. Junk, The Hague. 1977.

Bagolini, B. & N.M. Capobianco. Subjective space in comitant squint. Am. J. Ophthalmol. 59: 430 (1965).

Bagolini, B. & R. Tittarelli. Considerazioni sul meccanismo antidiplopico nello strabismo concomitante. Boll. d'Ocul. 39: 211 (1960).

Berard, P.V. Les prismes en thérapeutique ophthalmologique. Bull. Soc. Ophthalm. de France. 63: 626 (1963).

Bielschowsky, A. Congenital and acquired defects of fusion. Am. J. Ophthalmol. 18: 925 (1935).

Burian, H.M. Sensorial retinal relationship in concomitant strabismus. Trans. Am. Ophthalmol. Soc. 81: 373 (1945).

Burian, H.M. Discussion to the paper by B. Bagolini: Anomalous Correspondence: Definition and diagnostic methods. Doc. Ophthalmol. 23: 392 (1967).

Campos, E.C. Anomalous retinal correspondence. Monocular and binocular visual evoked responses. Arch. Ophthalmol. 98: 299 (1980).

Campos E.C. & T. Catellani. Perimetria binoculare nell'esotropia concomitante a piccolo angolo. Boll. Ocul. 55: 205 (1976).

Campos, E.C. & C. Chiesi. Perimetrie binoculaire dans l'exotropia concomitant. Bull. et Mem. Soc. Franç. Opht. 92° anné, Masson, Paris 1981.

Campos, E.C. & M.R. Zanasi. Die anomale Fusionsbewegungen: Der senso-motorische Aspekt der anomalen Binokularsehens. Albrecht v. Graefes Arch. Klin. exp. Ophthal. 205: 101 (1978).

Crone, R.A. Anomalous and normal motor fusion in esophoria and microesotropia. Trans. Ophthal. Soc. U.K. 100: 464 (1980).

Halldén, U. Fusion phenomena in anomalous correspondence. Acta Ophthalmol. Klin. Suppl. 37: 1 (1952).

Graefe, A. von. Über Doppelsehen nach Schieloperationen und Incongruenz der Netzhaüte Arch. für Ophthalmologie 1: 117 (1854).

Maraini, G. & L. Pasino. Variations in the fusional movements in cases of small angle convergent strabismus with harmonious anomalous retinal correspondence. Brit. J. Ophthalmol. 48: 439 (1964).

Pigassou, R. & J. Garipuy, Traitement du strabisme dans l'espace libre. Arch. Ophthalmol. 26: 445 (1966).

Pratt-Johnson, J.A. Sensory basis for prismotherapy in esotropia. Proc. 2nd Congress I.S.A. Edited by P. Fells, Diffusion générale du librairie, Marseille 1976.

Van der Hoeve, J. Über Augenmuskelwirkung und Schielen. Klin. Mbl. Augenheilk. 69: 620 (1922).

Author's address:
Department of Ophthalmology
University of Modena
Modena, Italy

SENSORIAL INTERACTIONS IN REEDUCATED STRABISMIC AMBLYOPIA

M. FOCOSI, G. SALVI & R. FROSINI

(Firenze, Italy)

Focosi & Parducci (1978) reported two particular cases: two children in whom the vision of their ambliopic eye had practically returned to normal after rehabilitation. They were subsequently operated on and strabismus was satisfactorily corrected.

When examined some years later, they showed a medium-slight mono-lateral myopia in the fixing eye. In order to have good visual acuity, both patients had to wear their monolateral correction.

The following observations were reported:

1. In binocular vision, without any correction, the visual acuity was equal to the non-corrected visus of the fixing eye.

2. As soon as the fixing eye was covered, the visual acuity immediately went back to normal as the fixation was taken by the ex-amblyopic eye.

3. Improvement would disappear with equal rapidity as soon as the non-corrected fixing eye was uncovered.

Nardi (in press) observed the same behaviour in two similar cases.

The following case is very similar to those mentioned above, and its features make it worth reporting.

A 27-year-old woman previously affected by right esotropia with aniso-metropia and very slight amblyopia. Right eye: visual acuity 9/10 with correction (+1.50 sf = +2.00 cyl at 100°). Left eye: it was originally the fixing eye, but at the examination the visual acuity had gone down owing to retinal detachment with macular involvement.

Surgery led to retinal reattachment, but also to a severe vitreo-macular retraction and the visus was reduced to 1/30. In binocular vision the patient went on reporting 1/30, whereas once the left eye was covered the visual acuity, with the correction on the right eye, immediately went up to 9/10.

Such an anomalous condition could be eliminated by applying a darkened glass on the left eye. This condition had been present for two years after surgery and was eliminated in binocular vision only when a 25 diopters external base prism was placed in front of the left eye.

A similar case was also reported by Focosi & Parducci (1978) for the appearance of a myopic macular lesion in the fixing eye.

This strange, constant behaviour leads to several considerations: a. We are evidently dealing with an active inhibition by the fixing eye; b. It confirms the observations reported by many authors who have investigated the inter-

© *1982, Dr W. Junk Publishers, The Hague. ISBN 90 6193 728 0*

ference of the fixing eye with the one affected by strabismus inasmuch as in binocular vision the visual acuity of the amblyopic eye is lower than when the fixing eye is completely occluded; c. The degree of inhibition by the fixing eye varies according to the situation experienced. Galassi (1978) noticed that the less dissociating the methods employed for the examination, the higher the decrease in visual acuity of the non-fixing eye (i.e. polarizing glasses versus haploscopic systems). This fully agrees with the observations reported by Focosi & Parducci (1978) and also by Nardi (in press). According to them the visual acuity with both eyes uncovered was equal to the non-corrected visus of the fixing eye whatever the degree of myopia was; d. The case reported confirms not only the above-mentioned findings, but also demonstrates that not even the practical abolition of the macular function (made worse also by metamorphopsies) in the fixing eye was sufficient to eliminate the inhibition and that only the shifting of the images by a high value prism into the periferal retina was able to avoid the incident; e. The persisting inhibition throughout the years demonstrates how deep-rooted the suppression can be mostly at the optional stage.

REFERENCES

Aulhorn, E. Die gegenseitige Beeinflussung abbildungsgleicher Netzhautstellen bei normalen und gestörtem Binocularsehen. Documenta Ophth. 23: 26–32 (1967).
Focosi, M. & F. Parducci. About a particular interaction of the fixating eye in strabismic amblyopia after treatment. Ophthalmologica 177: 109–113 (1978).
Galassi, F. Determinazione dell' acuità visiva nell'ambliopico recuperato in visione binoculare. Atti Fondazione Ronchi 33: 417–422 (1978).
Mackensen, G. Monokuläre und binokuläre statische Perimetrie zur Untersuchung der Hemmungsvorgänge beim Schielen. Graefes Arch. Ophthalm. 160: 573–587 (1959).
Nardi, M. In press.
Noorden, G.K. von & M.B. Leffler. Visual acuity in strabismic amblyopia under monocular and binocular conditions. Archs. Ophthal. N.Y. 76: 172–177 (1966).
Pigassou, R., L. Garipuy, M. Gorda & P. Sforrim. Amblyopic fonctionnelle. Annls Oculist. 202: 39–48 (1969).
Pugh, M.A. Foveal vision in amblyopia. Brit. J. Ophthal. 38: 321–331 (1954).

Authors' address:
Istituto di Clinica Oculistica
Università degli Studi di Firenze
Firenze, Italy

BINOCULARITY IN COMITANT ESOTROPIA AND EXOTROPIA

E.C. CAMPOS & C. CHIESI

(Modena, Italy)

ABSTRACT

With a series of experiments, it is shown that both in concomitant small-angle esotropia and exotropia, one can find wide areas of overlapping of the visual fields of the two eyes. This type of overlapping is defined as anomalous binocular vision. In this group of patients no suppression scotomas were detected. This is due to the fact that the test-targets were fusable stimuli, with appropriate controls for binocularity. The same patients, tested with more artificial (or 'dissociating') techniques, exhibited suppression scotomas in the identical areas where anomalous binocularity was found with our technique. In patients with large-angle exotropia, suppression scotomas were always present. However, their shape was strongly influenced by the testing technique.

It is concluded that reliable information on the quality of binocularity in strabismus can be obtained only with methods which alter as little as possible the everyday seeing condition of the patient.

INTRODUCTION

It has been clarified in the last twenty years or so, that any type of sensory testing in strabismus is strongly influenced by the technique employed by the examiner (Bagolini 1967; von Noorden 1979). Reliable qualitative results can thus be obtained only when the patient is tested in his/her casual seeing condition, i.e., fusable stimuli have to be used as test-targets (Bagolini 1958; Bagolini 1961; Bagolini 1967; Bagolini 1976; von Noorden 1979). On the basis of this principle, it was shown with horopter techniques that patients with small-angle esotropia enjoy an anomalous binocular vision, sustained by anomalous retinal correspondence (ARC) (Bagolini & Capobianco 1965).

Various studies have originated from this laboratory in recent years on the binocular visual field of patients with small-angle strabismus. These patients were examined using fusable stimuli as test-targets (Bagolini & Ravalico 1971; Campos & Catellani 1976; Bagolini & Campos 1977; Campos & Chiesi 1981). Results are summarized as follows:

(1) Patients with small-angle esotropia and exotropia show a wide area of binocular single vision sustained by ARC. (2) No suppression scotomas are

present. (3) The area of binocular single vision is more deeply rooted in the center than in the periphery of the visual field. These findings were further substained by objective methods (Campos 1980).

In the classical literature binocular visual fields are considered to exhibit at least one suppression scotoma of the deviated eye in the central area. The aim of this paper is to present data obtained by testing the same group of patients with our technique and with the one described by Harms (1937) in order to compare the results.

MATERIAL AND METHODS

Thirteen patients were included in this study. All had a small-angle non-alternating esotropia, ranging from 3° to 8° degrees. They showed an ARC as tested with the striated glasses. ARC was deeply rooted — never interruptable with filters ligher than n. 9 of Bagolini's red filters bar. Significant data on patients are summarized in Table 1.

Table 1.

Patient	Age	Visual OD	Acuity OS	Deviated eye	Angle of deviation in degrees	Diplopia with Bagolini's filter
1	12	6/6	6/7.5	OS	+5	12°
2	11	6/6	6/6	OD	+7	10°
3	16	6/6	6/7.5	OS	+3	10°
4	17	6/6	6/6	OD	+4	11°
5	15	6/9	6/6	OD	+8	12°
6	12	6/6	6/6	OD	+5	10°
7	11	6/6	6/6	OS	+4	11°
8	17	6/7.5	6/6	OD	+3	12°
9	12	6/6	6/6	OS	+4	9°
10	16	6/6	6/6	OS	+5	12°
11	8	6/6	6/6	OD	+6	12°
12	13	6/7.5	6/6	OD	+7	11°
13	10	6/6	6/6	OS	+8	13°

Experiment 1

Patients wore striated lenses and were at 1 m from a tangent screen (5 cd/m² luminance). They looked at a black fixation point (0.5° diameter), and were asked to indicate whether a white light source (0.3° diameter, 115 cd/m² luminance), moved perimetrically was seen single and crossed by one streak (suppression), crossed by two streaks (binocular single vision) or whether two lights were present, each crossed by one streak (diplopia). The experiment was repeated with the patients wearing a red filter (corresponding to n. 8 of Bagolini's bar) in front of the fixing eye, plus two striated glasses. Such obstacle to fusion was useful for assessing how deeply rooted the sensory adaptation was.

Experiment 2

Patients wore a pair of red-green glasses, with the red glass in front of the deviated eye. The Harms 'participation-perimetry' was performed using the same white light source as in Experiment 1. Subjects were asked to indicate whether the stimulus was seen green (suppression of the deviated eye), red (suppression of the fixing eye) or red and green (diplopia). For the 'exclusion perimetry', the stimulus was red. When it was not seen, it was assumed that the subject suppressed the deviated eye.

RESULTS

All 13 patients examined in Experiment 1 showed an anomalous overlapping of the visual fields of the two eyes, interpreted as anomalous binocular vision (Fig. 1A). No suppression scotomas were present in the area tested by us, which extended to 30° from the fixation point.

A significant restriction of the area of binocular single vision was caused by a red filter put in front of the fixing eye (Fig. 1B).

Results obtained with Harms participation and exclusion perimetry are summarized in Table 2. With the participation perimetry, two patients showed suppression of the deviated eye (case 6, 11) (Fig. 2); three had diplopia over the whole visual field (case 2, 3, 7); five had diplopia coexisting

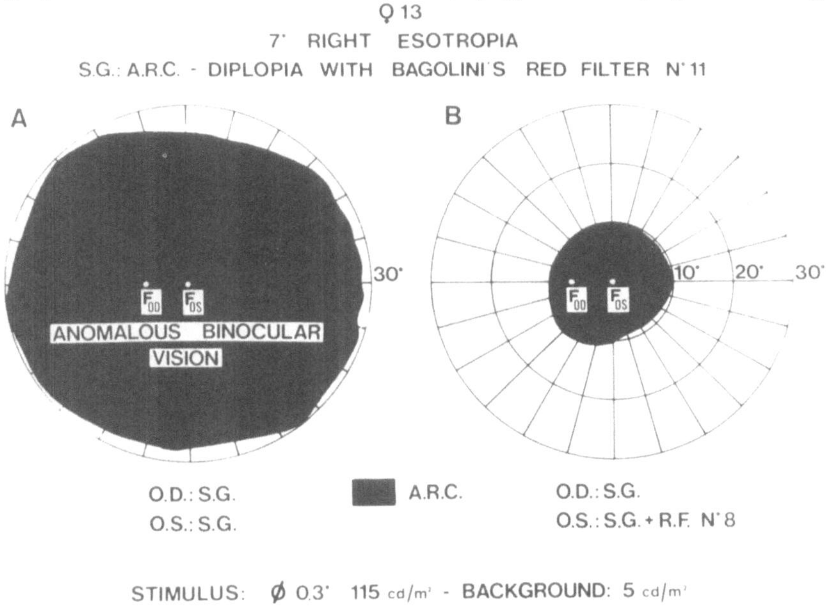

♀ 13
7° RIGHT ESOTROPIA
S.G.: A.R.C. - DIPLOPIA WITH BAGOLINI'S RED FILTER N°11
A
B
30°
F OD
F OS
ANOMALOUS BINOCULAR
VISION
10°
20°
30°
F OD
F OS
O.D.: S.G.
O.S.: S.G.
A.R.C.
O.D.: S.G.
O.S.: S.G. + R.F. N°8
STIMULUS: ∅ 0.3° 115 cd/m² - BACKGROUND: 5 cd/m²

Fig. 1. A: Using striated glasses as a control for binocularity and a white light source as a stimulus, a wide area of binocular single vision is detected in patients with small-angle esotropia. B: A red filter in front of the fixing eye causes a restriction of the area of binocular single vision.

Table 2

Patient	Participation perimetry	Exclusion perimetry
1	Suppression OS/Central diplopia	Fixation point and foveal scotoma OS
2	Diplopia	Fixation point scotoma OD
3	Diplopia	No suppression scotoma
4	Diplopia; suppression OD and OS	Foveal scotoma OD
5	Suppression OD/OS; Diplopia	Suppression scotoma including fovea and fixation point OD
6	Fixation and foveal scotoma OD	Sporadically suppression OD over the whole field
7	Diplopia	No suppression scotoma
8	Diplopia; suppression OD	Fixation point and foveal scotomas OD
9	Diplopia; suppression OD and OS	Foveal scotoma OS
10	Diplopia; scotoma including fovea and fixation point OS	No suppression scotoma
11	Fixation point and foveal scotomas OD	No suppression scotoma
12	Fixation point and foveal scotomas OD; Diplopia	Foveal scotoma OD
13	Fixation point and foveal scotomas OS; Diplopia	No suppression scotoma

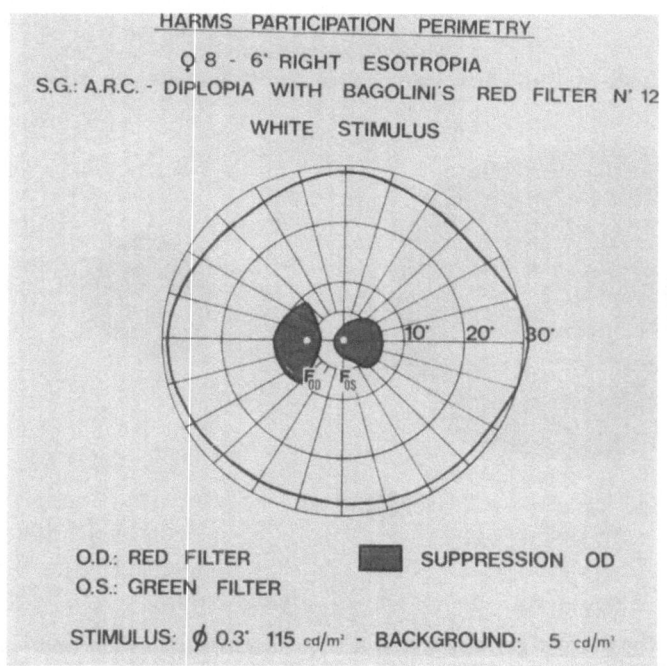

Fig. 2. Harms participation perimetry. Fixation point and foveal scotoma of the deviated eye. Note, with the Bagolini-Campos technique no scotoma was found in this patient.

with suppression of the deviated eye (case 1, 8, 10, 12, 13) (Fig. 3) and three had diplopia and suppression of the fixing and the deviated eye, according to the area which was tested (case 4, 5, 9) (Fig. 4B). With the exclusion perimetry no suppression scotoma was found in the deviated eye of five

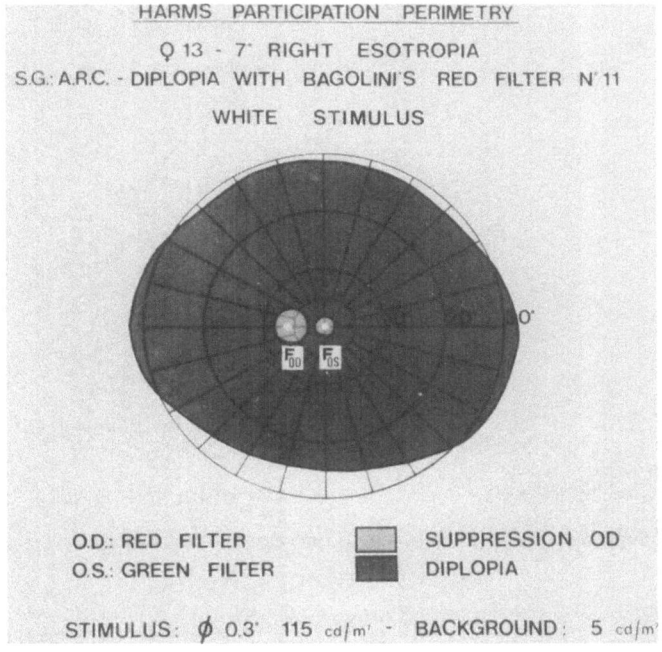

Fig. 3. Harms participation perimetry. Fixation point and foveal scotoma of the deviated eye centrally; diplopia peripherally.

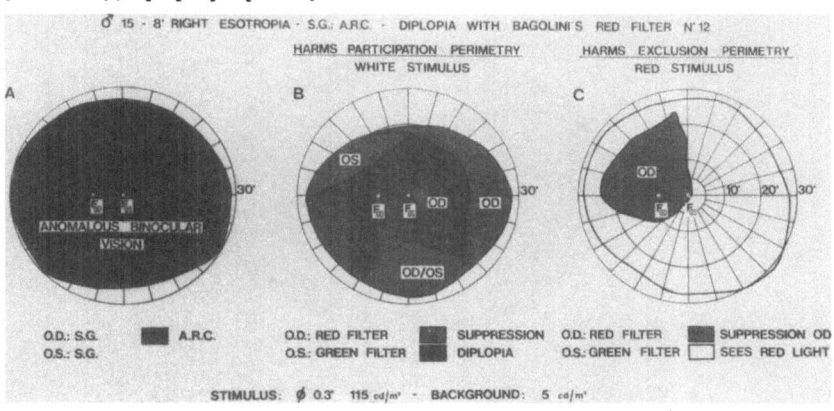

Fig. 4. A: Binocular single vision with the Bagolini-Campos technique. B: Harms participation perimetry: suppression OD and OS; alternating suppression and diplopia. C: Harms exclusion perimetry: scotoma including the fixation point and the fovea of the deviated eye.

Q 8 - 6' RIGHT ESOTROPIA
S.G.: A.R.C. - DIPLOPIA WITH BAGOLINI'S RED FILTER N° 12

RED STIMULUS

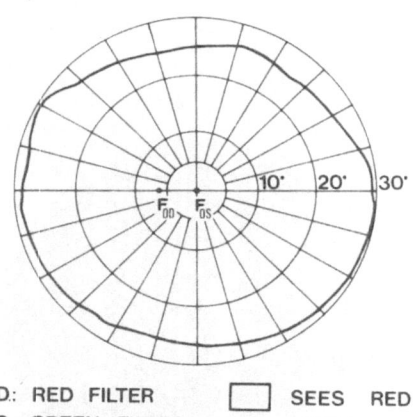

O.D.: RED FILTER   ☐ SEES RED
O.S.: GREEN FILTER   LIGHT

STIMULUS: ∅ 0.3' 115 cd/m² - BACKGROUND: 5 cd/m²

Fig. 5. Diplopia over the whole field with Harms exclusion perimetry.

HARMS EXCLUSION PERIMETRY

Q 13 - 7' RIGHT ESOTROPIA
S.G. A.R.C. - DIPLOPIA WITH BAGOLINI'S RED FILTER N° 11

RED STIMULUS

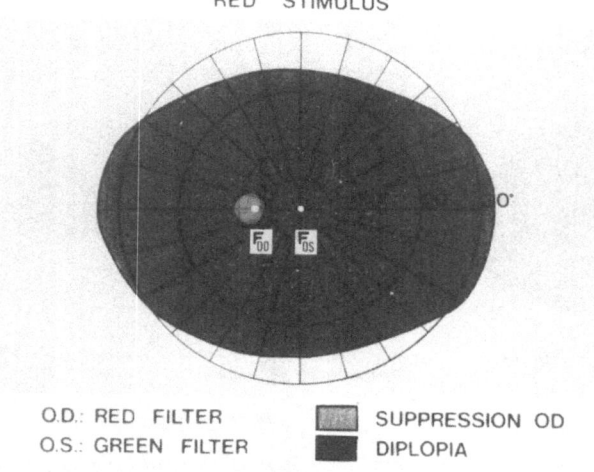

O.D.: RED FILTER   SUPPRESSION OD
O.S.: GREEN FILTER   ■ DIPLOPIA

STIMULUS: ∅ 0.3' 115 cd/m² - BACKGROUND: 5 cd/m²

Fig. 6. Foveal scotoma of the deviated eye and diplopia with Harms exclusion perimetry.

60

patients (case 3, 7, 10, 11, 13) (Fig. 5). A scotoma of the foveal area of the deviated eye was present in three patients (case 4, 9, 12) (Fig. 6); a fixation point scotoma alone was present in one patient (case 2). Finally, a fixation point scotoma associated with a foveal scotoma was detected in four patients (case 1, 5, 6, 8) (Fig. 4).

DISCUSSION AND CONCLUSIONS

This study confirms previous findings of this laboratory on the binocularity of strabismus. A wide area of binocular single vision was detected in 13 patients with small-angle esotropia. This anomalous binocularity is more deeply rooted in the center than in the periphery of the visual field. It is worthwhile to recall that recently we were able to demonstrate an identical behaviour in patients with small-angle non-intermittent exotropia, tested with our methods (Fig. 7). In large-angle divergent strabismus it is almost never possible to demonstrate hemianopic suppression scotomas; they can be found only by using dissociating techniques (Fig. 8).

Our group of patients showed constantly at least one suppression scotoma with the Harms participation perimetry. Data with Harms exclusion perimetry were more inconsistent, but often suppression of the deviated eye was detected.

Such discrepancy between the results obtained with our technique and that proposed by Harms should be attributed to the different testing conditions. We used fusable stimuli as test-targets and put the patient in his/her casual seeing condition. Harms, by utilizing red-green glasses elicited retinal rivalry. Such a phenomenon hampers fusion even in normals and has to be considered a cause of 'dissociation'.

It can thus be concluded that the high variability of results found in the literature concerning binocular perimetry in strabismus has to be attributed to the testing technique used by various authors. Suppression scotomas found only with dissociating techniques, need not necessarily to be present

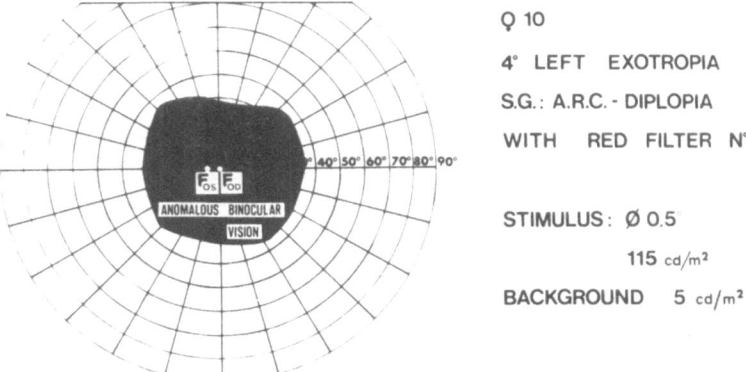

Q 10

4° LEFT EXOTROPIA

S.G.: A.R.C. - DIPLOPIA

WITH RED FILTER N° 12

STIMULUS: Ø 0.5

115 cd/m²

BACKGROUND 5 cd/m²

Fig. 7. Binocular single vision in small-angle exotropia.

61

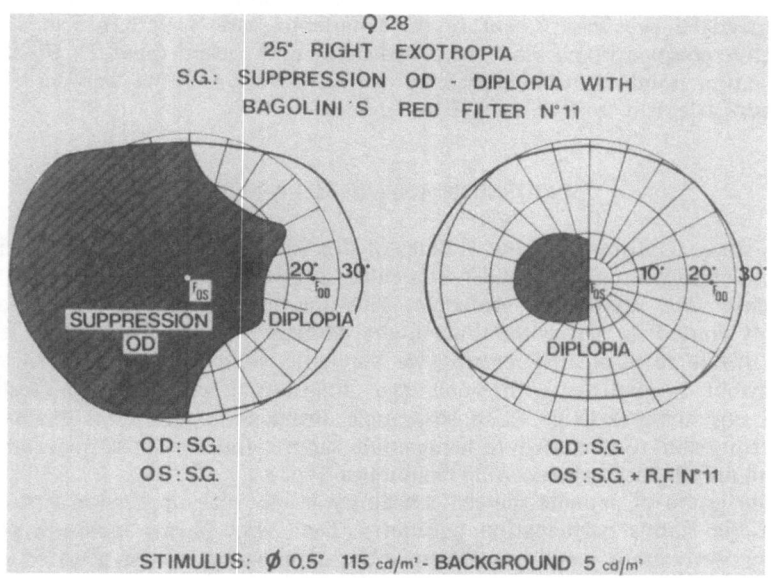

Fig. 8. Hemianopic suppression scotomas in large angle exotropia are found, only by using dissociating techniques.

in the everyday seeing condition of the patient. Reliable qualitative results can be obtained only by using non-dissociating techniques.

We suggest that a comparison of results of different authors is valid only if the testing techniques are superimposable, on the basis of the above mentioned concepts.

We hope that our comparative study may be of some use for clarifying conflicting data on this subject.

REFERENCES

Bagolini, B. Tecnica per l'esame della visione binoculare senza introduzione di elementi dissocianti: 'test del vetro striato' Boll. Ocul. 37: 195 (1958).

Bagolini, B. Diagnostic et possibilité de traitment de l'état sensorial du strabisme avec des instruments peu dissociants (test du verre strié et barre de filtres). Ann. Ocul. 194: 236 (1961).

Bagolini, B. Anomalous correspondence: definition and diagnostic methods. Docum. Ophthalmol. 23: 346 (1967).

Bagolini, B. Part I. Sensorial anomalies in strabismus (Suppression, anomalous correspondence, amblyopia). Docum. Ophthalmol. 41: 1 (1976).

Bagolini, B. & E.C. Campos. Binocular campimetry in small-angle concomitant esotropia. Docum. Ophthalmol. Proc. Series Dr W. Junk, The Hague. 14: 405 (1977).

Bagolini, B & . N.M. Capobianco. Subjective space in concomitant squint. Am. J. Ophthal. 59: 430 (1965).

Bagolini, B. & G. Ravalico. The binocular visual field in small angle strabismus. Proc. 2nd Int. Orth. Congr. Excerpta Medica, Amsterdam. 245: 43 (1971).

Campos, E.C. Anomalous retinal correspondence. Monocular and binocular visual evoked responses. Arch. Ophthalmol. 98: 299 (1980).

Campos, E. & T. Catellani. Perimetria binoculare nell'esotropia concomitante a piccolo angolo. Boll. Ocul. 55: 205 (1976).

Campos, E.C. & C. Chiesi. Perimetrie binoculaire dans l'exotropie concomitant. Bull. et Mem. Soc. Française d'Ophtalmol. 92° anné. Masson, Paris, 1981 p. 301.

Harms, H. Ort und Wesen der Bildhemmung bei Schielenden. Albrecht v. Graefes Arch. Ophthal. 138: 149 (1937).

Herzau, V. Untersuchungen über das Gesichtsfeld Schielender. Docum. Ophthalmol. 49: 221 (1980).

Jampolsky, A. Characteristics of suppression in Strabismus. Arch. Ophthalmol. 54: 683 (1955).

Noorden, G.K. von. Burian-von Noorden's Binocular Vision and Ocular Motility. Theory and Management of Strabismus. C.V. Mosby St. Louis, 1979.

Parks, M.L. Ocular motility and strabismus. Harper & Row, Hagerstown, 1975.

Pratt-Johnson, J.A. & A.L. MacDonald. Binocular visual field in strabismus. Canad. J. Ophthalmol. 11: 37 (1976).

Authors' address:
Pediatric Ophthalmology and Strabismus Service
Department of Ophthalmology
University of Modena
Modena, Italy

Requests for reprints:
E.C. Campos
Clinica Oculistica dell'Università
Via del Pozzo 71
41100 Modena, Italy

RESULTS OF THE FADENOPERATION IN ALTERNATING CONVERGENT STRABISMUS OF THE CONGENITAL TYPE

W. DE DECKER & W. HAASE

(Kiel, F.R.G.)

INTRODUCTION

It would not make sense to present the dry results without an idea of the conceptions behind. For this reason we shall introduce this communication with a few remarks on technical and indicational problems.

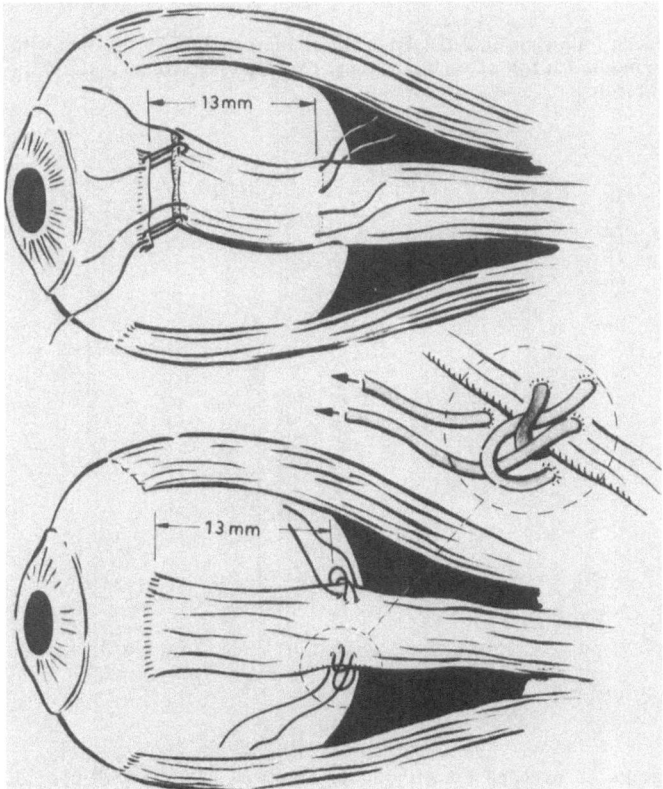

Fig. 1. Fadenoperation after Cüppers (top); own technique of choice (ground).

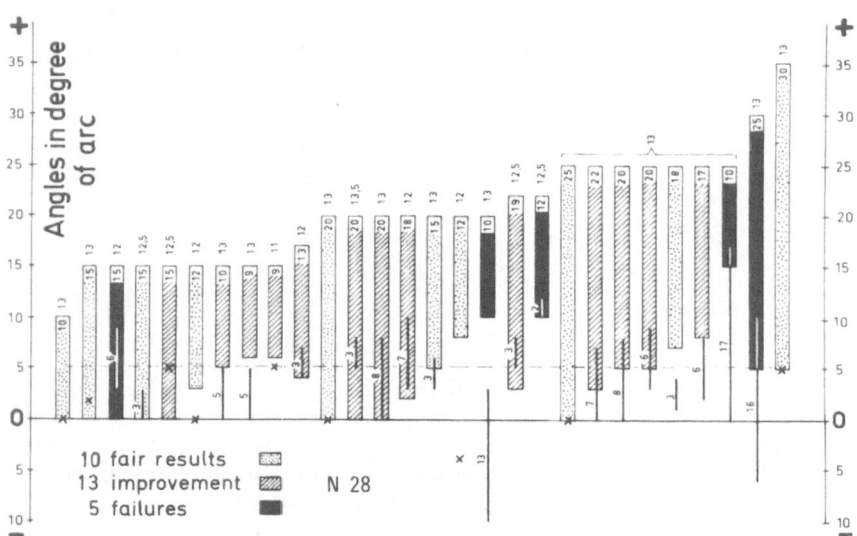

Fig. 2. Results following bimedial Fd without recessions in 28 patients with changing angles. Fd amount on top of each case vane. Black lines or crosses indicate the changing or constant results.

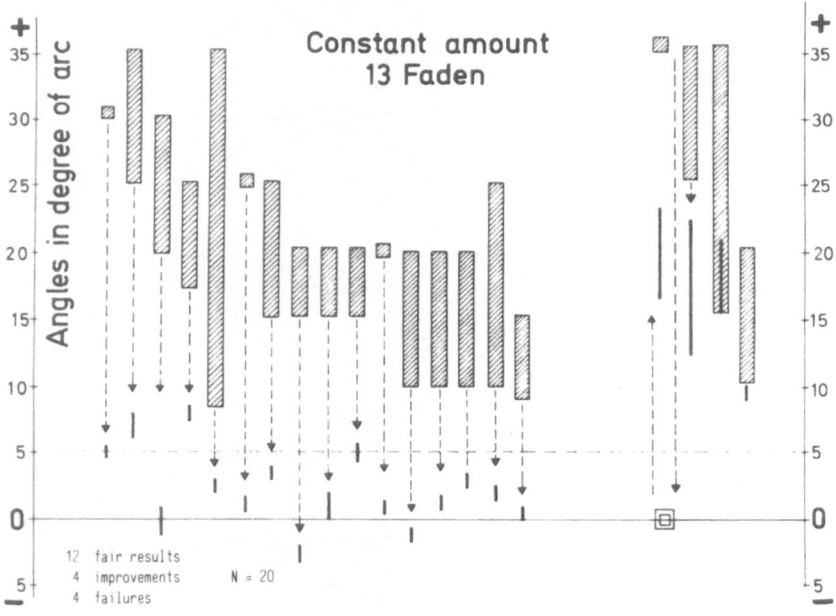

Fig. 3. Results of bimedial Fd without recessions in 20 cases with constant looking angles. Vanes show preoperative measurements, arrows indicate the postsurgical reduction of the maximum angles.

1. The original technique published by Cüppers (1974) contains an obligate disconnection and reposition of the muscle to the insertion (Fig. 1), which makes the operation easier but sacrifices the blood supply. It therefore had been our interest to save the vessels, which forced us to use a modification. We normally perform a posterior fixation on the edges only.

2. Many papers which present results of the Fadenoperation (Fd) display that the changing angle in congenital strabismus is composed of one constant, basic part and an additional, dynamic element (Mühlendyck & Linnen 1975; Quéré et al. 1978; Spielmann & Laulan 1978; Behrens-Baumann & Wölz 1978). The reader will find it logical that the favoured therapy should be a combination of recession and Fd. Like many others we began in this way, but in the course of time we reduced the number of recessions more and more, as we experienced that they often were unnecessary. As a first proof we operated on two groups of patients with Fd alone (Fig. 2, 3). One group

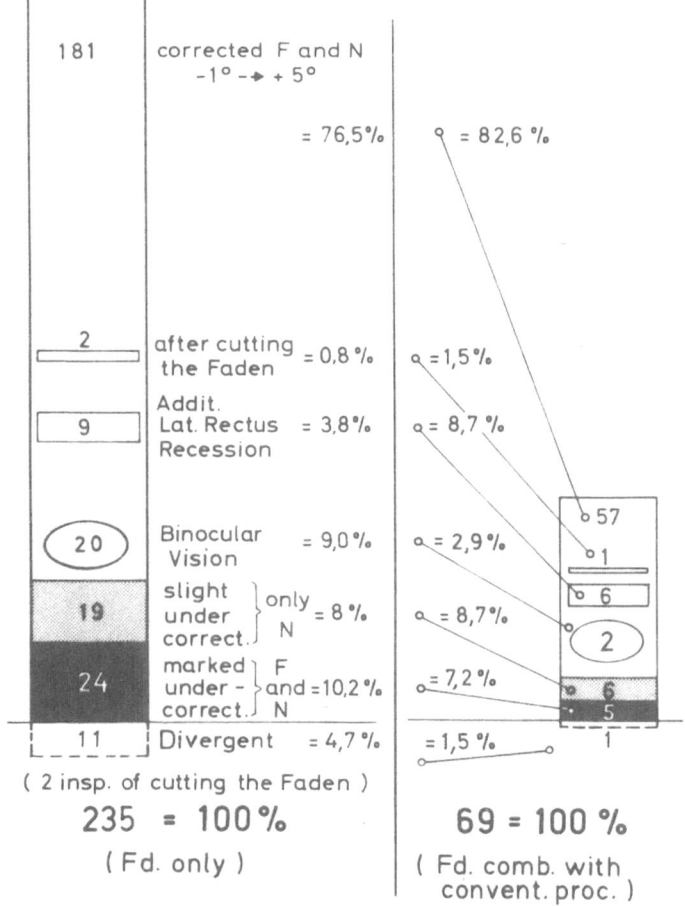

Fig. 4. Results of the Kiel clinic.

consisted of 28 children with angles which obviously changed between microtropia and maximum values, the other group of 20 patients showed socalled constant angles. The results were about the same!

3. The decision to perform a Fd only is made when the angle in all likelihood is not constant. This can be ascertained by: i. Careful observation. ii. Asking the parents, which we found very helpful. iii. Knowledge of a small sensorial angle. iv. Considering the other symptoms of congenital strabismus.

We come to the resolution to add a recession, when under general anaesthesia the eyes are not straight, and especially when passive abduction is limited.

RESULTS

The data we shall present are based on nearly 500 operations from 1978. Since that time we followed constant principles and can now analyse the results retrospectively. Any other problems, especially with the oblique muscles, had been operated upon separately, which must be ignored here. 235 patients of the Kiel clinic had bimedial Fd only, and 69 underwent combinations with recessions or resections (Fig. 4). In both groups the results look similar, 75 to 80% being successfully treated. The frequency of marked undercorrections exceeds the number of overcorrections. The

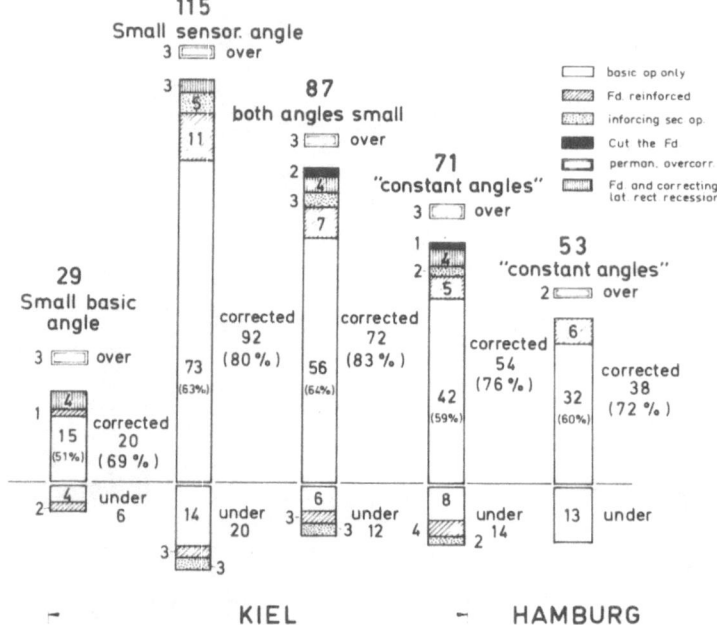

Fig. 5. Results of all patients from Fig. 4 and of a control group of the Hamburg clinic related to their preoperative motoric and sensoric data. See also the number and distribution of reoperations in particular. Standards of cure as shown in Fig. 6.

number of patients who reached true binocular vision is small in both samples, according to the congenital status. The consistency of the results in both groups is a good control for ourselves that in a majority the decision, whether or not to add a recession, had been correct. Fig. 5 shows, more in detail, the distribution to different preoperative conditions. It is not surprising that patients, who presented a small angle of anomaly had good results, but the two groups with obviously constant angles should be noticed. Their results have been not significantly worse than those of the others, which indicates that during childhood even extremely constant looking angles are not really fixated. Following Cüppers we would call this status 'permanently overinnervated'.

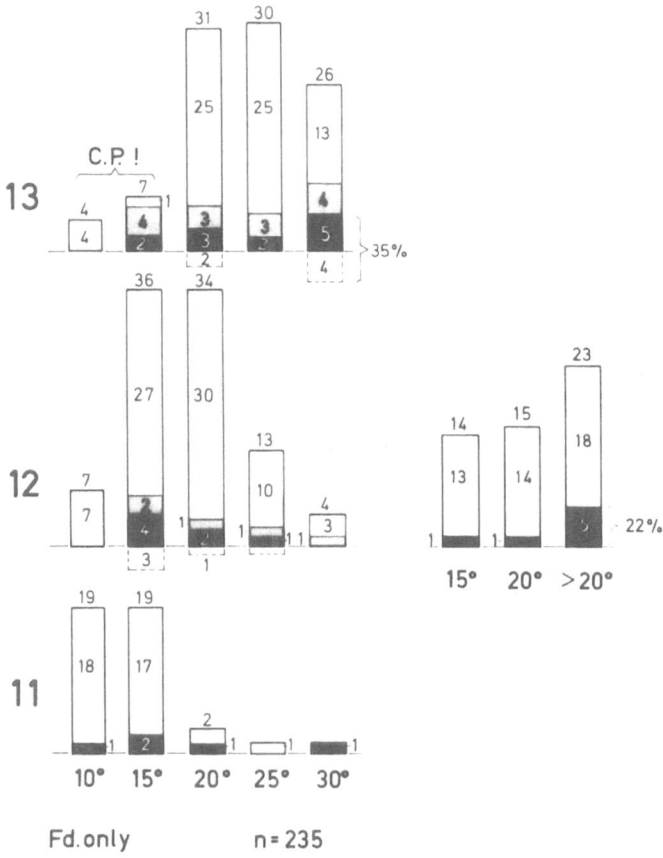

Fig. 6. Results of Fd without recessions, comparing the amounts of Fd to the maximum angles. clear: cured within −1° to +5°, dotted: slight undercorrections up to +7° (near dist.), black: serious undercorrections, lined: lasting overcorrections exceeding 1°(far dist.)

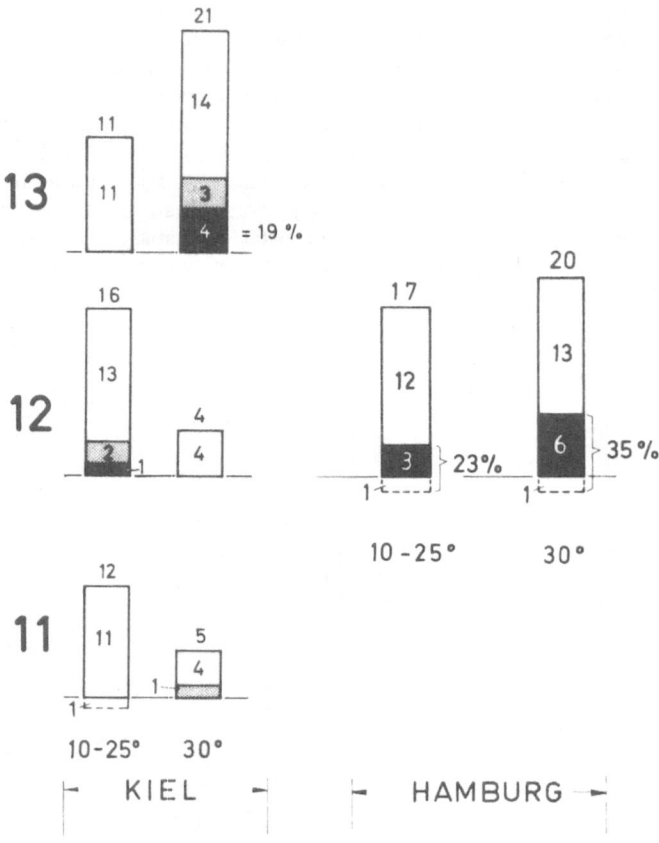

Fig. 7. Like Fig. 6, but with additional recessions.

Fig. 5 also shows the number and type of second operations in each group, and the lasting over- and undercorrections. It may be of interest for the surgical practice to give a distribution to the different amounts of the Fd (Figs. 6, 7). A bimedial Fa of 11 mm seems to be adequate for the correction of maximum angles of about 10° to 15°, 12 mm for 15° to 20°, and 13 mm is necessary for 25° maximum. When the angles exceed 25° an additional recession seems to be unavoidable; in cases with excessive angles on both medial recti, up to 4 mm. The control groups of the Hamburg clinic where mainly 12 mm amounts are in use show the same border, and again that Fd alone gives sufficient results only up to 20°, and larger maximum angles forces the surgeon to add recessions.

An unilateral Fd (Fig. 8) gives clearly poorer results and works sufficiently up to 15° only, and in addition the motility often shows the signs of an artificial palsy: Even many amblyopes use their dominant eye in

70

	Kiel			Hamburg		
	N$\underline{\underline{o}}$	failures	%	N$\underline{\underline{o}}$	failures	%
Total	81	22	27%	35	4	11.5%
Fd.only	39	9	23%	23	2	8.5%
Fd.comb. conv.surg.	42	13	31%	12	2	16.5%
Max.angle 10-20°	46	7	15%	31	4	13% !
20-30°	35	15	43%	4	0	–
Best condition: 1)Fd.only 2)Max.angle 15°	26	3	11.5%			

Fig. 8. Unilateral Fd gives much poorer results, except of small changing angles.

Table 1. Comparison of the results of professional surgeons and of residents.

Modus of surgery	Problem		Based on No. of pat.
	Solved	Unsolved	
Profess. surgeons, no reoperation	113 (84%)	22 (16%)	135 ⎫
Residents, no reoperation	73 (79%)	19 (21%)	92 ⎭ 75,5%
Profess. surgeons, reop. on own pat.	28 (67%)	14 (33%)	42 ⎫
Profess. surgeons, reop. on res. cases	26 (81%)	6 (19%)	32 ⎭ 24,5%
	240 (79,7%)	61 (20,3%)	301 = 100%

adducted position, which makes it easier to suggest a bimedial operation. We feel much comprehension for patients and colleagues who do not wish to operate on the only good eye, but with the agreement of the patient we prefer the bilateral procedure today.

One last remark brings us back to technical problems (Table 1). Even well trained residents had poorer results than professional surgeons, and the surgeons could reinforce the resident's failures more often than their own undercorrections.

REFERENCES

Behrens-Baumann, W. & U. Wölz. Ergebnisse der 'Fadenfixation' nach Cüppers bei Schielern mit schwankendem Winkel. Klin. Mbl. Augenheilk. 173: 814 (1978).

Cüppers, C. The so-called Fadenoperation II. Congr. I.S.A. Marseille 1974, Diff. Gen. Libr. Paris-Marseille, 1974, p. 395.

Mühlendyck, H. & H.J. Linnen. Die operative Behandlung nystagmusbedingter schwankender Schielwinkel mit der Fadenoperation nach Cüppers. Klin. Mb. Augenheilk. 167: 273 (1975).

Spielmann, A. & J. Laulan. Action of Recessions and Resections when associated with Cüppers Fadenoperation in Esotropia. Statistical Results. In: 'Strabismus' Edit. Reinecke (1978), Grune & Stratton N.Y.; S. Franc., London, p. 355.

Quéré, M.A., G. Chargeau & A. Pecherau. L'associtation chirurgie du filchirurgie classic dans le cure operatoire des esotropies. Bull. Soc. Ophthalm. de France 78: 373 (1978).

Authors' address:
University Eye Clinic Kiel
Orthoptic Department
Kiel, F.R.G.

POSSIBILITY OF CORRECT FUSION FORMATION
OF ADULTS

T. BARANOWSKA-GEORGE

(Szczecin, Poland)

It is generally accepted that a functional cure of long, persistent squint in adults is impossible. Employing the treatment according to principles of localization method (Baranowska-George et al. 1977; 1981) in a certain number of cases we did not obtain only positive constant cosmetic results but also functional ones.

We have treated 100 patients aged from 15 to 47 years, in whom the squint was evident from the early years of childhood. Complete functional cure and symmetry of the eyes were recorded in ten cases. These ten cases are found to have normal binocular distant and near vision, confirmed by the subjective test, by Bagolini's classical test and with the Starkiewicz modification, and by the visuscopic or with one or two filter's test, while the eyes are fixed parallel. In 61 patients we established poor, correct binocular vision, (in 23 patients we established a positive subjective test and in 38 patients Bagolini's classical test or visuscopic test was positive). We considered this as an introductory phase to normal binocular vision formation after a lapse of time. That is feasible, because, by resorting to localization exercises with prisms exactly compensating the squint angle, new cortical connections are slowly formed between the optic centres in occiput and the remaining parts of cerebral cortex, particularly with centres of kinesthesia and sense. The permanent symmetric or parallel fixation of the eyes is maintained by daily several-hours-long localization exercises, using hypercorrective prisms with alternate covering of the eyes of penalization, or in exceptional cases the covering of the eyes is abandoned (Berard 1969; Starkiewicz 1969). The exercises are given up only when the binocular vision appears to be stabilized. In the cases that failed to be cured functionally, we rely on peripheral binocular vision which sometimes is quite enough to obtain a durable cosmetic result and subjective positive test. Here the contribution factor, due to exercises is also the correct spatial localization with parallel eyes fixation or symmetrical excitation of both retinae by prisms compensating the angle of the squint.

An additional treatment is provided by euthiscopic dazzlement while the symmetry is preserved by exciting both retinae. The reduction of the squint angle and parallel fixation of the eyes are achieved thanks to localization exercises by means of hypercorrective prisms and surgical procedures performed step by step. The operations are mostly carried out on one extrinsic

Docum. Ophthal. Proc. Series, Vol. 32, ed. by A.Th.M. van Balen & W.A. Houtman   73
© 1982, Dr W. Junk Publishers, The Hague. ISBN 90 6193 728 0

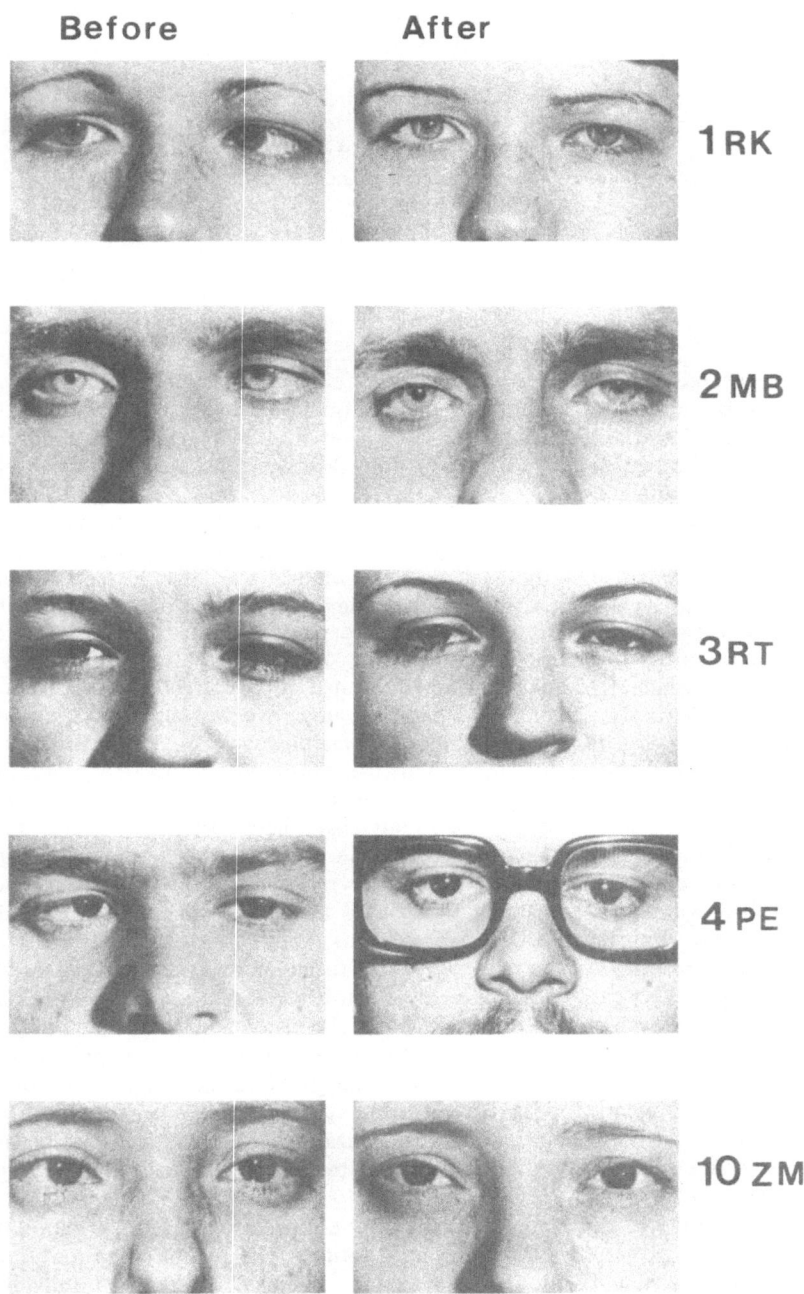

Before **After**

1 RK

2 MB

3 RT

4 PE

10 ZM

Fig. 1. Photographic documentation of five patients presented in Table 1 and 2. For the remaining patients there are no photos available.

74

Table 1.

Patient	Age	Time of squint onset	A. Before / B. After Treatm.	Visual acuity R. eye	Visual acuity L. eye	Squint angle	Binocular vision For distance	Binocular vision For proximity	Period of treatment	Period of the observation after treatm.
									(months)	(months)
1. R.K.	21	4	A	1,0	1,0	+30°	t. subj; c.Bt; suppr v-t; f-t: - dipl. cros 45°	suppr.	5	–
			B	1,0	1,0	0°	t. subj; c.Bt v-t; f-t (+)	as beside	–	12
2. M.B.	23	3	A	1,0	0,5	+40°	suppr.	suppr.	6	–
			B	1,0	0,5	0°	t. subj; c.Bt; m.Bt; v-t; f-t; dft. (+)	as beside	–	19
3. R.T.	17	3	A	1,0	0,5	+18°	t. subj; c.Bt; m.Bt. suppr. f-t; 1° v-t; -6° dipl. cros.	t. subj.–suppr. c.Bt; m.Bt; f-t-3° dipl. cros.	8	–
			B	1,0	0,6	0°	t. subj; c.Bt; m.Bt v-t; f-t; dft: (+)	as beside	–	23
4. P.E.	21	6	A	0,5	1,0	+35°	t. subj. (–) c.Bt; m.Bt; f-t-25° dipl. cros.	t. subj. (–) c.Bt; m.Bt; 10° f-t 30° dipl. cros.	5	–
			B	0,5	1,0	0°	t. subj; c.Bt; m.Bt v-t (+) f-t 0,5° dipl. cros.	as beside f-t (+)	–	7
5. W.K.	17	2	A	1,0	0,3	+25°	t. subj. (–) c.Bt; m.Bt; f-t-2° v-t-4° dipl. cros.	t. subj. (–) c.Bt; m.Bt; f-t-3° dipl. cros	4	–
			B	1,0	0,5	0°	t. subj.-c.Bt; m.Bt; f-t; dft. v-t (+)	as beside	–	24

t. subj. – test subjective
c.Bt; – classic-Bagolini's test
m.Bt; – modified-Bagolini's test
v-t; – visuscopic-test
f-t; – filter test
dft; – double-filter-test
suppr. – suppression
dipl. cros. – diplopia crossed

Table 2.

Patient	Age	Time of squint onset	A. Before B. After Treatment	Visual acuity R. eye	L. eye	Squint angle	Binocular vision For distance	For proximity	Period of treatment (months)	Period of the observation after treatm. (months)
6 G.H.	48	3	A	1,0	0,4	−35°	suppr.	suppr.	6	–
			B	1,0	1,0	0°	t. subj; c.Bt; m.Bt; f-t; v-t; (+)	as beside	–	36
7. Ch.A.	22	1	A	1,0	1,0	+30°	t. subj.-(−) c.Bt; m.Bt; f-t 10° dipl. cros.	t. subj; (−) c.Bt; m.Bt; f-t 7° dipl. cros.	21	–
			B	1,0	1,0	0°	t. subj; c.Bt; m.Bt; (+) v-t; 1° dipl. cros.	as beside	–	43
8. J.J.	22	1	A	1,0	1,0	+30°	t. subj; c.Bt; m.Bt; v-t suppr. f-t; 1° dipl. cros.	t. subj; c.Bt; m.Bt; supp. f-t; 7° dipl. cros. —	4	–
			B	1,0	1,0	0°	t. subj; c.Bt; m.Bt; v-t (+) f-t; 0,5° dipl. cros.	as beside	–	28
9. S.B.	15	5	A	1,0	1,0	+17°	t. subj; (−) c.Bt; m.Bt; v-t; f-t;-15° dipl. cros.	t. subj; (−) c.Bt; m.Bt; 10° f-t;20° dipl. cros.	7	–
			B	1,0	1,0	0°	t. subj; c.Bt; m.Bt; (+) v-t; 3° dipl. cros.	t. subj; (+) c.Bt; m.Bt; 2−3° f-t; 3° dipl. cros.	–	24
10 Z.M.	21	9	A	0,7	1,0	+22°	t. subj; (−) c.Bt; m.Bt;1° v-t; 10° dipl. cros	t. subj; (−) cBt; m.Bt; f-t; 2° dipl. cros.	9	–
			B	0.7	1,0	0°	t. subj. c.Bt; m.Bt; f-t; dift (+)	as beside	–	36

muscle of one eye at the time. Every operation is followed by treatment with hypercorrective and compensating prisms, simultaneously a gradual decrease in the strength of prisms compensating the squint angle. This diminution takes a slow course by one or two prismatic Dphr. In this way parallelly fixed eyes were recorded in 32 patients, there was also a reduction of the squint angle to the range of 2–5° in 33 patients, and to the range of 6–10° in 23 patients. In the latter the so-called prismatic orthotropia, according to Pigassou nomenclature, is found to be present. The squint angle ranging from 10–15° is still persisting in a group of 12 patients. We expect further gradual reduction of the squint angle during the stabilization of normal binocular vision in the course of time.

The mentioned treatment is conducted partly under clinical conditions and partly at the out-patients ward. The patients stay at the clinic from two to nine months, a complete treatment takes from one to four years. The clinical treatment is frequently accomplished step by step. The patient periodically resumes his daily work, permanently wearing the prisms compensating the squint angle, and during his free time he takes up the localization exercises with hypercorrective prisms for two to three hours daily. Since the treatment is systematic and above all exact, it leads to very positive cosmetic results. In the cases where the central nervous system is not too severely damaged we succeed, in this way in reconstructing correct cortical connections of the central parts of the retinae, which is the basis of correct fusion.

The patients are selected for this kind of therapy after a short preliminary treatment with prisms and after stating the absence of persistent diplopia with and compensating prismatic correction.

REFERENCES

T. Baranowska-George, E. Tokarz-Sawińska, M. Miszczak & J. Osiej. 'Traitement des strabismus alternants: méthode localisatrice par l'hypercorrection prismatique associée a une penalisation' Arch. Opht. Paris 11: 689–696 (1977).

T. Baranowska-George. 'Choroba zezowa: metoda lokalizacyjna leczenia zeza wg Starkiewicza i Baranowskiej-George', 'Okulistyka Wspólczesna' PZWL 1981 w druku.

Pr. V. Berard 'Le traitement du strabisme selon la méthode ortholocalisatrice de Starkiewicz-Baranowska-George', La clinique ophtalmologique revue medicale 6: 97–111 (1969).

W. Starkiewicz. 'Bases physiologiques du traitment du strabisme' La clinique ophtalmologique revue medicale 6: 73–81 (1969).

Author's address:
Clinic of Ophthalmology
Szczecin, Poland

EARLY ONSET ESOTROPIA

B. HARCOURT & J. MEIN

(*Leeds, United Kingdom*)

This paper is based on a study of 130 children with a history indicating an onset of convergent squint before the age of six months, who have been examined over a period of some years at Leeds General Infirmary. In order to ensure consistency and reliability of the data, as well as to make some longitudinal study of any changes in the findings, children who were less than two years of age at the final examination and those with less than 12 months follow up were excluded. The cases were then divided into those exhibiting nystagmus (group 1, 56 patients), and those not doing so (group 2, 74 patients). No attempt was made to analyse the nystagmus in detail, for even when it was mainly latent in character, there was usually a lateral version position in which it became manifest. Not only did the nystagmus vary in different directions of gaze and at different distances of fixation, but it also tended to change in character at successive examinations.

The principal features which were studied and compared between the groups are set out in Table 1. As expected, there was not a single instance of dissociated vertical divergence (DVD) among group 2 patients, and this confirms the widely held view that DVD is invariably associated with nystagmus (Mein & Johnson 1981). An A pattern of ocular movements (49 cases) was more common than a V pattern (37 cases) in the entire series of 130 patients, and was even more predominant in those children noted to have DVD (26 out of 43 patients, as against 11 with a V pattern). This again confirms the

Table 1.

	Group 1	Group 2
	56 patients	74 patients
nystagmus	+++	0
DVD	++	0
AHP	++	+/0
alternating	++	+
amblyopia	+	++
binocular vision	+/0	+/0
'A' pattern	++	+
presentation at age		
less than 1 year	++	+

common finding of an A pattern in patients with DVD which helps to differentiate this disorder from bilateral inferior oblique overaction, which is much more commonly associated with a V pattern of ocular movements.

The state of binocular vision was analysed in as much detail as was possible in these comparatively young patients, and in both groups was of very poor quality. There was evidence of stereoacuity in only 6 cases, and a cross with Bagolini glasses was seen and reported by only 11 children. Indeed, only 21 of the 130 patients demonstrated any evidence at all of worthwhile binocular vision, and there was no significant difference in these findings between the groups. Some aspects of the data are being subjected to further study and will be presented in a future communication. For instance, the group 2 patients had a smaller mean angle of squint than those in group 1, but the lack of any worthwhile binocular function even after surgery in both groups suggests that although on average the group 2 patients presented at a later age, this was on account of the less externally obvious nature of the squint and was not indicative of a later onset. The squint was less frequently an alternating esotropia in group 2, and this may account for the higher incidence of amblyopia in that group.

There are many striking similarities between the principal clinical features in our group 1 patients and those described by Lang (1968) in his study of a group of children with constant concomitant strabismus dating from birth or with early onset, although the 2 series are not strictly comparable as he included a few children with exotropia. The prominent features which he described were DVD (present in more than 90% of his patients), nystagmus (present in 55%) and an abnormal head posture (in 70%). He too noted an A pattern more commonly than a V pattern (21% of cases, compared with 17%). In the present group 1, nystagmus was by definition present in all patients, but only 73% exhibited DVD. We suspect that as some of our patients were still less than three years of age at their last examination, the final incidence of DVD in the series is likely to approach that reported by Lang. An abnormal head posture was noted in 66% of the group 1 cases, and although this is very similar to the incidence in Lang's series (70%), the type of compensatory posture was rather different. Lang noted that 19 of his 82 patients had a face turn towards the fixing eye (and this was always associated with nystagmus), but 29 patients had a head tilt towards or away from the fixing eye (*not* always associated with nystagmus) and 3 children exhibited abnormal chin elevation. By comparison, the overwhelming majority of the 37 of our 56 group 1 patients who had an abnormal head posture showed a simple face turn to adduct the fixing eye (33 patients).

Longterm follow up of our older patients made it clear that surgical treatment did not significantly affect the tendency to face turn, even after the eyes had been rendered mechanically 'straight'. The persistent compensatory head posture could still be seen, increasing when the patients concentrated hard on a near or distance fixation target with either eye occluded. We therefore conclude that the turn is not initially induced by the necessity to cross fixate on account of a large angle of concomitant esotropia, or of limited abduction, but is a purposive phenomenon to improve vision which persists even after surgery has rendered the eyes approximately parallel (while failing to produce really worthwhile binocular vision). A noticeable increase in the amplitude of the nystagmus when the eyes moved into an abducted position was not always observed, but nevertheless the stimulus to fix with the eye adducted does seem to have been an improvement in vision which this brought about. That is, it is a type of nystagmus compensation mechanism in patients not exhibiting all the features of the so-called 'nystagmus block' syndrome.

The observation that this type of abnormal head posture was common in our group 1 patients but absent in group 2 leads us to conclude that the presence of a face turn in a child with a history indicating an onset of constant esotropia before the age of 6 months is absolutely diagnostic of nystagmus, even, though the abnormal movements may be latent and subtle, requiring time and patience to elicit.

REFERENCES

Lang, J. Squint dating from birth or with early onset. In the First International Congress of Orthoptists, pp. 231–237. (1968) Kimpton, London.
Mein, J. & F. Johnson. Dissociated vertical divergence and its association with nystagmus. In Orthoptics, Research and Practice, ed. Mein, J. & Moore, S., pp. 14–16 (1981) Kimpton, London.

Authors' address:
Ophthalmic Department
Leeds General Infirmary
Leeds, England

A NEW HYPOTHESIS ON LATENT NYSTAGMUS AND ON THE CONGENITAL SQUINT SYNDROME

J. LANG

(*Zürich, Switzerland*)

Progress in strabology can only be made by careful differentiation of clinical entities. Such clinical entities are microtropia, the accommodative convergent squint, the normosensorial late convergent squint and the congenital squint syndrome.

Let us first hypothesise on the site of these different clinical entities.

In microtropia no motor factors are involved. Monocular fixation and binocular fusion do not exactly coincide. We therefore would localise the site of microtropia in the visual cortex.

Accommodative strabismus without high AC/A-ratio is the result of hypermetropia and therefore has its seat in the refraction of the globes.

Normosensorial late convergent squint can be cured completely by operation and therefore is most probably due to a convergent position of rest.

The congenital squint syndrome we once thought to have its seat in brain stem and to be due to an imbalance between vestibular and visual influence upon the oculomotor mechanisms. The congenital squint syndrome is characterised by strabismus since birth or dating from the first four months of life, having several signs which do not seem to be correlated with each other, namely latent nystagmus, dissociated vertical divergence, excyclorotation of the non fixating eye and anomalous head posture. In latent nystagmus, the fixation object in the non occluded eye very slowly moves from the foveola to the nasal side and then by a saccade returns to the foveola.

Crone (1954) and recently Mein & Johnson (1981) have believed that alternating hyperphoria or dissociated vertical divergence are the dominating feature in this syndrome.

For several reasons we believe that not D.V.D. but latent nystagmus is the main feature. Dissociated vertical divergence can be an acquired sign which we found in cases of unilateral aphakia or acquired unilateral blindness in the first few decades of life. We, however, have never seen latent nystagmus in an acquired condition.

Factors which may help us to gain insight into the pathogenesis of latent nystagmus and of the congenital squint syndrome may be divided into clinical observations and neuroanatomical facts:

1. Clinical observations show that in almost 99% of the cases with latent nystagmus there is a strabismus combined. Cases with orthotropia and latent nystagmus are extremely rare.

Docum. Ophthal. Proc. Series, Vol. 32, ed. by A.Th.M. van Balen & W.A. Houtman   83
© 1982, Dr W. Junk Publishers, The Hague. ISBN 90 6193 728 0

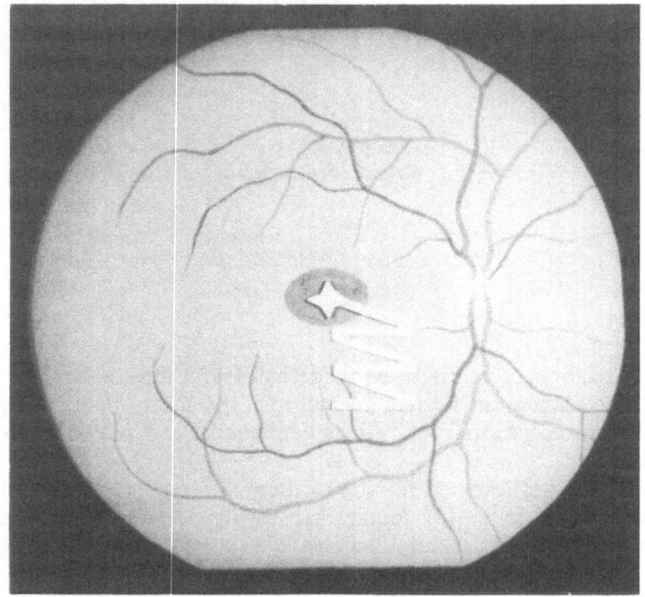

Fig. 1. Latent nystagmus.

2. In infants with the congenital squint syndrome both eyes are in a convergent position. The fixation object does not lie in the foveola but in both eyes on the nasal border of the fovea. Gradually fixation moves into the foveola. We got the clinical impression that only when the fixation has moved to the foveola latent nystagmus can manifest itself.

3. In some cases one can see that in binocular vision the leading eye does not fixate exactly with the foveola.

4. In a case of very pronounced latent nystagmus and high amblyopia we found that the leading eye had two possibilities of fixation: one at the nasal

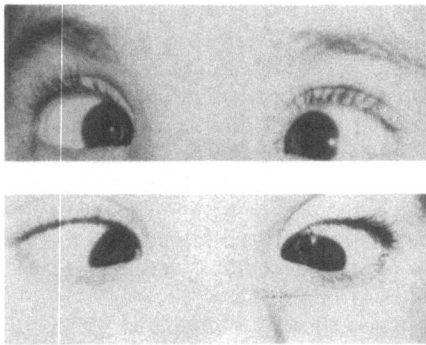

Fig. 2. Congenital convergent strabismus: both eyes in convergent position.

84

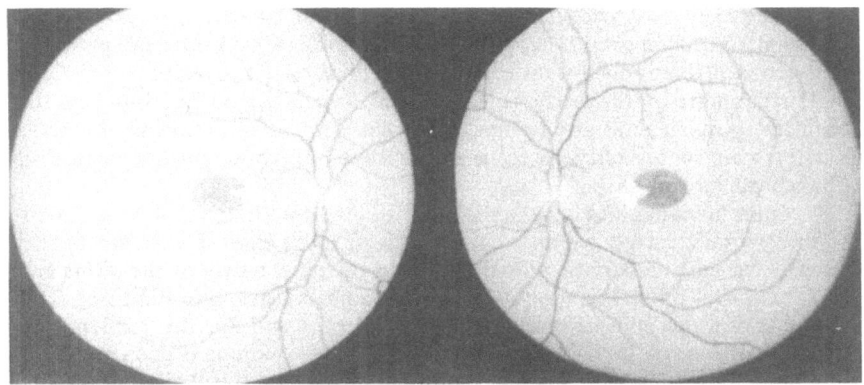

Fig. 3. Eccentric fixation in both eyes.

border of the fovea and the other on the nasal side of the papilla. In the nasal position fixation was almost steady, whereas by fixation on the border of the fovea a latent nystagmus was seen. We have made similar observations in other cases.

Concerning the neuro-anatomical facts, one must bear in mind that beside the retino-geniculo-striate system there exist other pathways, the most important being the extra-geniculo-striate pathway to the colliculus superior and from there to the pulvinar and then to the cortex, as shown in the diagram by Trevarthen & Sperry (1973). This second visual pathway is claimed to be responsible for ambient vision.

Bernheimer (1961) has demonstrated that 20–30% of the fibres of the

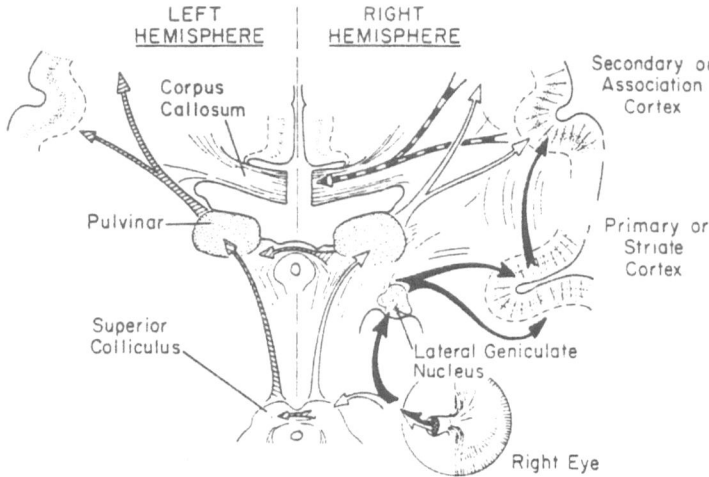

Fig. 4. Extra-geniculo-striate pathways to the colliculus superior and to the pulvinar (Trevarthen & Sperry 1973).

85

optic nerve do not reach the corpus geniculatum laterale, but pass to the pretectal and tectal area. According to Minkowsky (1961) these are probably only crossed fibres which stem from the nasal halves of the retina.

Furthermore in the early stages of the human foetal development the primitive phylogenetic arrangement of a *complete* decussation of the nerve fibres occurs in the chiasma. It is not until the 11th week that uncrossed fibres begin to appear.

Keeping in mind that congenital squint is often seen in cases of prematurity or of cerebral damage, we may expect that in these cases the phylogenetical older extra-geniculo-striate system, based on the nasal halves of the retina and on the crossed optical fibres and subserving ambient vision, is dominant. This accounts for the convergent position of the eyes and for the tendency to fixate in the nasal part of the retina. As visual development goes on in the first months of life, fixation moves into the fovea to fulfill the task of discriminating forms.

When both eyes are open, no nystagmus is seen since opposite movements of the eyes are counterbalanced. When one eye is occluded, counterbalance does not exist any more, and fixation slowly glides from the fovea into the nasal part of the retina due to the tendency of ambient vision, and then quickly returns to the foveola again, bringing back the object in the area of discrimination. This may explain the mechanism of latent nystagmus.

We are fully aware that this hypothesis is based only on clinical impressions and on possibly insufficient neuroanatomic facts. So there is no need to rush into brain surgery for congenital squint!

REFERENCES

Crone, R.A. Alternating Hyperphoria. Brit. J. Ophthalm. 38, 591 (1954).

Bernheimer, see St. Duke-Elder, System of Ophthalmology, Vol. II, H. Kimpton, London. (1961).

Lang, J. Squint dating from Birth or with early Onset. Transactions of the First International Congress of Orthoptists, H. Kimpton, London. (1968).

Mein, J. & F. Johnson. Dissociated Vertical Divergence and its Association with Nystagmus. Transactions of the Fourth International Orthoptic Congress, H. Kimpton, London. (1981).

Minkowsky, see St. Duke-Elder, System of Ophthalmology, Vol. II, H. Kimpton, London. (1961).

Trevarthen, C.B. & R.W. Sperry. Perceptual unity of the ambient visual field in human commissurotomy patients. Brain 96, 547–570 (1973).

Author's address:
Freiestrasse 47
CH-8032 Zürich, Switzerland

STRABISMUS IN CEREBRAL PALSY

K. WYBAR
(*London, England*)

The term cerebral palsy denotes a bilateral affection of the brain with a lack of any uniform aetiology or pathology: sometimes there is an arrested development or an infective process in intra-uterine life so that the condition is determined pre-natally; sometimes there is some factor which is related to the birth particularly when there is a significant degree of prematurity or following a period of profound neonatal anoxia; in other cases there may be a post-natal influence such as an infective agent causing an encephalitis or meningitis, or even a degenerative condition. However, it is now considered that this interpretation of cerebral palsy is too diffuse and the term should be reserved for conditions in which the motor deficits stem from an injury to the brain during the birth process or immediately thereafter. Cerebral palsy represents a heterogeneous group of conditions which manifests a wide variety of paralytic and spastic features, associated with abnormal movements which tend to be choreiform or athetoid in nature, and there is almost invariably some degree of mental defect.

Sometimes cerebral palsy may not be clear-cut, but it should be suspected when the history reveals difficulties in the perinatal stage, such as a prolonged labour, a significant period of hypoxia, neonatal hypoglycaemia, kernicterus, or when the infant is slow in reaching the various recognised milestones of development in the absence of any other obvious condition.

It is common for disorders of ocular motility to occur in cerebral palsy. Sometimes this takes the form of a persistent conjugate deviation of the eyes in a particular direction so that there is a supranuclear lesion, and nystagmus may also be a feature, but most commonly there is a straight-forward squint which rapidly acquires concomitant features so that the squint tends to be concomitant when the first examination takes place, but in the early stages it is almost certain that there is an incomitant element, particularly some degree of unilateral or bilateral VIth nerve paresis.

It is the purpose of this paper to emphasise the peculiar difficulties in the management of the type of squint which occurs in cerebral palsy. As a general rule in my opinion, it is important to operate as soon as possible in a manifest squint which develops in early childhood in order to achieve a useful form of binocular association even if this is of an anomalous nature in the presence of a small residual deviation (secondary microtropia), provided any significant refractive error is corrected, and provided also any amblyopia is dealt with as far as possible. However, the squint which occurs in cerebral palsy is an exception to this rule and frequently it is wise to defer the operation until the child is older.

This delay in engendered by the characteristically poor results of surgical treatment in such cases from a long-term point of view, largely because of an absence of any form of fusion even of an anomalous type. This lack of fusion is difficult to interpret in precise terms, and, although a congenital absence or defect of the fusion faculty in the aetiology of squint (Worth 1915) is no longer tenable, it is evident that the fusion faculty becomes disrupted in cerebral palsy.

The anatomical union of the two separate afferent visual pathways which results in a physiological union represents a summation of the two independent visual stimuli in a psychical manner at a higher level. It must be assumed, therefore, that in cerebral palsy the peculiarly refined higher cerebral mechanisms are unduly susceptible when there is a disruption of various parts of the neurological mechanism, and this concept also explains the notorious loss of fusion which occurs in an incomitant squint as the result of a head injury which causes considerable neurological disruption with usually a profound initial period of unconsciousness, despite previous normal binocular function.

There is general agreement that in manifest squint in early childhood a satisfactory result, even after extremely careful surgical treatment, is seldom achieved, particularly from a long-term point of view, unless there is a restoration of some form of fusion and whether this is of a normal or anomolous nature is largely of academic importance. Unfortunately a functional result is seldom possible in cerebral palsy, and when surgical treatment is carried out at an early stage, there may be a poor relief of the squint at a time the patient is becoming socially increasingly conscious of the squint, and it may be more difficult then to obtain a satisfactory result particularly when the early surgery has been of a repeated nature. Perhaps ideally the surgical treatment should be carried out during the adolescent period, but this does not take into account the morale boosting effect to the parents when the squint is 'straightened', so that apparently there is one less handicap, and I suggest as a compromise that the ideal age for the surgical interference is around 6–8 years.

REFERENCE

Worth, C. Squint: Its Causes, Pathology and Treatment. John Bale, Sons and Danielsson, London. 4th Edition 1915, p. 59.

Author's address:
The Hospital for Sick Children
Great Ormond Street
London WC1, England

COMPARATIVE STUDY OF THE ANAESTHESIA TEST IN NORMAL AND STRABISMIC CHILDREN

M.A. ZATO, J.C. CASTIELLA & J. GARCIA SÁNCHEZ

(*Madrid, Spain*)

ABSTRACT

The authors studied the eye position in different periods of anaesthesia in normal and strabismic children in order to compare the response of strabismic and normal children and to differentiate the innervational component of strabismus from the static component.

INTRODUCTION

As everybody knows, anaesthesia changes the eye deviation of the strabismus subject, which to some authors is of no value (Isemberg 1975, 1979) while to others it is diagnostically valuable (Quere 1978; Gomez de Liaño et al. 1977; Castiella et al. 1978; Gomez de Liaño 1979). It is also stated that in normal children under anaesthesia, eyes tend to converge (Breining 1957), whereas in grown-ups they tend to divergence.

In 1977, after having talked to Prof. Quere, who is also interested in this matter, we began this study introducing a preliminary communication which we entitled 'Anaesthesia test on blocking strabismus'. Two years later we did a second communication on this subject in which we added Zato's forced duction test, intended to be used on surgical indication of blocking-strabismus, closely related to the anaesthesia test (Castiella et al. 1978).

Finally, we had to assess what happened in normal children from the ophthalmological point of view, with the same anaesthesia technique compared with the information obtained from the strabismus subject. We believed that in every strabismic deviation there were two components: one innervational and able to be changed (dynamic component of deviation) and one peripheral, due to muscle contracture.

We proposed as a work hypothesis that, under anaesthesia, the innervational or central components disappear, with only the peripheral component or rest muscle tone being left. Thus, we first needed to take a look at what happens in normal subjects and compare it to strabismic ones.

Docum. Ophthal. Proc. Series, Vol. 32, ed. by A.Th.M. van Balen & W.A. Houtman   89
© *1982, Dr W. Junk Publishers, The Hague. ISBN 90 6193 728 0*

MATERIAL AND METHOD

In close collaboration with the anaesthesia and reanimation service of the Hospital del Nino Jesus (Jesus Christ Child Hospital) of Madrid we studied 335 unselected children in the anaesthesia files nos. 80/323 through 80/ 2.575 who were operated on for the most diverse ailments, ophthalmological and central nervous systems diseases excluded. Age groups are shown in Table 1.

Also the response was studied in 656 unselected anaesthesias done for convergent strabismus operation among the same group of files, with the same technique, anaesthesia personally and freely chosen also with respect to the age as shown in Table 1.

Table 1.

Age (Years)	Number of cases	
	Normal children	Strabismic children
2–4	186	331
5–7	126	292
8–10	24	33
	336	656
	$\bar{X} = 4{,}56$	$\bar{X} = 4{,}63$
	$S = 1{,}88$	$S = 1{,}79$

TECHNIQUE

Anaesthesia induction was done by the following steps: (Martinez Jaraiz et al. 1969; Martinez Jaraiz 1976; Uemera 1974).

Anaesthesia technique

Induction

5% 5 mg/kg = 0,1 ml/kg	Pentotal
Total dose Atropine	
0,4 mg	Lactants
0,5 mg	up to 7 years old
0,6 mg	more than 7 years old
1,0 mg	grown-ups
	Succinil-Dicoline
0,8 mg/kg	Lactants
0,7 mg/kg	Children

Intubation

Thus we have four drugs, three of them (Pentotal, Fluothane and N_2O) with no or nearly no action on neuromuscle level and highly active on central level (Gomez de Liaño et al. 1977); and the fourth one, succinil-dicoline, with a strong action on muscle level and very slight on central level.

Anaesthesia keeping-on
1) 1% Fluothane vaporized by a N_2O-O_2 mixture at 2/1 ratio; 2) Three minutes after the beginning of spontaneous breathing 'check eye position'.

The angle is measured: a) before the anaesthesia; b) pentotal; c) with succinil-dicoline; and d) after three minutes of spontaneous breathing, writing it down on the standard file card (Table 2).

The angle was measured by the corneal reflex with prismethod (Krimsky's method), the subject lying under a light perpendicular between the two eyes. Measurement was done by the same person who did not know the preanaesthetic value. Only more than five degree (10 diop.) variations were written down to prevent us from error when using the angle measurement method.

RESULTS

Normal children

%	Cases	Eye position

Pentotal

%	Cases	Eye position
78	260	No change — Orthotropia
19	64	Below 15 degrees divergence
22		
3	11	Convergence

Succinil-Dicoline

%	Cases	Eye position
90	301	No change — Orthotropia
5	18	Below 5 degrees divergence
10		
5	16	Up to 20 degrees convergence

Keeping-on state

%	Cases	Eye position
99,7	334	No change — Orthotropia
—	—	Divergence
0,29	1	10 degrees convergence

Strabismic children

%	Cases	Eye position

Pentotal

38,10	250	No change — the same angle
13,87	91	Orthotropia
45,42	298	Up to 15 degrees divergence
2,59	17	The angle decreases its convergence

Succinil-Dicoline

92,2	605	The angle increases or remains the same
2,74	18	Orthotropia
5,03	33	Below 15 degrees divergence

Keeping-on state

40,24	264	No change in angle deviation
50	328	The angle decreases under anaesthesia
9,7	64	Orthotropia or below 10 degrees divergence

If we study the results according to the type of strabismus, we obtain:

a. No blocking strabismus clinically tested 238 cases in the period we studied according the afore-shown schemes, that is to say, in the keeping-on period which is where there are highly significant differences between the response of normal children and strabismic ones, resulted in the following ways:

198 cases keep the same angle
 36 cases diminish the angle
  4 cases of orthophoria?
  0 cases of divergency

b. Major blocking strabismus 228 cases

  2 cases keep the same angle
162 cases diminish the angle
 62 cases of orthophoria
  2 cases of divergency

c. Medium blocking strabismus — 190 cases

 66 cases with no angle variation
122 cases diminish the angle
  2 cases of orthophoria
  0 cases of divergency

COMMENT

If we first study the results on normal children we note first that eye position under pentotal action could be slightly significant perhaps but not very valuable because the deviation percentage is 22, being 19% of it divergent and only 3% convergent.

Along with succinil-dicoline, we can only state that it decreases the tendency to divergency and increases, but not significantly, the presence of convergence (this being very logical due to the action of this drug) 10% of children showing variations of eye deviation being 5% convergent and 5% divergent. Amount of orthophorias is high but this too is not very valuable.

In the period of keeping-on, it is when statistic results become clearer, because orthophoria was found in 99% of cases. This fact is highly significant and allows us to state some conclusions about the variations of angles with this standard anaesthesia method.

But, what happens with strabismic subjects? We also see that with pentotal, at large, there exists nearly the same percentage of divergence variations as no-variation-and-very-slight-tendency-to-convergence one. This was seen before in normal subjects from which no statistic conclusion could be derived.

%	Cases	Eye position

238 Cases without blocking syndrome

%	Cases	Eye position
83,19	198	No change angle deviation
15,12	36	The angle decreases
1,68	4	Orthotropia
—	—	Divergence

228 Cases major blocking syndrome

%	Cases	Eye position
0,87	2	No change in angle deviation
71,03	162	The angle decreases
27,19	62	Orthotropia
0,87	2	Divergence

190 Cases medium blocking syndrome

%	Cases	Eye position
34,73	66	No change
64,21	122	The angle decreases
1,05	2	Orthotropia
—	—	Divergence

As in normal subjects, with succinil-dicoline, the divergence tendency decreases and sometimes even induces increase of angle. No statistical conclusion can be drawn.

However, it is in the keeping-on period that conclusions can be drawn. Compare the response in this period of non-strabismic children with strabismic children. In this period 40% of the cases keep the same angle, 10%

orthophoria and the angle decreases in 50%. These results differ significantly from the results in normal children from which 99% did not change the angle.

The different response to this test of three types of strabismus is also significant. The cases with no blocking did not change the angle in 83%. This very closely resembles the normal children. In major blocking cases the angle changed in 98%. In medium blocking cases the response is irregular, 34% had no angle change and only 64% showed a decrease of angle.

Thus we think that in most cases, eye position during anaesthesia in children in the keeping-on period helps us to differentiate between strabismus with an innervational component and one which is only static.

EPILOGUE

With this technique, we think that the eye position during 3 minutes of spontaneous breathing period of anaesthesia allows to draw some conclusions with respect to diagnosis and surgical indications. Although it is not a clinical proof of blocking the anaesthesiatest can be used as a diagnostic tool next to Zato's forced duction test.

REFERENCES

Aptl. Isemberg, S. Eye position of strabismus patients under general anesthesia. pp. 471/422 B. Internt. Orthop. Congress Boston (1975).

Aptl. Isemberg, S. Eye position of strabismus patients under general anesthesia. Amer. Jour. Ophthal. 574–579 (1977).

Breining, G. The position of rest during anesthesia and sleep. Arch, Ophthal. Ama. 1957–57 (323–327).

Castiella, J.C., M.A. Zato & M.J. Hernani. Indicacion quirurgica a partir del diagnostico de bloqueo Acta estrabologica. 107–114 (1978).

Gomez De Liaño, F., M.A. Zato & J.C. Castiella. Analisis de los movimentos oculares bajo narcosis (Arch. Soc. Esp. Oftal. Tomo 37 No. 12 1145–1158 (1977).

Gomez De Liaño, F., M.A. Zato & J.C. Castiella. Der diagnostische wer der anästhesie für die chirurgie des strabismus (Klin. Mbl. Augenheink 175, 355–359 (1979).

Martinez Jaraiz, J., et al. Analisis de 484 casos de anestesia para estrabismo Rev. Exp. Anestesia 16–76 (1969).

Martinez Jaraiz, J. Anestesia en cirugia estrabologica Acta estrabologica 1–15 (1976).

Ohmi, E., et al. Eye position of squinting eyes during general anesthesia. Acta Soc. Ophthal. Jap. (1975).

Quere, M.A. et al. Operation du fil et chirurgie clasique dans les estropies fontionelles, le signe de l'anesthesie. La Cliniq. Ophtal. 2, 125–145 (1978).

Uemera, Y. Ocular movements during induction of general anesthesia in children Vol. II, 215–219, XXII Concilium Ophtal. Paris (1974).

Weiss, J.B. Spasme et contracture spasmodique chez les strabismes convergent Bull. Mem. Soc. Fran. Ophtal. 548–558 (1967).

Zato, M.A. La divergencia post-quirurgica Arch, Soc. Esp. Oftal. XLI 6, 685–690 (1981).

Authors' address:
Clara del Rey 50–33
Madrid 2, Spain

UNILATERAL TRAUMATIC APHAKIA

J.H. PAMEIJER

(*Rotterdam, The Netherlands*)

Unilateral traumatic aphakia is often a great obstruction for binocular and stereoscopic vision. Even after repair of the focusing power, binocular rehabilitation can be delayed by many factors. In order to investigate the long term results of the binocular functions, all cases of unilateral traumatic cataract over the last eight years, treated in the Eye Hospital Rotterdam, were traced in the medical archives. Before sending them an invitation for re-examination, the patients had to fulfill the following requirements: – no ocular abnormality before the accident; – the age at the time of the accident had to be between 8 and 50 years; – the traumatic lesions had to be limited to the anterior segment; and – the visual acuity after the accident had to be recovered up to, at least, 50%.

165 patients fulfilled these requirements and 61 of them were willing to cooperate the orthoptic re-examination.

The orthoptic results were arranged according to the following four classifications:

I: Binocular single vision (B.S.V.) with good stereoscopic vision (S.V.): these patients had no orthoptic abnormalities and they recognised the circles of the Titmus stereotest.

II: Binocular single vision with moderate stereoscopic vision: these patients had no orthoptic abnormalities, but they recognised only the fly of the Titmus stereotest and they had stereoscopic vision in the synoptophore too.

III: Binocular single vision without stereoscopic vision.

IV: No binocular vision, but diplopia, suppression or confusion was present.

Of the 61 unilateral traumatic aphakia patients, 27 eyes were corrected with an intra-ocular lens, while 34 eyes were fitted with a contact lens. From these 34 patients, fitted with a contact lens, 19 patients did wear their lens the whole day, whereas 15 patients did not wear their lens at all or did wear their lens incidentally.

When the binocular functions, arranged in the afore mentioned classes, are plotted against the interval between the trauma and the fitting of the contact lens (Fig. 1), is obtained for the 19 patients, who wear their lens more than 10 hours a day. The X-axis represents the interval in months, while on the Y-axis the four classes of binocular rehabilitation are plotted. Every dot represents one patient. This figure demonstrates, that about 84% of these patients have a good to moderate binocular rehabilitation. A correlation between the interval and the rehabilitation cannot be found.

The results of the 15 contact lens patients, who did not wear their lenses, plotted in the same way, are presented in Fig. 2. This figure demonstrates, that only 26% of the patients have a good to moderate binocular rehabilitation and that delay of fitting a contact lens decreases the chance of binocular rehabilitation.

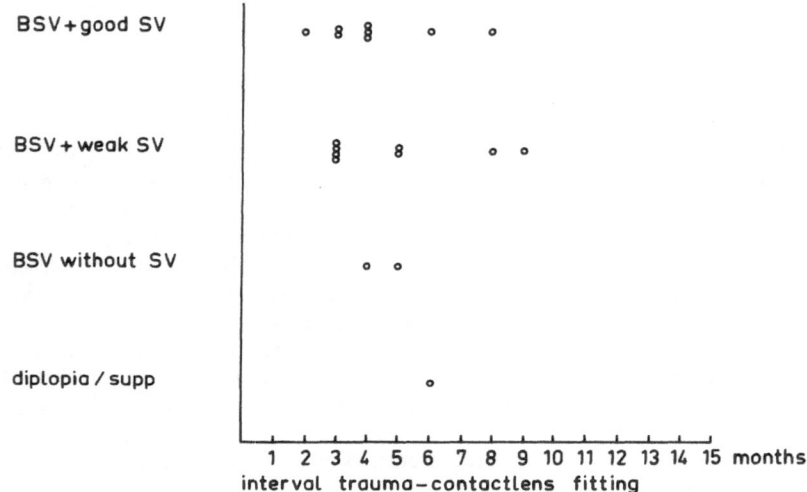

Fig. 1. B.R. of 19 patients fitted with a contact lens with a wear time >10 hours daily.

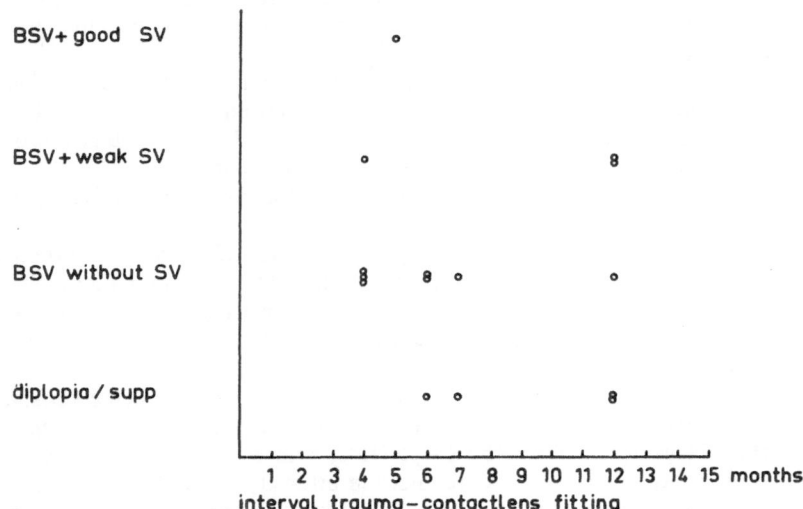

Fig. 2. B.R. of 15 patients fitted with a contact lens with a wear time <2 hours daily.

96

Another important factor that can influence binocular functions badly is the aniseikonia. This factor plotted against the binocular functions is shown in Fig. 3. The X-axis now represents the aniseikonia. In this figure no correlation appears to exist between the binocular functions and the aniseikonia. Even with an aniseikonia of 11%, good stereoscopic vision was possible. The average aniseikonia for the whole contact lens group was 6%.

Let us now have a look at the patients, where the traumatic aphakia was corrected with the implantation of an intraocular lens. This group consisted of 27 patients; 8 of them received an intraocular lens primarily, within four months after the accident; while 19 patients received the lens secondarily, with an average of 7 years after the accident. Since refusal of the contact lens was the indication for secondary implantation, this interval of 7 years may be considered as a period of binocular interruption. The relation between binocular rehabilitation and the interval between trauma and implantation for the 8 primarily implanted eyes is demonstrated in Fig. 4. 87% of these patients have a good to moderate binocular rehabilitation.

Less favourable is the binocular rehabilitation in the 19 patients, who received an intraocular lens secondarily, as is shown in Fig. 5. Delay of secondary implantation reduces the chance of good binocular rehabilitation. The average aniseikonia for the patients, who received an intraocular lens, was 2.8%.

If we compare now the binocular rehabilitation of the two groups of contact lens patients and of the two groups of patients with an intraocular lens, Table 1 is obtained. The best results are scored by the primarily implanted group; 87% of these patients have good to moderate binocular rehabilitation, followed by the contact lens group with a wear time longer than 10 hours a day: 84%. The next group is the secondarily implanted group: 70%. The worst results are obtained from the contact lens group with a wear time less than 2 hours a day: 26%.

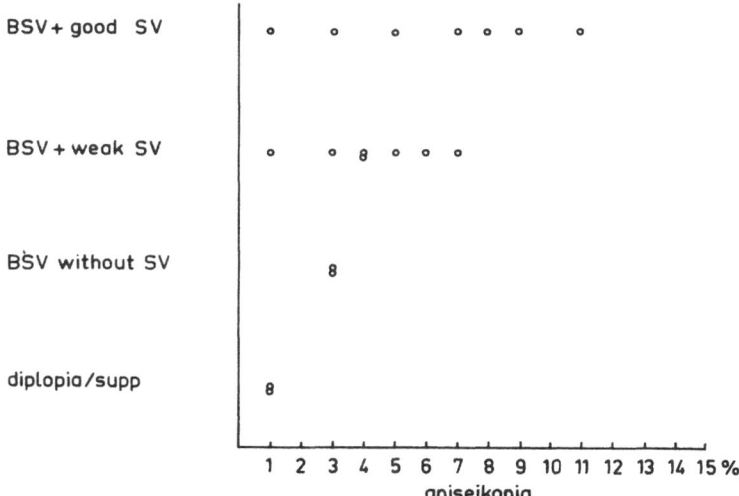

Fig. 3. B.R. of 19 patients with a contact lens related with the aniseikonia.

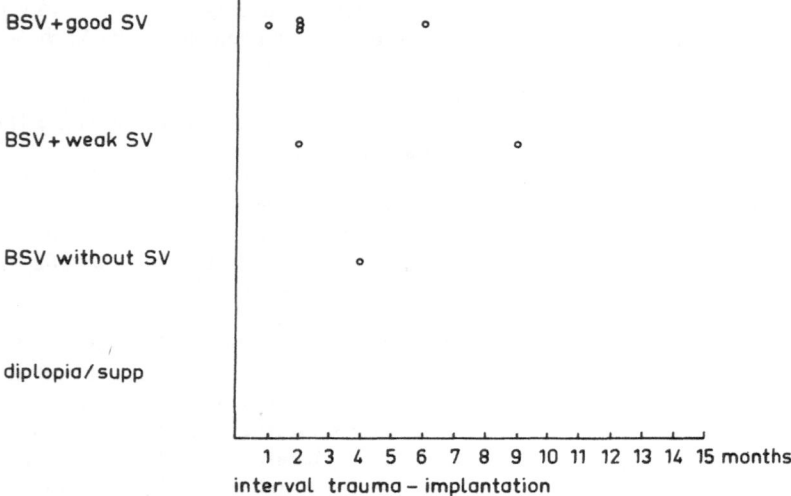

Fig. 4. B.R. of 8 direct-implanted eyes.

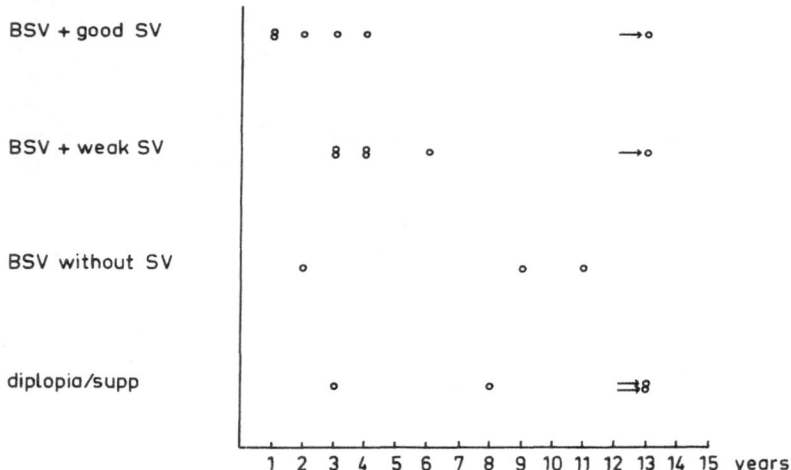

Fig. 5. B.R. of 19 secondary implanted eyes.

A very interesting detail of this examination was the comparison of binocular functions before and after secondary implantation of an intraocular lens. Fig. 6 demonstrates the binocular functions before (with contact lens) and after the implantation.

The binocular functions improved in 7 out of 11 patients. Reasons for this improvement are continuous focusing and absence of the prismatic side effect of the moving contact lens. In 4 out of 11 patients no improvement was observed. Two of them maintained total suppression, while the

Table 1. Binocular rehabilitation-comparison.

	cl >10 hrs	cl < 2 hrs	pr.impl.	sec.impl.
	19 pat.	15 pat.	8 pat.	19 pat
B.S.V. + good S.V.	42%	6%	62%	38%
B.S.V. + weak S.V.	42%	20%	25%	32%
B.S.V. without S.V.	10%	46%	13%	10%
diplopia/suppr.	6%	28%	-	2 %

BEFORE   AFTER

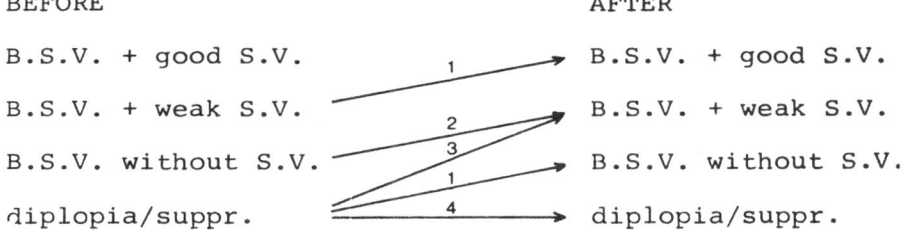

Fig. 6. B.R. before (with contact lens) and after implantation.

last 2 patients complained of diplopia after implantation. This diplopia was caused by absence of fusional amplitude.

In conclusion: the binocular rehabilitation in unilateral traumatic aphakia may succeed if the focusing power, by preference an intraocular lens, is repaired as soon as possible.

REFERENCES

Balen, A.Th.M. van. Binkhorst's method of implantation of pseudophakoi in unilateral traumatic cataract. Ophthalmologica (Basel) 165, 490–494 (1972).

Balen, A.Th.M. van. Four years' experience with Binkhorst lens implantation. Amer. J. Ophthal. 75, 755–763 (1973).

Binkhorst, C.D. & M.H. Gobin. Injuries to the eye with lens opacity in young children. Ophthalmologica (Basel) 148, 169–183 (1964).

Binkhorst, C.D. & M.H. Gobin. Pseudophakia after lens injury in children. Ophthalmologica (Basel) 154, 81–87 (1967).

Binkhorst, C.D., M.H. Gobin & P.A.M. Leonard. Post-traumatic artificial lens implants (pseudophakoi) in children. Brit. J. Ophthal. 53: 518–529 (1969).

Dannheim, E. & H.U. Retzlaff. Fusions- und Aniseikonieprobleme bei einseitiger Aphakie. Klin. Mbl. Augenheilk. 174, 629–634 (1979).

Enoch, J.M. Physiology of monocular aphakia. Ophthalmology 86, 391–398 (1979).

Flick, H. Die einseitige Aphakie im Kindesalter. Klin. Mbl. Augenheilk. 167, 664–669 (1975).

Frey, T., D. Friendly & D. Wyatt. Re-evaluation of monocular cataracts in children. Amer. J. Ophthal. 76, 381–388 (1973).

Gernet, H. The binocular confusion in unilateral aphakia. Ann. Ophthal. 11, 617–621 (1979).

Haghfelt, T. & E. Goldschmidt. Social and medical aspects of unilateral traumatic aphakia. Acta Ophthal. 55, 401–408 (1977).

Highman, V.N. Stereopsis and aniseikonia in uniocular aphakia. Brit. J. Ophthal. 61, 30–33 (1977).

Percival, S.P.B. & K.M. Yousef. Treatment of uniocular aphakia. A comparison of iris clip lenses with hard corneal contact lenses. Brit. J. Ophthal. 60, 642–644 (1976).

Rubinstein, K. Management of unilateral aphakia. Brit. Orthopt. J. 17, 82–86 (1960).

Sjølie, A.K. & K.K. Mortensen. Unilateral traumatic cataract in children. Acta Ophthal. 55, 395–400 (1977).

Author's address:
Eye Department
Erasmus University
Eye Hospital
Schiedamsevest 180
3011 BH Rotterdam, The Netherlands

MOTOR TONUS ADAPTATION IN SQUINT

S. RÉTHY & S. GÁL
(Duisburg, F.R.G.)

Adaptations to the deviation are considered to be responsible for some constant symptoms of squint. We just heard from Bagolini's interesting data on the anomaly and suppression as supposedly binocular adaptations at the sensorimotor level. He also mentioned the sensory adaptation as monocular adjustment in squint.

We now turn our attention to symptoms owing to the less known motor tonus adaptation. We are familiar with the difficulties arising from the wear of full correcting glasses since the time of Donders. (Fig. 1).

It is a pity that Donders cannot discuss with Gobin the dubious correctness of those glasses which can align so little of the convergent squint angle. Donders described the necessity of cycloplegia in optic correction of hypermetropia. But there is still no explanation for the failure of cycloplegia in not always revealing the full extent of latent hypermetropia. The resistance of latent hypermetropia against manifestation and of the rest angle

The first sound theory on the etiology of convergent squint was put forward by DONDERS about a hundred years ago (1864).

The treatment was obvious from this theory: the wearing of a hypermetropia correction.But ... in the majority the deviation is not even corrected by wearing spectacles.

GOBIN M.H. [1969]

(Something seems to be wrong with these spectacles.... or with the theory ?)

DONDERS did not elaborate on the tonus stabilization and on
the resistance to therapy created by the
central adaptations adjusting to the deviation and
developing sensory and motor impulse-patterns...

Fig. 1.

Docum. Ophthal. Proc. Series, Vol. 32, ed. by A.Th.M. van Balen & W.A. Houtman
 ISBN 90 6193 728 0

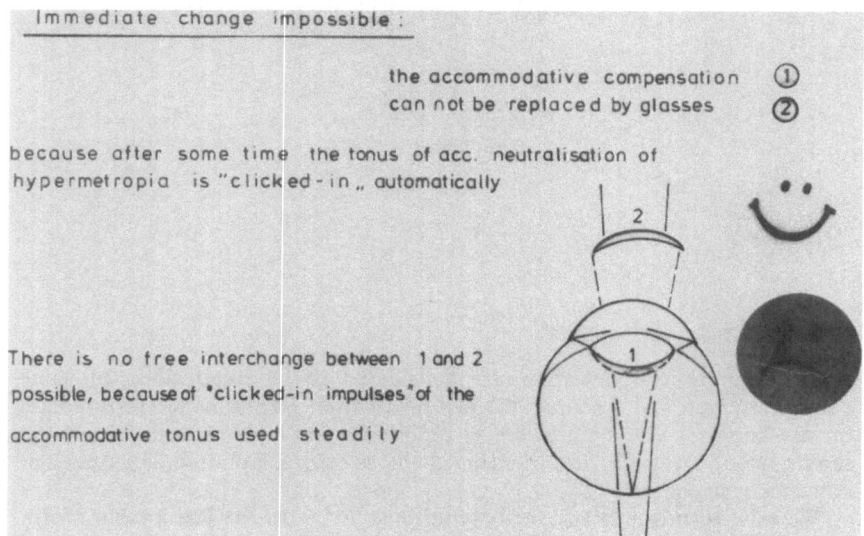

Immediate change impossible :

the accommodative compensation ①
can not be replaced by glasses ②

because after some time the tonus of acc. neutralisation of
hypermetropia is "clicked-in „ automatically

There is no free interchange between 1 and 2
possible, because of "clicked-in impulses"of the
accommodative tonus used steadily

Fig. 2.

against relaxation occurs often. Let us take a look at practical aspects. (Fig. 2).

The steadily used tonus of accommodation neutralizing hypermetropia cannot be relaxed immediately. The free choice of sharp focusing by glasses or by the necessary accommodative tonus is not possible. The accommodative impulses fluctuate for some time before they stabilize the tonus, more and more neutralizing the hypermetropia. (Fig. 3).

The motor tonus, clicking in gradually at a constant level of activity, needs neither attention nor voluntary effort, as before. The automatic tonus activity

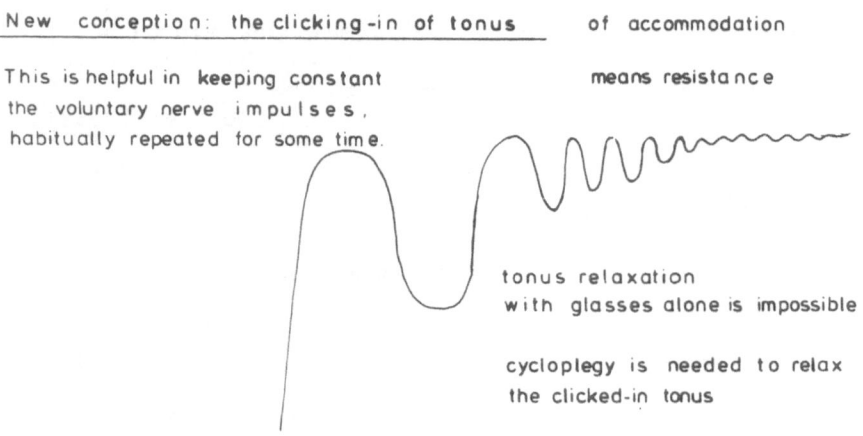

New conception: the clicking-in of tonus   of accommodation

This is helpful in keeping constant
the voluntary nerve impulses,
habitually repeated for some time.

means resistance

tonus relaxation
with glasses alone is impossible

cycloplegy is needed to relax
the clicked-in tonus

Fig. 3.

cannot be stopped voluntarily. The cause can be local muscle spasm or central impulse pattern activity, repeated steadily by the brain (Fig. 4).

We performed a simple experiment with short-acting cycloplegy in order to differentiate between them. It has shown that the latter is true. In hypermetropic children from seven years of age the manifested refractive error under cyclopent (1%) was fully corrected immediately. Vision for distance was 1.0 with the full correction. Some five hours later, with the glasses constantly worn, the vision became blurred. The blur with the glasses was due to an overcorrection owing to the recovering tonus of accommodation. After seven to eight hours the situation was the same as it was before the cyclopent instillations. Vision is much better without the glasses. The hypermetropia is sometimes fully latent. Glasses are not accepted at all, until a new cycloplegia is given. After half an hour the vision becomes blurred, glasses are accepted readily. In another six hours time the images are out of focus again until new cyclopent drops are given. How often are they needed until the tonus does not recur automatically in spite of the glasses?

In our experience cycloplegia was needed over a period of 7 to 50 days, depending upon the severity of the motor tonus adaptation. A certain time is needed until the dynamic phase of the clicked in impulses relaxes immediately with the glasses. This means that the sensitivity for focus-defocus stimuli is recovered when the light as the generalized stimulus is abolished. (Fig. 5).

Without treatment the generalization of stimuli continues. Relaxation is no longer achieved in darkness as it was in the first phase of clicking in of impulses. The tonus relaxation in dim light can be studied by the infra-red

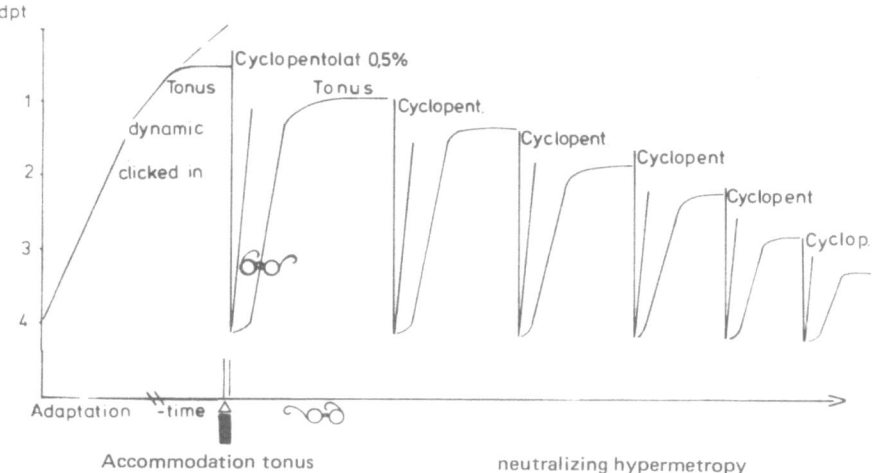

Fig. 4.

103

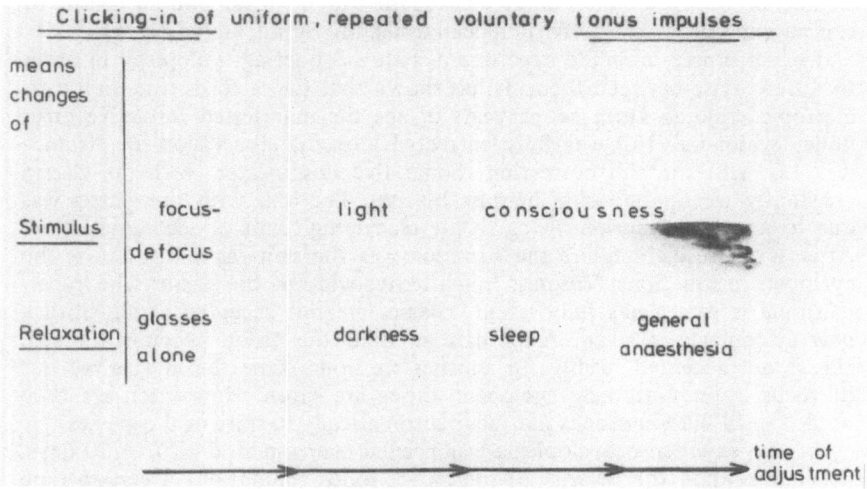

Fig. 5.

Topcon refractometer. At the next stage the relaxation can be achieved during sleep; later under general anaesthesia only. The stimulus becomes more generalized, it is consciousness itself. The impulses are activated at a subcortical level, relaxed in deep anaesthesia. (Fig. 6).

At this static stage of clicked in impulses a new feature of latent hypermetropia can be recognized: the stabilized latent form. The well-known triade of Donders, namely the total h. made up of the manifest and the latent h. can be completed by the new term of stabilized latent hypermetropia. Atropine

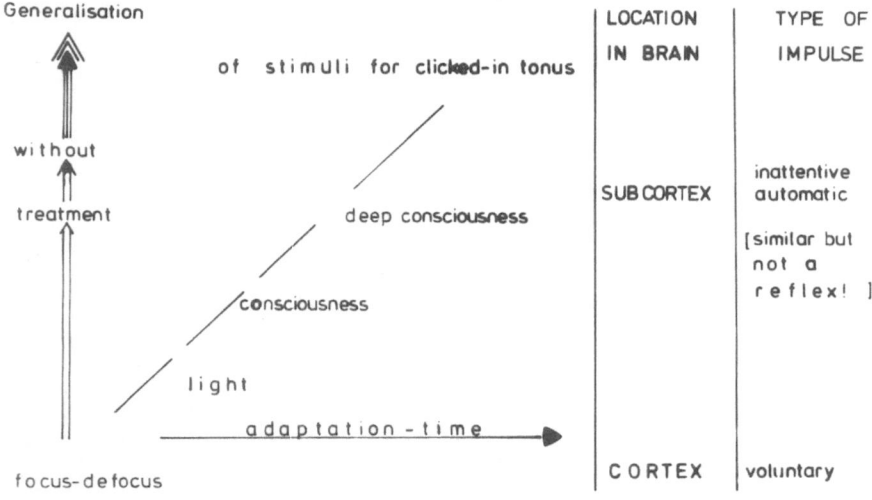

Fig. 6.

104

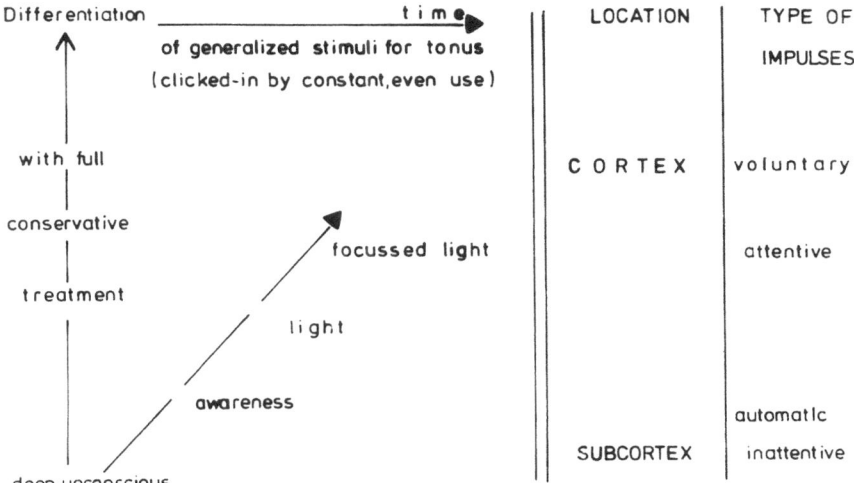

Fig. 7.

instillations can no longer reveal the full amount of latent hypermetropia. Time is needed to relax the clicked in tonus. By repeatedly giving atropine instillations (after some time of the wearing of the full correction) the strength of the glasses can be augmented. The gradual manifestation of the stabilized latent hypermetropia can last up to one or two years with the wear of fully correcting or slightly overcorrecting glasses. In some cases a pseudoemmetropic state may reveal itself half a year later as stabilized latent hypermetropia of 1 or 3 dioptres. (Fig. 7).

The differentiation of stimuli under treatment is the reverse of the generalisation process established without treatment. It is not very sensible to give prolonged atropinization without optic correction as help for the relaxation. The generalized stimulus is differentiated gradually by the wearing of glasses adjusted from time to time to the more relaxed tonus and higher manifested h. The regulation of the impulse pattern becomes more cortical again needing more attention as the focus defocus system of stimuli regains its effectiveness.

The adaptations to the deviation as well as the motor tonus adjustment take place regularly early in life. At the third or fourth month of life hypermetropia can already be latent. Cycloplegia is necessary to reveal it, especially in the lower grades of hypermetropia. If we dare to draw the logical conclusions from the facts of adaptation stabilizing the deviation we have to treat squint cases immediately from the onset by full correction even from the second month of life.

Authors' address:
Am Grünen Ring 21
D-41 Duisburg 18, F.R.G.

THE SUBJECTIVE ANGLE AS A BASIS FOR THE SURGERY OF THE ANATOMICAL DEVIATION

A. SPIELMANN

(Nancy, France)

SUMMARY

Esotropia is dissociated into its two components: the anatomical deviation (minimal deviation in principle) and the dynamic deviation (functional esotropia). The value of the Subjective Angle (Striated glasses test) is compared with the value of the minimal objective deviation (and not as it is usually done with a global deviation) before and after surgery. The surgical suppression of the spasm allows an interesting control of the diagnosis of anomalous correspondence.

When an angle of anomaly is found its average value is always 6 diopters in small and in large deviation. In many cases, the surgical suppression of the spasm causes an immediate disappearance of the angle of anomaly even if orthophoria is not established. In these cases of 'false' A.R.C., the angle of anomaly is thus part of the spasm embodied in the measure of the minimal deviation. The 'angle of anomaly' in true A.R.C. is still 6 diopters (before and after surgery). It could be the same part of the spasm (unable to carry on a proper localization) totally fixed.

Practically, the value of the subjective deviation always has to be taken into account in our surgery since it is the closest to the anatomical deviation. In adults a surgery of relocation based on the value of the subjective angle, plus a Fadenoperation for the value of the angle of anomaly, gives in many cases an orthophoria with binocularity, suggesting those closed relations existing between the angle of anomaly and the spasm.

For the past few years, the horizontal deviation in variable squint has been dissociated clinically and surgically by Cüppers into its two components: the anatomical deviation and the functional Esotropia. By functional Esotropia, I mean this reflex motor answer to a sensorial anomaly (ametropia, occlusion) or to a motor anomaly (alphabetic syndrome, microstrabismus), which causes a defect of the monocular or binocular perception in children.

The subjective angle determined with the Bagolini striated glasses test, has usually been equated with the global angle of squint. I have studied its connection with a minimal objective deviation (which is supposed to represent the anatomical basic deviation), before and after surgery. Because it is so difficult to isolate totally the anatomical deviation, the surgical cure of the innervational component of the Esotropia allows for an interesting control of the pre-operative diagnosis of the retinal correspondence. This gives a better understanding of the role of the 'spasm' or 'hyperadduction' in the pre-operative misdiagnosis, when it is often confused with the angle of anomaly, and of its possible role in the genesis of some 'Anomalous Retinal Correspondence (A.R.C.).

MATERIAL

Two hundred cases of convergent squint have been studied.

One hundred cases in cooperant children from four to eight years old whose spasm has been cured by surgery (even if orthophoria was not obtained)

50 with a subjective angle = 0 had only a Fadenoperation (mono or bilateral) because of a minimal deviation always found $\leqslant 8^{\triangle}$

50 with a subjective angle $\neq$ 0.

One hundred cases in adults from 18 to 50 years old. The spasm was not taken into account in the selection of adult patients.

50 cases had a subjective angle = 0

50 cases had a subjective angle $\neq$ 0

In these four groups, the selected cases were the most recent ones answering the criteria.

METHODS

Measures

The Maximal Objective Angle (M.O.A.) was determined in space, elicited by a slow alternate cover test, for far and near fixation, with and without glasses.

The Minimal Objective Angle (m.O.A.) was determined by a light cover-uncover test with glasses.

The Subjective Angle (A.S.) was determined with the Bagolini Striated glasses test before the cover test, in normal fixation first and then with prism starting from an over-correction of the supposed minimal deviation. (The strias are traced directly on the patient's glasses.)

Repetition of the tests is essential. A scotoma without changes in the spatial localization is considered as normal correspondence.

Surgery

The oblique or vertical defects is always corrected.

A conventional surgery was applied to the minimal deviation (which is supposed to be the closest to the anatomical deviation). A Fadenoperation was applied to the spasm (M.O.A. – m.O.A.).

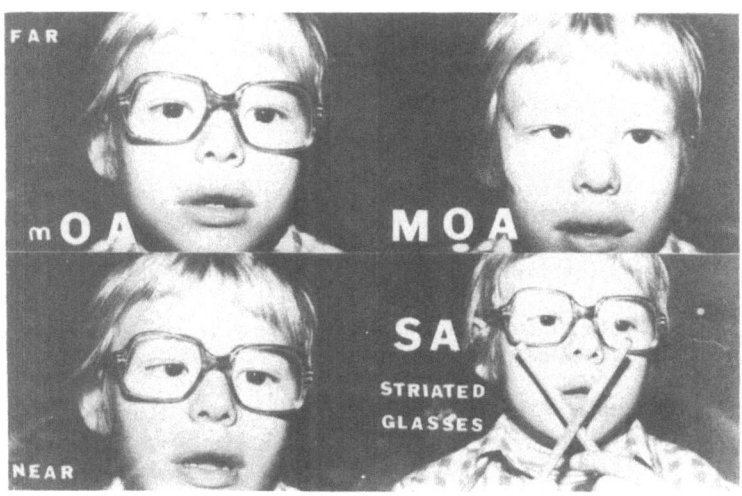

Fig. 1. m.O.A. = Minimum Objective Angle. It is determined by a rapid Cover-Uncover test with glasses. Here *m.O.A. = 6 diopters.* M.O.A. = Maximum Objective Angle. It is determined by a slow cover test with and without glasses. Here *M.O.A. = 50 diopters.* S.A. = Subjective Angle. The Bagolini strias are traced on the spectacles. Here *S.A. = 0.*

RESULTS Table 1 and 2

Table 1: S.A. = 0. 100 cases:
Children = 50 cases; Adults = 50 cases.

   a) In those squints with a small angle of deviation always found ≤8 diopters) and a subjective angle equal zero, a Normal Retinal Correspondence (N.R.C.) is found in 40% of the cases in adults as well as in children.

   b) In 40% of the cases (44% of children, 34% of adults) the angle of anomaly disappears if the spasm is suppressed surgically. Its average value is always 6 diopters (False A.R.C.).

   c) In 16% of the children, this angle of anomaly of 6 diopters persists

Table 1.

SA = 0		100 Cases		
		cases	spasm	A of A
NRC	ch	20 = 40%	$35^{\triangle}$	
	a	20 = 40%	$35^{\dagger}$	
F. ARC	ch	22 = 44%	$35^{\triangle}$	$6^{\triangle}$
	a	17 = 34%	$40^{\triangle}$	$6^{\triangle}$
ARC	ch	8 = 16%	$35^{\triangle}$	$6^{\triangle}$
	a	13 = 26%	$30^{\triangle}$	$10^{\triangle}$

after surgery. The cases of 'true' A.R.C. with microstrabismus are more numerous in adults 26% (as it was stressed by Lang).

Table 2: S.A. ≠ 0. 100 cases:
Adults = 50 cases; Children = 50 cases.
In children
a) In those cases where the minimal deviation is larger (AS ≠ 0), the percentage of N.R.C. is 56% and of F. A.R.C. is 30%. The total percentage of N.R.C. is thus 86%, the same as in small deviations.
b) The average value of the angle of Anomaly, real of false, is still 6 diopters.
c) The angle of anomaly disappears after surgery in 75% of the cases (the 30% of F. A.R.C.) and persists in 25% of the cases (the 14% of A.R.C.).
In adults
a) The percentage of N.R.C. is only 14% while the A.R.C. is now 56%. The spasm diminishes to $20^\triangle$ – as the angle of anomaly elevates to $12^\triangle$. Nine cases of pseudo 'strabismus fixus' had a peripapillar fixation and formed a special group.
b) Only 3 cases without a spasm have been found in adult patients, all belonging to the cases of N.R.C.

Table 2.

SA ≠ 0		100 Cases		
		cases	spasm	A of A
NRC	ch	28 = 56%	$30^\triangle$	
	a	7 = 14%	$25^\triangle$	
F. ARC	ch	15 = 30%	$30^\triangle$	$6^\triangle$
	a	15 = 30%	$25^\triangle$	$6^\triangle$
ARC	ch	7 = 14%	$25^\triangle$	$6^\triangle$
	a	28 = 56%	$20^\triangle$: 19 ST. FIX. 9	$12^\triangle$

COMMENTS

a) When the answer to the striated glasses test is compared to the minimal deviation in children, the average value of the angle of anomaly, true or false, is always 6 diopters, whether it is a strabismus with a small deviation or with a larger one. This value is still 6 diopters in adults with F. A.R.C. It is equal to $12^\triangle$ only in A.R.C.
b) In 55% of the cases (73% in children) the surgical suppression of the spasm gives an immediate disparition of the angle of anomaly. It could be an immediate adaptation to the new motor conditions as described by Bagolini (1961). But the normalization happens even if an orthophoria is not established, provided the spasm is cured. It could be a normalization of the localization by the Fadenoperation. But the normalization is far too fast. Thus it

110

appears logical to admit an error in the pre-operative diagnosis due to the difficult approach of the anatomical deviation as long as the spasm exists (Cüppers & Thomas stressed the necessity of tests studying the O.A. and the S.A. at the same time). This may explain the approximation of 6^Δ found statistically in my surgery.

c) The angle of anomaly, in the cases of False A.R.C. seems thus to be a part of the spasm, the average value of it being 6^Δ, embodied in the measure of the minimal deviation. This fact is perfectly illustrated by the correspondence 'variable in time' when repeated tests, succeed in finding a N.R.C. Moreover, as far as these gross measurements are concerned diagnosis of A.R.C. in space may only reflect our inability to measure correctly the basic anatomic deviation. A study with afterimage has to be done. But the cases of afterimage normalized when the eyes are closed i.e. when there is no spasm it is interesting to notice.

d) Certainly the subjective measures are less dissociating and give a better approach of the anatomical deviation as stressed by Urist. One can even wonder if the subjective angle is not the real initial anatomic angle (innate N.R.C.) on which a spasm, unable to carry on a proper immediate localization(?) is superimposed. If the spasm is totally releasable the retinal correspondence would be normal. If part of the spasm is tightly linked to the basic deviation but released by surgery, for instance, there is a false A.R.C. When this part of the spasm is fixed, 'anatomised' the Retinal Correspondence is really abnormal. The angle of anomaly is a little more important in adults where it reaches 12^Δ to the prejudice of the spasm (20^Δ).

e) Contrary to popular opinion, the spasm exists in adults as well as in children (94% of the cases). But it is more difficult to be provoked or released. (Spasmodic contracture of Weiss and Pigassou.) Then it is still more easily mistaken with an angle of anomaly.

CONCLUSION

A spasm of an average value of 6 diopters seems to be included very often in the objective measure of the minimal angle. It is often mistaken with an angle of anomaly of the same value but it may become a real, anatomical angle of anomaly if fixed.

In practice, when the determination of the anatomical deviation is so difficult, it is advisable to take into account the value of the subjective angle in the determination of one's surgery. The subjective angle tested with the Bagolini Striated glasses test gives in variable squints the closest value of the basic deviation in 84% of the cases in children. In the other cases it leads to the comfortable situation of microstrabismus. A negative subjective angle must forbid any surgery other than a careful Fadenoperation.

In adults where the spasm is as frequent as in children but more difficult to be released, I have operated for some years in the anomalous correspondences, on the basis of the subjective deviations by a conventional surgery and a Fadenoperation for the angle of anomaly (+ the spasm). This technique has provided me, in many cases, with good results of restoration of a binocularity in the primary position of gaze, suggesting then the closed relations existing between the angle of anomaly and the spasm. Interesting results obtained with the same technique in divergent squint with A.R.C. evoke the problem of the existence of the spasm of divergency.

REFERENCES

Bagolini, B. Diagnostic et possibilité de traitement de l'état sensoriel du strabisme concomitant avec des instruments peu dissociants (test du verre strié et barre de filtres). Ann. Ocul. 00: 194–236 (1961).
Spielmann, A. Les strabismes Variables. Année Thérapeutique et clinique en Ophtalmologie. Vol. XXXI: 207–231 (1980).
Spielmann, A. Action of Recessions and Resections when associated with Cüppers' Fadenoperation in Esotropia Strabismus. Reinecke Ed' Grune et Stratton, New York. (I.S.A. meeting – Kyoto) pp. 355–369 (1978).

Author's address:
11 rue de la Ravinelle
F-54000 Nancy, France

INFLUENCE OF PROGRESSIVE PRESS-ON-PRISMS ON CHANGING SQUINTING ANGLES

H. AICHMAIR

(*Vienna, Austria*)

INTRODUCTION

A wrong position of the eyes may prevent light beams of a fixation object from falling on normally corresponding areas of the retina. This can be remedied only by correction of the eye's position or by a change in the direction of incidence of the beams (Flick 1975). In order to apply the second method the use of a prism is recommendable (Aichmair 1978).

There are dispersion prisms that split up visible light into its spectral colors; deviation prisms are preferred in ophthalmology. They can be either wedge-shaped or Fresnel prisms. In the latter case only the spikes of several prisms are arranged one directly after the other (Fig. 1). This ensures that too much weight is avoided while the optical principle of deviation is maintained. Because of the many wedge-shaped spikes arranged one after the other, an increased scattering of light develops at their base, inducing vision loss. Nevertheless, modern prism therapy has become possible only after the invention of Fresnel prisms (Schäfer 1976).

If a prism is held in front of each eye, base outwards, the pair of eyes has to turn into a convergent position in order to still see the fixation object as single; consequently, bases turned inwards induce a divergent position. Difficulties with prisms always result when variable squinting angles exist, for instance, when after an operation the globes are parallel or almost so for distant vision but there is still a considerable convergence excess for near vision, or, when the squint occurs mainly at near vision and cannot be equalized by refractive correction, not even with bifocal glasses.

Unfortunately, orthoptic training cannot always eliminate this condition; not every patient responds to it nor is every patient, because of age, profession or distant residence, able to train sufficiently. Therefore, we have searched for a possible way to treat these patients also with prisms. The prisms generally used up to now can influence only one squinting angle. We believed that press-on-prisms of different strengths (according to the results of a prismatic cover test (Aichmair 1978)) that are cut into strips and pressed on spectacles in the order of their diopters should induce a prismatic effect of different grades depending on the angle of looking through them. We have named such prisms 'progressive press-on-prisms', analogous to progressive spectacles.

Docum. Ophthal. Proc. Series, Vol. 32, ed. by A.Th.M. van Balen & W.A. Houtman 113
© *1982, Dr W. Junk Publishers, The Hague. ISBN 90 6193 728 0*

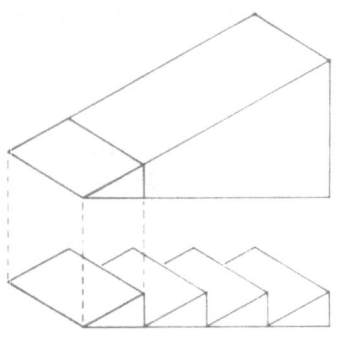

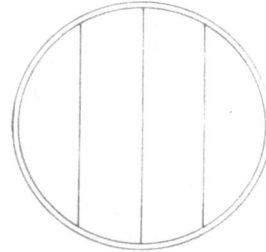

Fig. 1. Principle of Fresnel prisms.

METHOD

The individual strips of press-on-prisms are glued on a 1.0 occlusion foil (Fig. 2), cut out in the shape of the spectacles and fixed on the glass by adhesion (Fig. 3).

It is important not to cut them too narrow so that they can adhere; it is better to omit one strength if necessary. The prism is always adjusted in front of the better eye. When the glasses were put on we checked to see whether the strips were oblique since this would create problems for the patient. For the same reason, the border of the strips should not pass through the pupillary area.

In two children, shortly after fitting the prism, the results were worse than before. At first we could find no explanation but after close examination of the progressive press-on-prism that had been cut out by hand we discovered that some of the spots were not completely straight (Fig. 4). Since then all foils have been cut by machine and vision is now almost unimpaired.

114

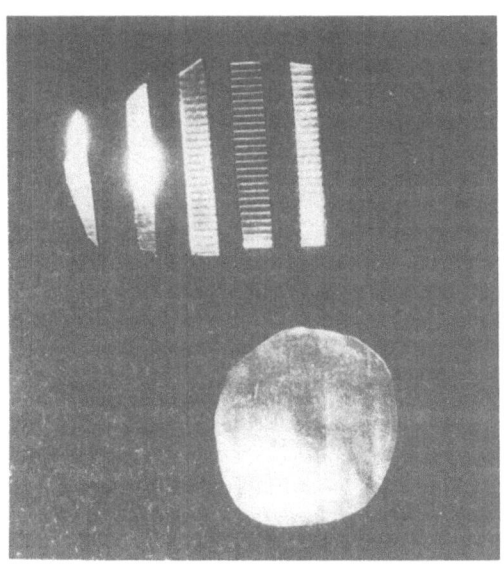

Fig. 2. Strips of press-on-prism of different strength and 1.0 occlusion foil.

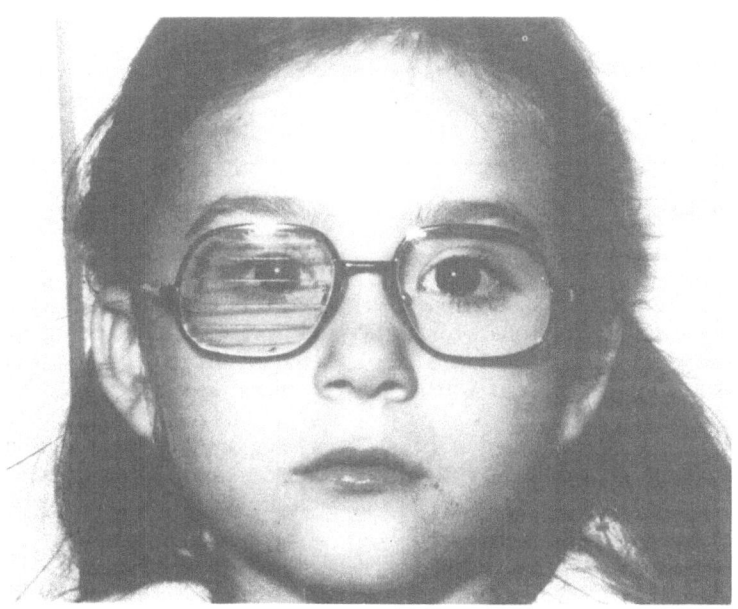

Fig. 3. Patient with progressive press-on-prism on her glasses.

115

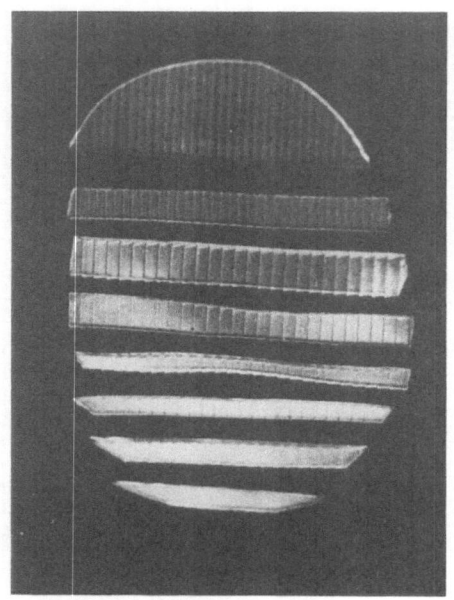

Fig. 4. Progressive press-on-prism with poorly cut strips.

RESULTS AND DISCUSSION

Results of treatment with progressive press-on-prisms in 25 patients.

Squinting angle:	Better	Unchanged	Treatment stopped	Total
Primary	9	2	3	14
Post-operatively	10	1	–	11
Total	19	3	3	25

Patients were between ages 4 and 11 years; only one patient was 30-years-old. Treatment lasted from one week to 17 months and has also been continued in some cases. The evaluation is based on the prismatic cover test, range of fusion and stereotest after Worth; 'better' means success in one or more of these criteria.

Three patients achieved a parallel position, one of them temporarily without a prism, as long as 7 months after discarding it. The grownup wears the prism some hours per day and has practically normal binocular vision with it.

Treatment was stopped in three cases because the parents did not co-operate (the children lost their prisms or did not wear them, had them fitted obliquely or in front of the wrong eye), although the results at the onset of the therapy would have been most promising.

116

In three cases the therapy showed no change in the patient's condition or after a short-lived amelioration a return to the former results occurred.

One child wore the prism only for one week, then it was discarded because of a beginning convergence excess for near vision. Nevertheless, its sensoric functions have improved considerably — from +10 and +30 prism diopters the child has turned to practically parallel position in free space; the range of fusion has doubled. These results have remained stable for 7 months.

Two patients had a divergent strabismus: in one the angle could be reduced to half of what it had been before and the formerly totally lacking fusion could be established; in the other patient the divergent angle for near vision could be changed into a convergent one and is now treated with a weaker prism.

In most of the patients the range of fusion could be improved or for the first time built up at all; in some patients the angle for distant vision could be totally eliminated and the angle for near vision decreased or near- and distance-angle could be approximated so that the starting situation for regular therapy has been created.

In conclusion we can state that of our rather small number of 25 patients more than three-fourths (19) could improve their condition of changing squinting angles by therapy with progressive press-on-prisms. Therefore, it seems advisable to try this new method. Our experiments continue; should the results still prove to be promising after some time, we will try to ensure the manufacture of progressive press-on-prisms.

REFERENCES

Aichmair, H. Die Binokularuntersuchung mit besonderer Berücksichtigung der Prismenkorrektur. Augenärztl. Fortbild. 5/2, 217–228 (1978).

Flick, H.J. Das Schielen des Kindes. Diagnostik, Therapie, Prognose. Dtsch. Ärzteverlag GmbH., Köln-Lövenich (1975).

Schäfer, W.D. Strabismus in der Praxis. Untersuchungstechnik und Behandlungsablauf. Springer Verlag. Berlin. (1976).

Author's address:
2nd University Eye Clinic
Alserstr. 4
A-1090 Vienna, Austria

BINOCULAR VISION IN TREATED SQUINTS

F. POLYCHRONIADIS & S. POLYCHRONIADIS-SCOUROS

(Athens, Greece)

The goal of this paper is to show that some form of binocular vision can be achieved by correction of refraction anomalies and orthoptic treatment.

From the beginning of our trial we approached the treatment of squint from a binocular point of view which included most aspects of the treatment of amblyopia (Polychroniadis 1960; 1969).

PHYSIOLOGY

Binocular vison is built up from about the age of three to four months through successive stages of development of reflexes, which are in the one part of conditional and in the other part of unconditional nature.

In the past it was assumed that if a squint became manifest during the period of development of binocular vision, it was unlikely that any binocular vision could develop (Plicque 1946; Crone 1980; Bredemeyer & Bullock 1963).

In a series of 237 patients we started treatment as early as possible. The treatment afforded the patient the opportunity to develop a kind of binocular vision which was within his reach, either it was binocular single vision or abnormal retinal correspondence. Some of these patients were observed during a ten years period. We believe that the results will be better in treated cases than in those cases which lack the benefit of the treatment. The results will show improvement in visual acuity, binocular vision and angle of deviation (Polychroniadis & Polychroniadis 1975).

COURSE OF TREATMENT

1. *Full correction of any refractive error.* As early as possible a prescription was made for refractive errors. Astigmatism was fully corrected. The power of + sphere lenses was gradually increased. The youngest patients treated in this way was of the age of eight months.

Penalisation, by means of a slight overcorrection of the fixing eye, was used as a part of the binocular treament of amblyopia. If necessary, the glasses were readjusted for best visual acuity and optimal alignment of the eyes (Polychroniadis 1960).

Docum. Ophthal. Proc. Series, Vol. 32, ed. by A.Th.M. van Balen & W.A. Houtman 119
© *1982, Dr W. Junk Publishers, The Hague. ISBN 90 6193 728 0*

2. *Treatment of amblyopia.* In young patients we tried to overcome amblyopia with a minimal amount of occlusion. Occlusion appears to have harmful effects on the normal functions of the occluded eye as well as on the normal development of binocularity. But vision appears to improve most rapidly at the age below 2 to 3 years (Ikeda & Tremain 1980). Penalisation (as outlined above) was used in the older patients, together with exercises with binocular Haidinger brushes in the Synoptophore, combined with the presentation of real objects for the non amblyopic eye. Monocular reading or watching the television during short periods was also advised to most patients (Stanworth & Naylor 1955).

Alternate fixation was not demanded as a criterium for the reestablishment of visual acuity. However, it was noticed temporarily during the period of penalisation (Thomas 1958).

3. *Stimulation of binocularity* with the aid of the Synoptophore, exercises in free space by prisms, and exercises of convergence and relative convergence (stereograms included) were found very important tools in the course of the treatment.

The treatment was usually given in 20 to 30 sessions, which were spread over a period of two months or when the patients were very young over a period of more than one year. Our experience was that a daily treatment during a period of two weeks (or up to one month) was more effective than one weekly session.

After the end of the treatment follow up was carried out after one month and later after three or six months as the patients grew older.

Cases with results

In 237 cases which were not lost from follow up, the average age was between two to three years. In the youngest patients of the material the treatment started from the age of eight to nine months. Five to six years was the maximum age for starting the treatment.

Improvement of vision in the younger age group was between 65 and 85 percent (depending on the previous treatment), and in the oldest group between 45 and 64 percent. Binocular vision was present in 25 to 40 percent of the cases. Eighty to 90 percent of the cases in which binocular vision improved, showed a diminution of the angle of deviation.

CONCLUSION

We aimed at an improvement of binocular single vision, where it was present, together with a good visual acuity in both eyes, and a stable position of the eyes which was acceptable from a cosmetic point of view.

In our mind there are still a lot of questions concerning the development of binocular vision. Why equals the fusional range, and the relative positive and negative convergence in many microtropic patients the values of those with normal binocular vision? What are the causes that the fovea of the squinting eye never realigns to the other fovea? Why are the cells of the periphery so elastic and adaptable as compared to those of the fovea? We believe that this special type of binocular vision in strabismus is based on the physiological properties of the extra-foveal cells. These cells do not appear to withstand the enforced coordination, the task which we impose to them.

This as well as the big problem of amblyopia, we are sure, will soon be answered by the excellent work of all of them who are concerned with the problem, clinicians and researchers, ophthalmologists, physiologists and orthoptists.

ACKNOWLEDGEMENT

We would like to thank Mrs. Cicely Freeman and Mrs. Jackie Berrow and Mrs. Anne Madeod for all the help and encouragement which they gave us.

REFERENCES

Bredemeyer, H. & K. Bullock. Orthoptics, Theory and Practice, St. Louis C.V. Mosby Co. (1968).
Crone, R.A. Anomalous and normal motor fusion in esophoria and micro-estropia. Trans. Opht. Soc. U.K. 100, 464 (1980).
Ikeda, H. & K. Tremain. Amblyopia and cortical binocularity. Trans. Opht. Soc. U.K. 100, 450 (1980).
Plicque, J. Analyse de la vision binoculaire. An. d'Ocul. Févr. (1946).
Polychroniadis, F. Contribution au traitement de l'amblyopie par la methode des posteimmage Thèse pour le Doctorat, Athènes Traduction aux Annales d'oculistique Févr 1961, p. 161 (1960).
Polychroniadis, F. Conclusions tiréss de notre expérience sur les problèmes de traitement de l'amblyopie. Arch. Un. Med. Balcan. T VII no. 3, p. 272 (1969).
Polychroniadis, S. & F. Polychroniadis. The Confrontation of Cases of Strabismus with Small Angles of Deviation Int. Cong. Orthoptics (Past, Present, Future) Boston (1975).
Stanworth, A. & E.J. Naylor. The measurement and clinical significance of the Haidinger effect. Trans. Opht. Soc. U.K. 75, 67–73 (1955).
Thomas, Ch. L'occlusion monoculaire dans la thérapautique du strabisme et de l'amblyopie. Soc. d'Opht. de l'Ouest de France. 7, 12 (1958).

Author's address:
8 Merlyn Street
Athens, Greece

CAUSES AND TREATMENT OF CONSECUTIVE EXOTROPIA

M.H. GOBIN

(*Antwerp, Belgium*)

SUMMARY

In a series of 785 esotropic patients which were treated by surgery a consecutive exotropia occurred 172 times. An analysis of the results revealed that this overcorrection often was due to a vertical deviation and/or a limitation of adduction. Out of the 172 cases of consecutive exotropia 134 were re-operated: in addition to a bilateral 5 mm recession we carefully dealt with any vertical deviation and in case of a large angle or a limitation of adduction we added a monolateral or a bilateral loop to the recession of the lateral rectus muscle.

CAUSES AND TREATMENT OF CONSECUTIVE EXOTROPIA

A consecutive exotropia has always been a difficult problem. It has a strong tendency to recur so that extensive surgery is needed. An extensive surgery in turn may result in the reappearance of the original esodeviation so that the patient looses his confidence in the surgeon.

As a consequence many ophthalmologists become cautious: they rather aim at an undercorrection in order not to create an overcorrection. An undercorrection however is as much a failure as an overcorrection. Therefore we decided not to avoid this problem in the hope to find an adequate therapy for a consecutive exotropia.

In a series of 785 esotropic patients which were treated by a bimedial recession of at least 5 mm combined with an oblique muscle surgery a consecutive exotropia occurred 172 times (Gobin, in press). An analysis of different parameters was made in order to detect the causes of those consecutive exotropias.

The preoperative angle of esotropia was considered and contrary to what one would expect the largest preoperative esotropias presented the strongest tendency to turn into an exotropia (Gobin, in press). We think that this may be due to a limitation of adduction the larger preoperative angles requiring a loop recession of the medial rectus muscle (Fig. 1). When a loop was used 26,9% of the cases presented a consecutive exotropia and only 19% when no loop recession was performed.

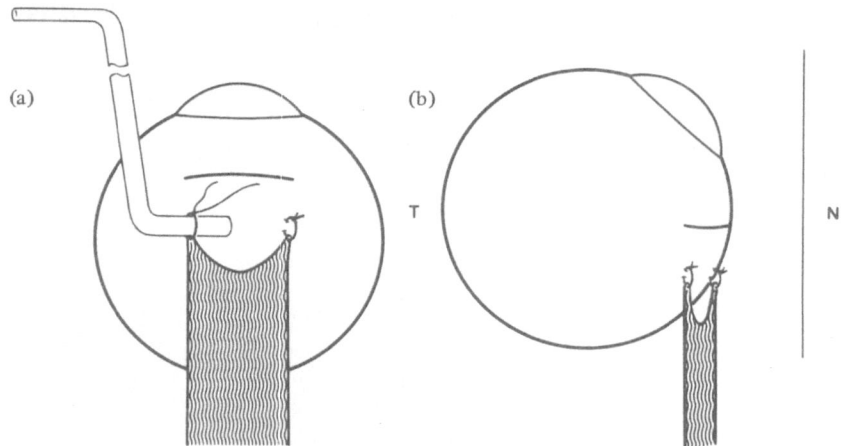

Fig. 1. Recession with a loop of a horizontal rectus muscle. The suture is placed over a probe (a), thus resulting in a loop which allows the muscle to retract further backwards without limiting the arc of contact (b). In order to obtain a large loop we use a probe with a diameter of 2 mm and for a small loop we use a probe of 1,5 mm.

The smallest angles presented the best prognosis: 49 cases of microtropia were operated on because of marked vertical incomitances or because of an intermittent decompensation into a larger unesthetic esotropia and a consecutive exotropia occurred less frequently than in larger angles (Table 1). Probably the peripheral fusion reflexes were strong enough to compensate for the surgical overcorrection. This is confirmed by the high percentage of good results we find in this group: after the 9 overcorrections were reoperated, 46 out of the 49 patients were straight.

We always take the angle as measured without wearing glasses into account the so called accommodative component of the squint being only partially of accommodative origin. The fact that we operated on the accommodative component did not enhance the risk of overcorrection. The cases of intermittent squint which correspond approximately with the fully accommodative cases present half as much overcorrections as the constant ones where as the number of straight cases is much higher in the first than in the second group (Table 2). This table contains the final results after reoperation.

It might be surprising that we operate on the accommodative component of the squint but we must stress the fact that we have the experience that binocular vision spontaneously reappears and that the accommodative com-

Table 1. Results after a bimedial 5 mm recession in microtropia.

Straight	38	77,6
Eso ≤ +7°	0	0,0
Eso > +7°	2	4,1
Exo	9	18,4
Total	49	%

Table 2a. Results in constant esotropia.
After 113 reoperations for exotropia.

Straight	431	68,0
Eso ≤ +7°	122	19,2
Eso > +7°	35	5,5
Exo	46	7,3
Total	634	%

Table 2b. Results in intermittent esotropia.
After 21 reoperations for exotropia.

Straight	131	86,8
Eso ≤ +7°	8	5,3
Eso > +7°	6	4,0
Exo	6	4,0
Total	151	%

ponent of the squint disappears after a successful combined horizontal and oblique muscle surgery (Gobin & Bierlaagh 1976). After all, as surgery to measure is illusive it is impossible for the surgeon to limit his operation to the non accommodative component of squint. If he obtains straight eyes with glasses he probably created an overcorrection which has been compensated by the peripheral fusion reflexes which can act even when no sensorial fusion is demonstrable.

A postoperative vertical deviation has also a great influence on the results (Table 3). The overcorrections are doubled when a vertical deviation is present and a recurrence of the esodeviation is nearly tripled. This means that a vertical deviation prevents the fusion reflexes from straightening the eyes but not that it favours the appearance of a consecutive exotropia. However as we systematically aim at a horizontal overcorrection counting on the fusion reflexes to compensate for it, a vertical deviation will prevent this compensation consolidating the surgical overcorrection.

In order to determine the causes of failure of our treatment of consecutive exotropias we analysed the results of our operations. Until 1969 we treated a consecutive exotropia by undoing the recession of one or both medial rectus muscles. Two inconveniences frequently occurred: an unesthetic aspect of the medial canthus which gives the appearance of a pseudostrabismus and even worse, an alternation of eso- and exotropia which puts the surgeon in check.

Therefore we changed our approach and performed systematically a bilateral 5 mm recession of the lateral rectus muscle. An analysis of 117 cases revealed that in 16,2 percent an exotropia reappeared (Table 4). The main causes of failure were: an amblyopia, a vertical deviation, a large exotropia and a limitation of adduction of the dominant eye (Gobin 1981). An amblyopia and a vertical deviation resulted more often in a recurrence of the original esodeviation where as a large preoperative angle and a limitation of adduction led to a residual exodeviation.

Table 3. Relationship of the results with the absence (RVD−) or presence (RVD+) of a real vertical deviation.

Results	RVD−		RVD+	
Straight	385	71,0	77	31,7
Eso ≤ +7°	35	6,5	52	21,4
Eso > +7°	35	6,5	29	11,9
Exo	87	16,1	85	35,0
Total	542	%	243	%

The amount of hypermetropia did not influence the results and the age at which the child was operated on as well as the interval between the first and the second intervention had little effect, except in younger children where the exotropia had some tendency to recur (Gobin 1981).

As a consequence of this analysis we adapted our surgical management by carefully dealing with any vertical deviation and in case of a large angle and/or a limitation of adduction by adding a unilateral or a bilateral loop to the 5 mm recession of the lateral rectus muscle.

According to these rules we operated 134 out of the 172 consecutive exotropias of our group of 785 esotropic patients (Table 5). If we compare the results with those of the first series we can see that the number of residual exotropias has decreased but at the cost of a recurrence of an esodeviation. In order to find out the cause of this recurrence we divided our cases into two groups: one where a limitation of adduction was present after the first operation and one without a limitation of adduction (Table 6). In the first group 66% of the patients became straight versus 45% in the second group; moreover the recurrence of an unesthetic esotropia ($> +7°$) is far less frequent when a limitation of adduction is present.

In our opinion the good results in group I are due to a progressive resistance to adduction and abduction which is produced by the tightened check-ligaments and by adhesions (Fig. 2). This resistance or brake effect on the medial rectus muscle prevents the esodeviation from reappearing and the brake on the lateral rectus muscle which is realised by adding a loop to the recession saves the patient from a residual exotropia. Both progressive brakes balance each other and keep the eyes nearly straight allowing the fusion reflexes to compensate the residual deviation (Fig. 3).

A cause of failure of our surgical management is thus the absence of an adequate progressive brake on both the medial and the lateral rectus. A vertical deviation however represents also a major cause of failure: out of the 11 cases of recurrence of an exotropia 9 showed a vertical deviation after the reoperation.

Table 4. Results after a 5 mm recession of both lateral rectus muscles.

Straight	67	57,3
Eso ≤ +7°	23	19,7
Eso > +7°	8	6,8
Exo	19	16,2
Total	117	%

Table 5. Results of 134 out of 172 exotropes we reoperated on.

Straight	67	50,0
Eso ≤ +7°	33	24,6
Eso > +7°	23	17,2
Exo	11	8,2
Total	134	%

Table 6a. Group with a limitation of adduction.

Straight	22	66,7
Eso ≤ +7°	6	18,2
Eso > +7°	3	9,1
Exo	2	6,1
Total	33	%

Table 6b. Group without a limitation of adduction.

Straight	45	44,6
Eso ≤ +7°	27	26,7
Eso > +7°	20	19,8
Exo	9	8,9
Total	101	%

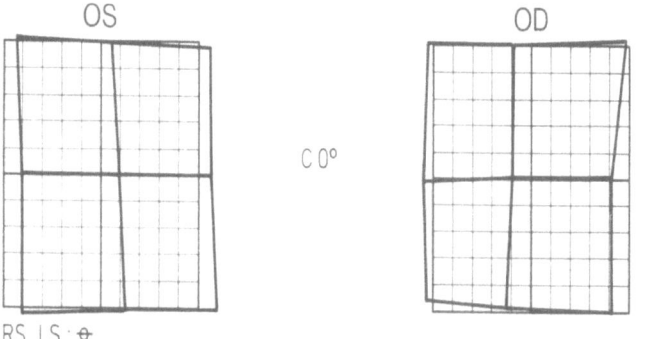

Fig. 2. When a medial rectus muscle is recessed the checkligaments are tightened and offer a progressive resistance or brake against adduction.

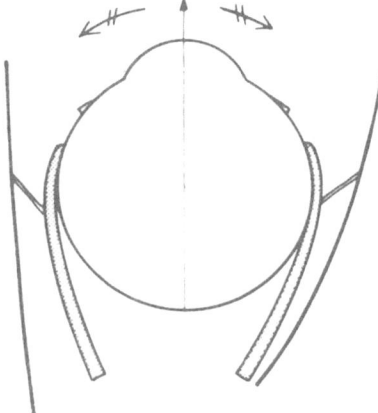

Fig. 3. When the lateral rectus muscle is recessed the progressive brake introduced by the tightened checkligaments of this muscle will balance the progressive brake on the medial rectus.

In order to determine the best method to deal with the vertical deviation we analysed the influence of a reoperation in the 81 patients who showed a vertical deviation after the first operation (Table 7). Surgery on the vertical recti alone seems to be unpredictable and a bilateral surgery of the oblique muscles leads to a vertical overcorrection if associated with a weakening of a vertical rectus muscle and to a vertical undercorrection if performed without a vertical rectus added. It is a unilateral operation on an oblique muscle combined or not with a vertical rectus which gives the best results. A pure horizontal muscle surgery is also capable to reduce a vertical deviation on condition that it is a small one.

In the light of our results we can now propose the following rules for the management of consecutive exotropias. In order to reduce the number of operations we must continue to aim at an overcorrection at the first opera-

127

Table 7. Effect of different types of surgery on the vertical deviation (RVD): pure vertical muscle surgery, surgery on 1 or 2 oblique muscles with a vertical rectus (+vert.) or without a vertical rectus (−vert.) and pure horizontal muscle surgery.

RVD	Pure vert.	1 oblique		2 obliques		Pure horiz.
		+vert.	−vert.	+vert	−vert.	
eliminated	3	11	7	2	7	4
undercorr.	4	2	4	2	15	1
overcorr.	2	7	1	8	0	1
Total	9	20	12	12	22	6

tion. In case of doubt we have to add a loop to the recession of the medial rectus muscle a limitation of adduction preventing a recurrence of the original esodeviation after the correction of a possible consecutive exodeviation. On the contrary, if we are more cautious we risk a horizontal undercorrection which needs further surgery; this surgery in turn can lead to a consecutive exotropia which necessitates a third intervention.

With regard to the treatment of a consecutive exotropia we do less in small horizontal angles when they do not exceed 5° and when no limitation of adduction is present: we replace the recession of the lateral rectus of the dominant eye by a central tenotomy. When a limitation of adduction is present we always perform a bilateral 5 mm recession and in angles which exceed 5° we add a loop on the hyperactive lateral rectus muscle especially if the limitation of adduction is localised on the dominant eye (Table 8). If the limitation of adduction is marked we even use a loop when no exodeviation is present in the primary position.

Concerning the vertical deviation we may neglect a small one especially if it is expected to disappear after the correction of exodeviation (Table 9). A hypertropia indeed decreases when a depression in adduction is present and a hypotropia decreases when there is an elevation in adduction (Fig. 4).

Table 8. Treatment of a consecutive exotropia.

A. Horizontal deviations without lim. of add. (CT = central tenotomy)		B. Horizontal deviations with lim. of add.	
Small angles : (<−5°)	CT of the LR of the fixing eye + 5 mm rec. of the other LR.	Small angles : (<−5°)	5 mm rec. of both LR.
Medium angles: (−5°/−15°)	5 mm rec. of both LR.	Larger angles: (>−5°)	5 mm rec. of both LR + uni- or bil. loop.
Larger angles : (>−15°)	5 mm rec. of both LR + uni- or bil. loop.		

Table 9. Management of vertical deviations

Small real vertical deviation	: no vertical surgery
Medium real vertical deviation	: surgery of an obl. muscle
Large real vertical deviation	: surgery of a vert. rectus

128

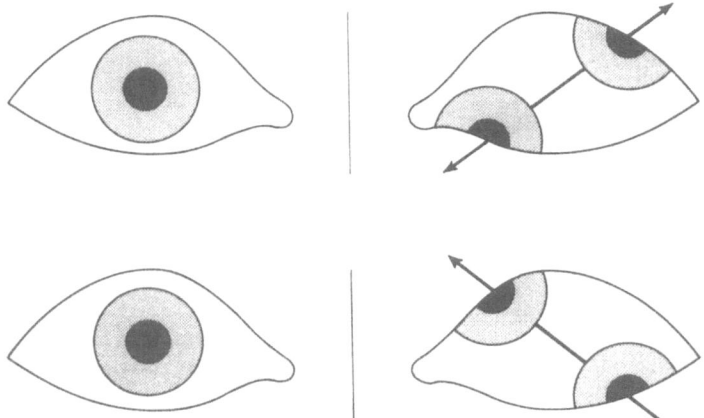

Fig. 4a.

Fig. 4b.

When the vertical deviation is moderate surgery will more likely be done on one oblique muscle without adding a vertical rectus muscle.

When the vertical deviation is more marked surgery will preferably be limited to a vertical rectus muscle adding an oblique muscle only in large angles as this combination greatly enhances the effect.

To conclude we may say that we have to remove all obstacles against fusion in order to avoid a consecutive exotropia. We must cure an amblyopia preoperatively by an adequate treatment and prevent it from recurring post-operatively by an occlusion of one or several hours a day during many years. The horizontal and cyclovertical deviations must carefully be searched for and it is essential to reduce them in one operation session taking care not to induce new obstacles such as adhesions. Therefore a quick and atraumatic surgery is required which depends largely on the dexterity and the experience of the surgeon; as a consequence the ophthalmologist has to adapt his indications to his results.

In order to cure a consecutive exotropia we must not undo what has been done except in rare occasions. A recession of both lateral rectus muscles is the treatment of choice whilst any remaining cyclovertical deviation and limitation of adduction is carefully dealt with.

REFERENCES

Gobin, M.H. Résultats de la chirurgie verticale et horizontale simultanée. J. Fr. Ophtalmol. (in press).

Gobin, M.H. & J.J.M. Bierlaagh. Four-muscle surgery in V-esotropia with long-term orthoptic follow-up. Transactions of the Third International Orthoptic Congress. Symposia Specialists, Miami, U.S.A, 427–440 (1976).

Gobin, M.H. Nouvelles conceptions sur la pathogénie et le traitement du strabisme. J. Fr. Ophtalmol. 4, 1, 7–18 (1981).

Author's address:
Orthoptic department
University Clinic of Leiden
Leiden, The Netherlands

Centre of Strabology
44, Karel Ooms Street
Antwerp, Belgium

130

POSTERIOR FIXATION SURGERY IN PARETIC STRABISMUS INDICATIONS AND TECHNIC

W. DE DECKER

(*Kiel, F.R.G.*)

SUMMARY

By seven clinical situations the author shows how Fd as a tool can be used to improve palsies by counterpareses (artificial palsies to yoke muscles). Fd should not be mistaken as a kind of recession, and the surgeon should be always aware that this technique is only one among others. Fd opens a second door in the treatment of incomitant strabismus, but raises new problems, as it produces artificial palsies which do not always harmonize with the accidential palsies to be cured!

INTRODUCTION

Planning this paper I became aware that the 30 cases we operated on since 1974 were so different that any trial to present a statistic evaluation would be not worthwhile. For this reason I shall demonstrate seven specific clinical cases, from whom I hope that they contain the main perspectives. But I should first remind you to two facts which may not be neglected, and refer to a few technical problems.

A Fadenoperation (Fd) or posterior fixation should be performed nearly bloodless, under excellent view and the surgeon must be able to reach at least 13 mm (caliper) or 14 mm (circumferential angle) beyond the insertion. 12 mm on the inferior rectus equal 13 to 14 mm on a medial rectus, or 17 to 18 mm on a lateral rectus.

A Fd causes an artificial palsy with a slight exponential increasing effect but does not change the basic position of an eye very much. Cüppers (1981) stated repeatedly that its influence to the primary position should be zero, while in our own experience it is small but not neglectable. Suppose that the Fd would be set to the posterior pole. The lever arm of the fixed muscle would become null, and the antagonist could rotate the globe until the balance of forces would find a new equilibrium. The same happens in minor amounts, but this can be ignored as the amount does not exceed 12 mm on the medial, 16 mm on the lateral and 11 mm on a vertical rectus muscle. In contrast recessions on the vertical recti cause marked shifts of the primary position, about $2°/mm$ (Conrad & De Decker 1975), while large recessions in addition also cause pareses. In practice we therefore have to decide, which kind of counterparesis might be adequate in each case, according to the basic angle in primary position. Counterparesis is a straight translation from the German and means a weakening procedure to a yoke muscle (contralateral synergist).

In cases of comitant strabismus of the congenital type a Fd only can be the adequate tool. But paretic cases normally need combinations with conventional procedures, i.e. operations on other muscles, which does not ordinarily mean combinations of Fd with recessions on the yoke muscle which we are to weaken.

CLINICAL DEMONSTRATIONS

Let me try to demonstrate the mentioned principles, beginning with simpler cases and proceeding to the more complicated situations.

VI Nerve palsy
The Turkish patient suffered from an injury 10 years ago. An old VI N. palsy became fixed into a convergent strabismus without any abductional ability. Fig. 1 shows the result of a previous Hummelsheim operation combined with lateral rectus resection, which set the involved right eye straight in primary position. We abandoned with a recession of the right medial rectus

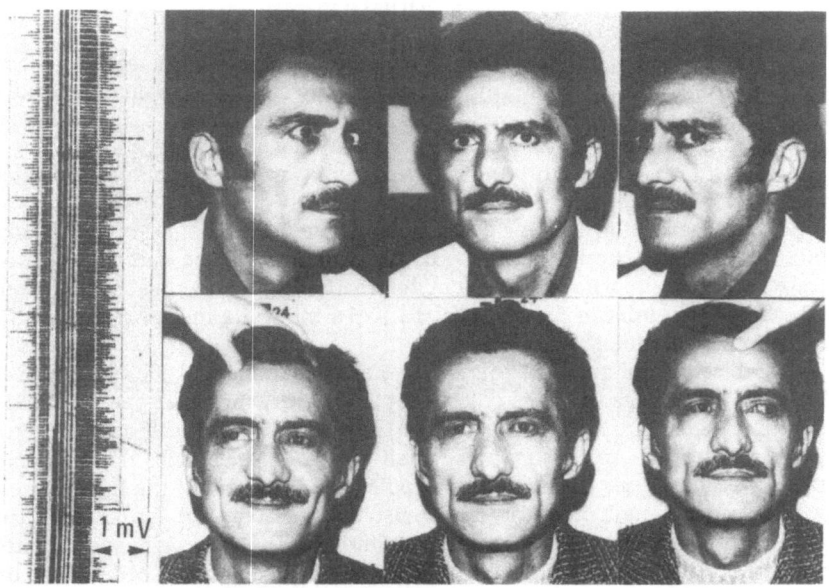

Fig. 1. Top: VI N. palsy; primary position achieved following a Hummelsheim procedure to the right eye. Bottom: After adding a Fd to the left medial rectus the patient was able to abduct the right eye. The gaze motility to left has not been disturbed.

132

as we feel in many cases that this procedure might ruin the only range of comitance, i.e. to sacrifice the motility for an improvement in the primary position. As a second step we added a Fd to the left medial rectus, which created a fair abductional ability of the right eye.

IV N. palsy
The patient, a male aged 55, had undergone a tuck to the left, paretic superior oblique and a recession to the left inferior oblique. As we still found a basic right hypertropia we decided to recess the right inferior rectus, and had good success. In this case the Fd would have overcorrected the slight incomitance, but undercorrected the basic vertical angle.

Underdeveloped superior oblique
The girl showed both the symptoms of a IV N. palsy and of a congenital strabismus. While trying to tuck the left superior oblique we found a missing connection of its tendon to the globe (De Decker & Conrad 1977). The tendon was detected in front of the trochlea. We formed a loop which we connected with the natural insertion, and recessed the ipsilateral inferior oblique. Fig. 2 shows that after this intervention there was no vertical deviation, but a convergent strabismus with inconstant angle and left depressor deficit. Subsequently we performed Fd's to both medial recti and to the contralateral right inferior rectus, as the vertical deviation increased in down gaze. Finally we had a good motor result (Fig. 3) and a microtropia with some binocular function.

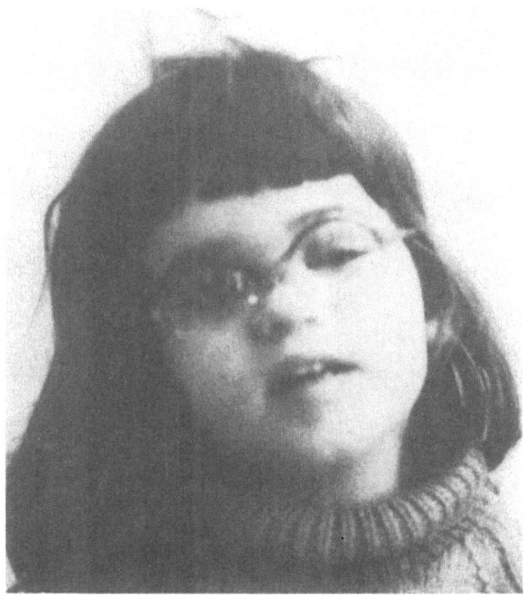

Fig. 2. See text.

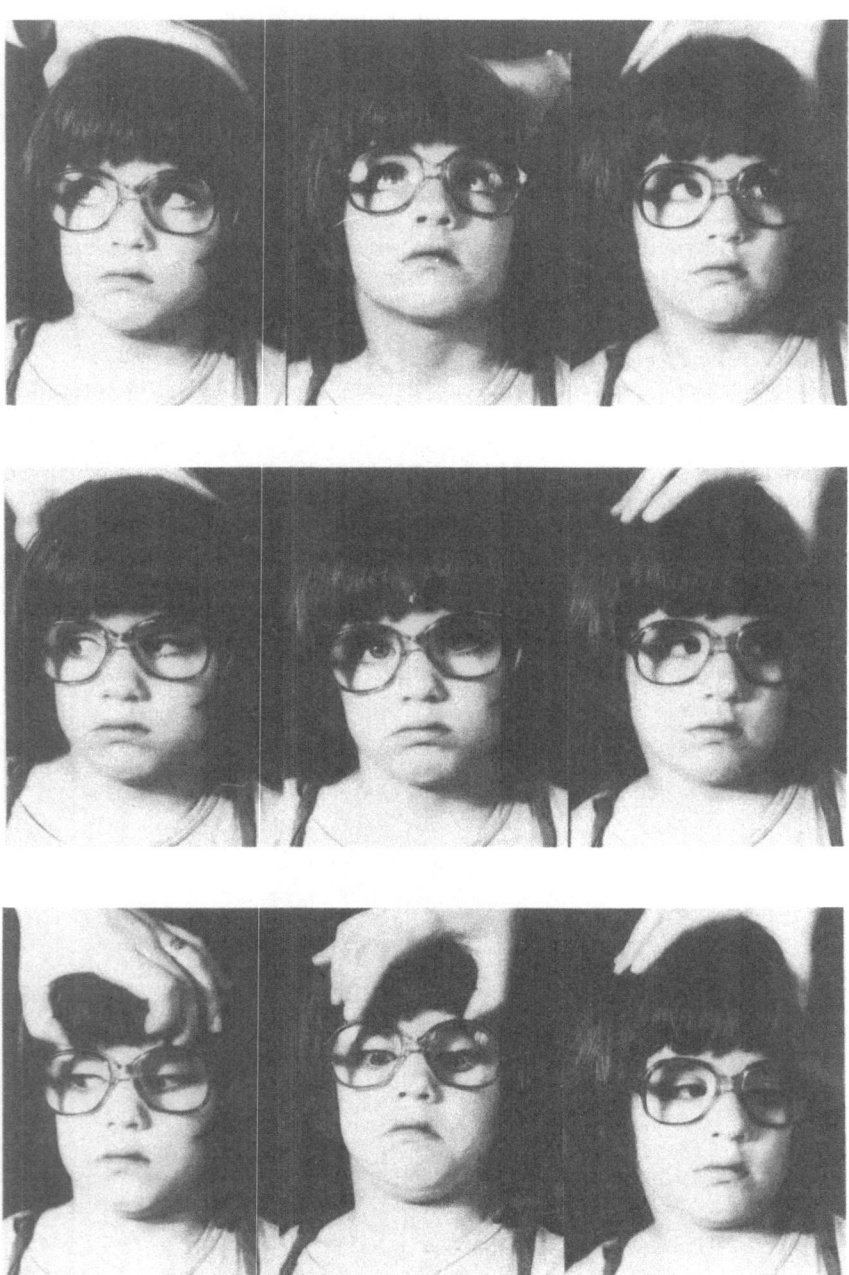

Fig. 3. Girl with underdeveloped left superior oblique. Following Fd to the right inferior rectus as a final step she achieved a fair eye position and motility.

134

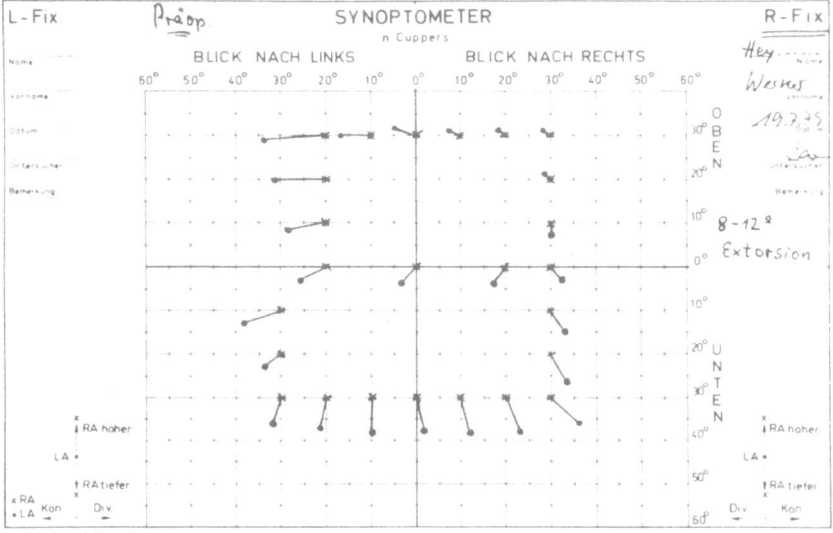

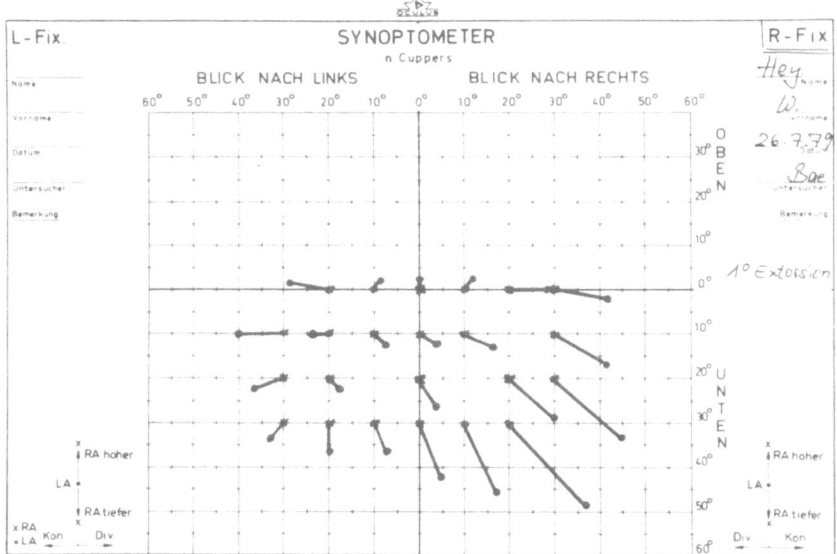

Fig. 4. Top: Synoptometer readings show the inhibition of the depression of the right eye due to a stiff superior rectus (1) and recessed superior oblique (2). Bottom: After recessing (1) and advancing (2) the muscles the primary position was improved, but diplopia in down gaze had increased.

135

Vertical imbalance following detachment surgery
The retinal surgeon cut the right superior oblique in order to place a big implant. Subsequently the superior rectus shrunk, and we had to advance the one, due to a marked extorsion, and to recess the other. After this basic step the eye position became better, but there was still an enormous lack of de-

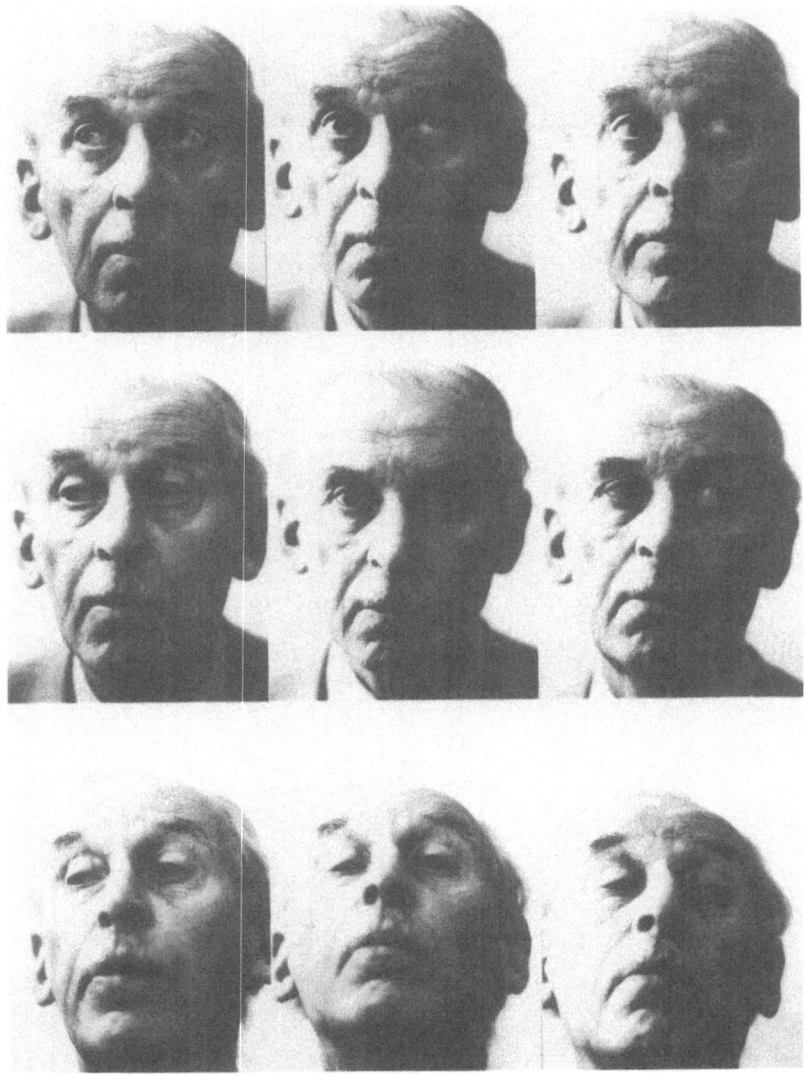

Fig. 5. Same patient as in Fig. 4. A Fd to the left inferior rectus normalized fairly the motility in down gaze, while primary position and up gaze had been cured before by conventional surgery.

pression (Fig. 4). So we added a Fd to the contralateral left inferior rectus. This operation nearly normalised the position and the motility (Fig. 5).

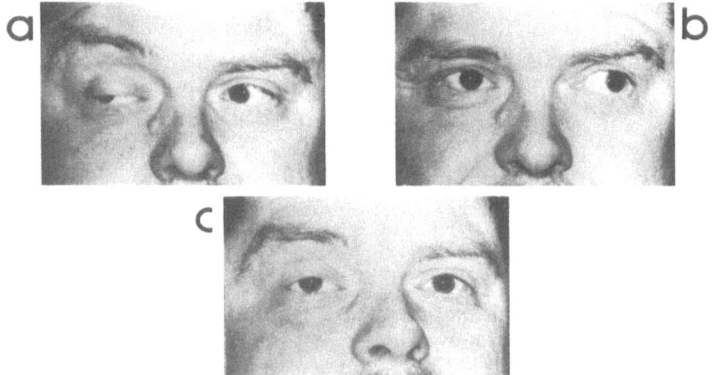

Fig. 6. a. Paretic right levator palpebrae. b. Misdirected fibers of the right medial rectus raising lid when patient looks to the left side. c. Improvement of the levator function following Fd to the left lateral rectus.

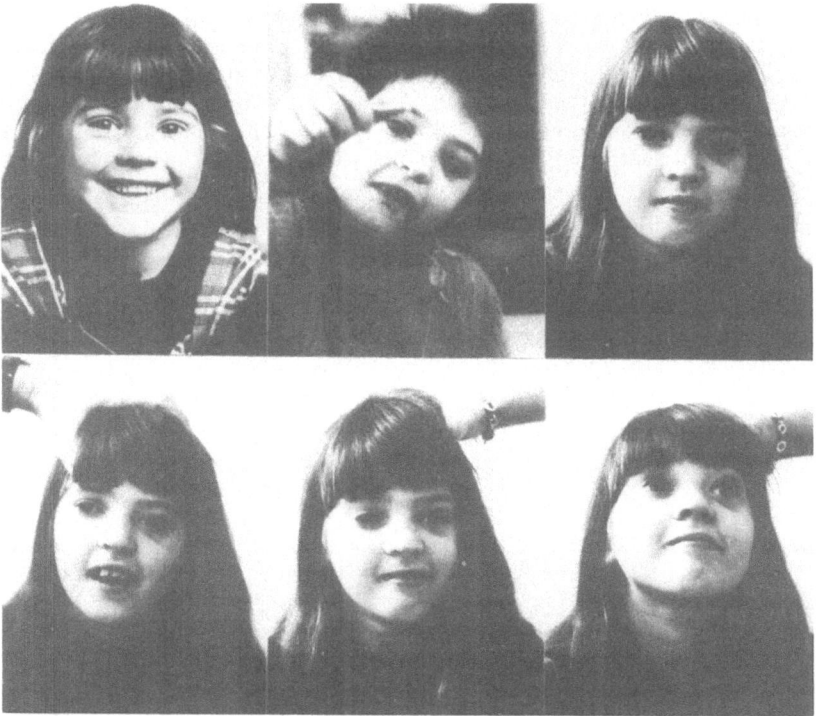

Fig. 7. Top left: before accident; top middle: after accident, before treatment; top right: after therapy, in primary position; bottom: after therapy, looking into different gaze directions.

137

III. N. palsy with ptosis

Frequently a misdirected reinnervation follows a III. N. palsy. Very often the upper lid can be raised only when the paretic eye adducts (Fig. 6). In this situation a Fd to the contralateral lateral rectus, with or without a recession, not only reduces both the horizontal angle and the incomitance, but also forces the patient to increase the innervation of this lateral rectus. This stimulates the paralysed medial rectus, following Hering law, and the lid will rise.

Severe bilateral III. N. and right IV. N. palsy

The poor child (Fig. 7), presented with an exodeviation and a complete ptosis of the left eye, while EMG showed that both eyes were paretic. Our surgery consisted of 4 steps (Table 1), in order to compensate for the excyclodeviation, the incomitant exotropia and the ptosis, which again depended on the amount of adduction. As a final step we added a suspension of the lid by a strip of fascia lata, but not before a counterparesis to the contralateral lateral rectus had activated all the innervation power of the left medial rectus and, due to misdirected reinnervation, of the levator also.

Destruction of the pretrochlear part of the superior oblique

This is one of the burdens a strabologist has to cope with. Following Parks (1979) there is no tendon sheath, whereas the surrounding tissues invaginate or exvaginate as the tendon moves. A serious destruction of this apparatus cannot become restituted at all. So we usually will find a dysfunction in up and down gaze (Fig. 8), which after a recession of the resting superior

Table 1. Clinical data of a child with bilateral III. N. palsy, and steps of surgical restoration.

April 1978:	Accident with complex brain damage	
31st July 79: (1)	right medial rect. resection	5 mm
	right sup. obl. tuck	6 mm
	left medial rect. resect.	6 mm
	left lateral rect. recession	7 mm
4th Dec. 79: (2)	right lat. rect. Fd	19 mm
	right sup. obl. re-tuck	7 mm
	left med. and lat. rect. res.	4 mm
	and transpos. upwards	9 mm
6th Nov. 80: (3)	right inferior obl. recession	6 mm
	right superior rectus Fd	12 mm
31st March 81: (4)	Ptosis Oper. by Fascia lata	
12 May 81:	lid fissure right eye: 9 left eye:	6–7 mm
	lid lag (left eye)	1 mm
	visual acuity r. eye 1.0 l. eye 0.6 (partly)	

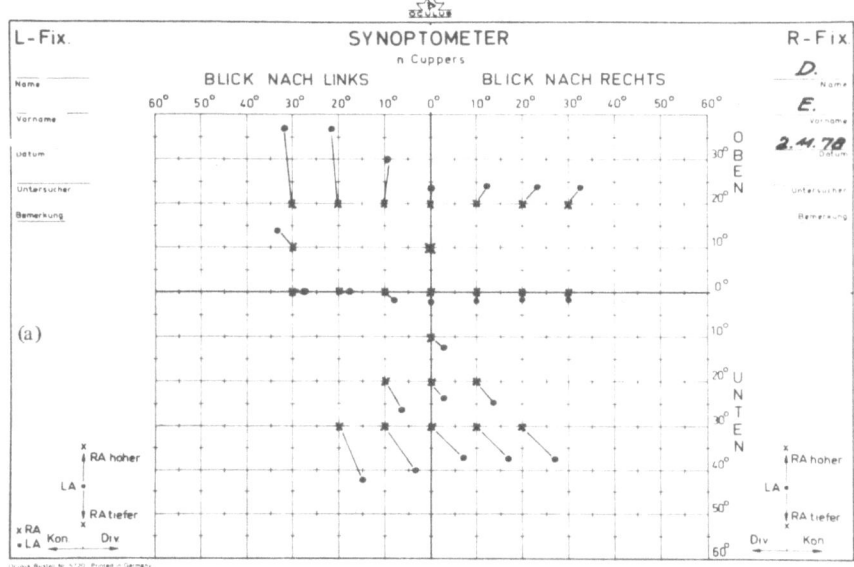

Fig. 8a.

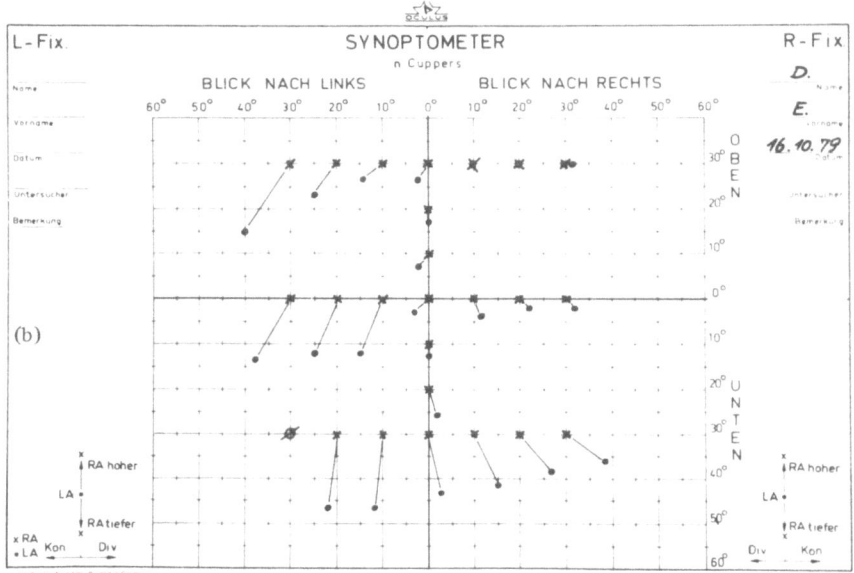

Fig. 8b.

139

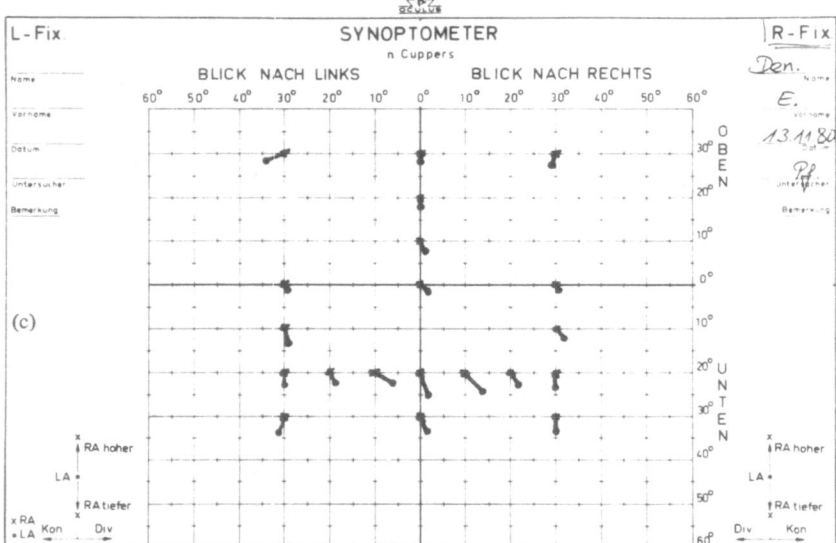

Fig. 8c.

Fig. 8. a. Inhibition of the right eye in up and down gaze following destruction of the tendon of the superior oblique. b. Transformation into a depressor palsy by recession of the injured muscle. c. Reduction of the latter by a Fd to the contralateral left inferior rectus.

oblique looks like a severe IV nerve palsy. A Fd to the contralateral inferior rectus (12 mm) sometimes can smoothen the incomitance, as it did in our example.

CONCLUSIONS

In clinical practice a Fd together with conventional operations may be beneficial, but there is one problem open to further investigations which has been brought up recently by Cüppers (1981) and by my coworker Conrad. (Conrad & Treumer 1981). As the Fd causes an artificial palsy, there must be a definite curve which describes the subsequent motility. If this curve equals the curve of functional loss of the paretic muscle, the result will be sufficient, if not, another complicated incomitance will be established. Here a wide field of investigation is still open!

140

REFERENCES

Conrad, H.G. & W. de Decker. Zur Klinik und Nomenklatur des nichtparetischen Verti-
kalschielens. Klin. Mbl. Augenheilk. 166, 775 (1975).

Conrad, H.G. and H. Treumer. Zum Wirkungsprofil der Fadenoperation. Klin. Mbl. Augen.
heilk. 178, 174 (1981).

Cüppers, C. Contribution au problème de l'arc du contact. Present Soc. Ophth. Belge,
Brüssel, June, 1981.

De Decker, W. & H.G. Conrad. Surgical Transposition of the Insertion of the Superior
Oblique in Cases of Pseudoaplasia and Traumatic Disturbances. Symp. DOG Freiburg
1977, Bergmann, München 1978, 111.

Parks, M.M. The Superior Oblique Tendon. Doyne Mem. Lecture Trans. Ophthal. Soc.
U.K. 97, 288 (1977).

Author's address:
University Eye Clinic
Orthoptic – Pleoptic Department
Kiel, F.R.G.

RESULTS OF CÜPPERS FADENOPERATION
(POSTERIOR FIXATION SUTURE)

H. KAUFMANN

(Giessen, F.R.G.)

Cüppers described the principle of the Fadenoperation or posterior fixation suture for the first time in 1971.

Probably the mechanical principle (Fig. 1) is mainly based on decreasing the arc of contact by an artificial attachment behind the tangential point. The result is a reduction of globe rotation in favour of a retraction. This effect can be demonstrated geometrically. It is easy to calculate, how great is the proportion of muscle action which is no longer available for rotation, that is, the extent of the artificial paresis.

A second effect arises from the fact that the operation puts out of action a part of contractile muscle. Some years ago we believed this effect to be essential and as long ago as 1976 we performed a similar operation by ligation and cauterisation in 13 cases. The improvements in the squint angle were not significant and we have once more abandoned the technique which has recently been resurrected under the name of 'le faux-fil'.

The third effect (Fig. 2) is the result of a relative shortening of the muscle because the distance T—F—O is longer than the physiological distance T—O.

Another effect (Fig. 3) is based on the fact that the muscle is embedded in

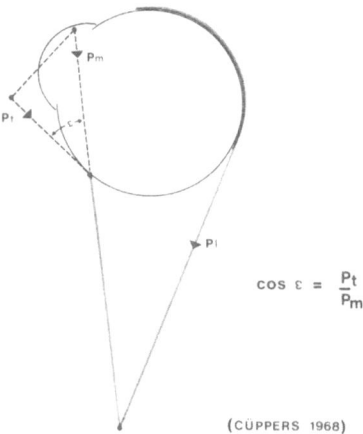

$$\cos \varepsilon = \frac{P_t}{P_m}$$

(CÜPPERS 1968)

Fig. 1.

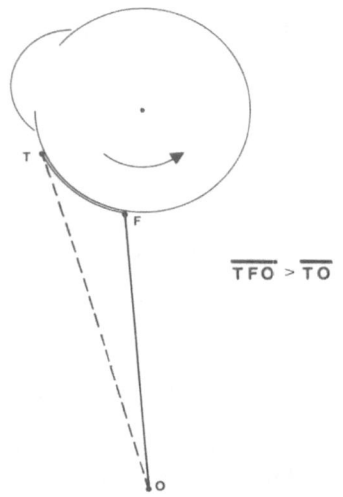

$$\overline{TFO} > \overline{TO}$$

Fig. 2.

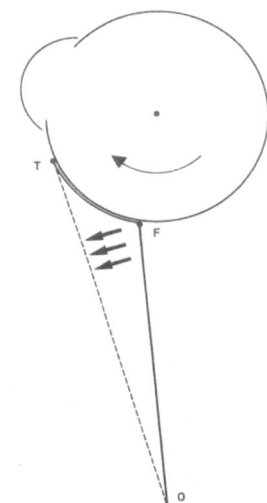

Fig. 3.

different connective tissue structures which endeavour to maintain the physiological course of the muscle, and draw the point of the posterior fixation suture to the straight line T–O. These different effects of the posterior fixation suture sometimes work together but also partly contrary to each other. At the moment we see no rational and mathematically reliable possibility to produce a model of the action of the posterior fixation suture.

Until this problem is clarified we have only one possibility, namely to examine the effect of the posterior fixation suture in a homogeneous series of patients as strictly defined as possible.

Since 1974 we have performed about 2.000 posterior fixation sutures, first in Bonn and since 1979 in Gießen. Since that time this corresponds to an almost unchanged 20% of all muscle operations performed. We have already reported in 1979 on the effect of bilateral posterior fixation suture on the medial rectus in 100 patients.

We have now undertaken a new investigation with a total of 157 patients who were selected from the total clinical patients according to the following criteria:

1. All patients showed a non-accommodative convergence excess. For this clinical picture I prefer the term adduction excess. Characteristically, these patients have esophoria, a small angle esotropia or a microstrabismus at distance fixation and a squint angle usually about twice as large at near fixation without relaxation by bifocals.

29% of these patients had, moreover, a squint angle with a variability of more than 5° in the alternate cover test at 5 m. The variability averaged 10,7°.

2. All patients underwent operations in 1980 by two surgeons using the same technique. In all 157 patients a bilateral posterior fixation suture was carried out without any other simultaneous intervention.

144

The results in relation to the angle reduction were as follows:
You see the reduction of the squint angle at distance fixation and near fixation (Fig. 4). For example, bilateral posterior fixation sutures of 13 mm reduced the distance angle by 7,5° and the near angle by 13,7°. The basis of this is the squint angle in the alternate cover test on the last day before the operation and on the first or second day after the operation in order to exclude as far as possible binocular influences. The standard deviation at 12 mm was 3,6° and rose to 7° at 15 mm.

These mean values differ from those we published in 1979 by less than 1°.

These effects unfortunately do not remain so big. We have reexamined all patients 3 to 9 months (average about 6 months) later (Fig. 5). You see that after this time the effect has become less and particularly at the higher adjustments. The angular variations were barely present immediately postoperatively and after 6 months and amounted to only 1,5° on the average.

In order to check whether the refraction and size of the eye had any influence on the effect of the posterior fixation suture, all the operations were analysed in three groups with different refractions. There were no significant differences. We cannot decide whether the size of the eye had any influence on the effect of the operation or whether the refraction was not sufficiently correlated with the size of the eye in our patients.

The results on binocular functions were classified as follows: Normal binocular vision, if the Bagolini test is positive without deviation and without amblyopia. Microstrabismus, if the Bagolini test is positive with a little deviation in the cover test. Strabismus, if the Bagolini test is negative.

Before surgery 95% had strabismus for distance and near fixation, 5% already had microstrabismus or normal binocular vision at distance fixation and a greater deviation at near fixation (Figs. 6, 7). After surgery 9% had normal binocular vision for distance and near fixation, 50% had microstrabis-

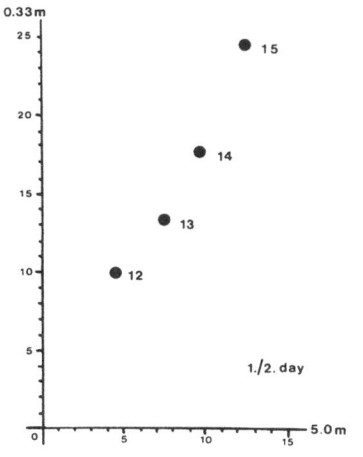

Fig. 4.   Fig. 5.

145

mus at distance and near fixation, 15% had a microstrabismus or a strabismus less than 5° for distance and near fixation. That is a total of 74% which we consider successful. 26% still had strabismus with an angle of less than 10° at any distance.

The majority of these 26% were satisfied with the operation because the squint angle was considerably less than before the operation; we, however, were not always satisfied. Some of these patients underwent a second operation which is not, of course, included in these statistics.

A comment on surgical overcorrections: Immediately after the operation 3 patients were divergent on distance and near fixation, another 4 only on distance fixation. These angles decreased during the observation period, but they still remained. Three patients who were convergent or straight became divergent by the sixth month, all below 5°. After 6 months 10 patients altogether (= 6,3%) were divergent, usually only at distance fixation or below 5°, none of them were above 10°. What conclusions can be drawn from these results?

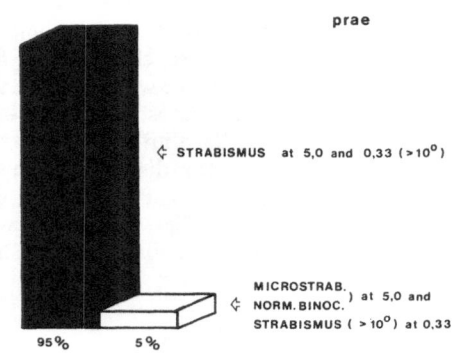

Fig. 6.

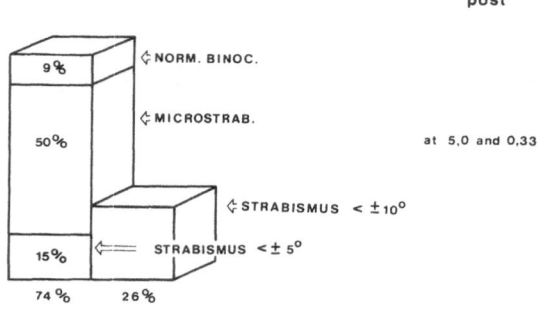

Fig. 7.

146

A few years ago we analysed the effects of over 1.000 conventional operations for horizontal squint (Fig. 8). It was shown that with combined recession-resection procedures near and distant squint angles are about equally influenced. The near squint angle is distinctly more reduced by bilateral recessions. Unfortunately a great many squint angles lie in the shaded area before the operation and could not be satisfactorily corrected by conventional surgery. Now this area is covered by Cüppers' posterior fixation suture. This procedure cannot replace conventional surgery. The two surgical principles supplement each other to an outstanding degree.

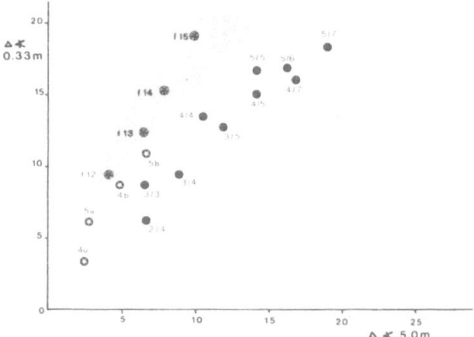

Fig. 8. ● Recession-resection (mm). ✪ Unilateral (u) or bilateral (b) recession (mm). ✪ Fadenoperation (f) (mm).

Author's address:
Klinik für Bewegungsstörungen der Augen und Neuroophthalmologie
Friedrichstrasse 18
D-6300 Giessen, F.R.G.

147

BASIC MOTOR MECHANISMS IN PARETIC SQUINT

G. KOMMERELL

(Freiburg, F.R.G.)

ABSTRACT

The review includes the following topics: Variability of incomitance patterns caused by predominant damage to low- or high-threshold motor units; slowed saccades in the on-direction, and twitch saccades in the off-direction of a paretic muscle; contracture of the ipsilateral antagonist; absence of brainstem reflexes in the ipsi- and contralateral eye muscles; adaptive correction of saccades and of latent incomitance; neurapraxia and neurotmesis; misdirected regeneration; muscular neurotization; Duane's Syndrome.

PHYSIOLOGICAL INTRODUCTION

A detailed analysis of eye muscle palsies has to take into account the mechanisms by which the CNS normally increases a muscle's tension. Let us take the right lateral rectus (LR) as an example (Fig. 1). Most of the muscle's motor units are at rest in the off-position, that means, in extreme adduction. While the eyeball approaches the mid-position, some of the motor units reach their threshold and begin to fire. We call these units 'low-threshold' units. The 'high-threshold' units are still silent and do not begin to work before the eye is abducted beyond the midline.

The forces between the muscle tendon and scleral insertion have been measured in situ (Fig. 2). We can see that the force of the LR increases only very little when the eye is moved from adduction to the midposition. But with further abduction, the force of the LR rises steeply. In the antagonistic MR, the change of forces is reversed.

Shifts of eye position from adduction to the midposition are accomplished predominantly by the relaxation of the MR, and not by the pull of the LR. However, to reach positions of abduction, the pull of the LR becomes the dominant factor, and near the endposition, the MR is stretched beyond its relaxation capability, so that its tension is increased passively.

Variations of paretic incomitance

In the case of a complete LR paralysis, the remaining horizontal eye movements are exclusively due to contraction and relaxation of the MR. This

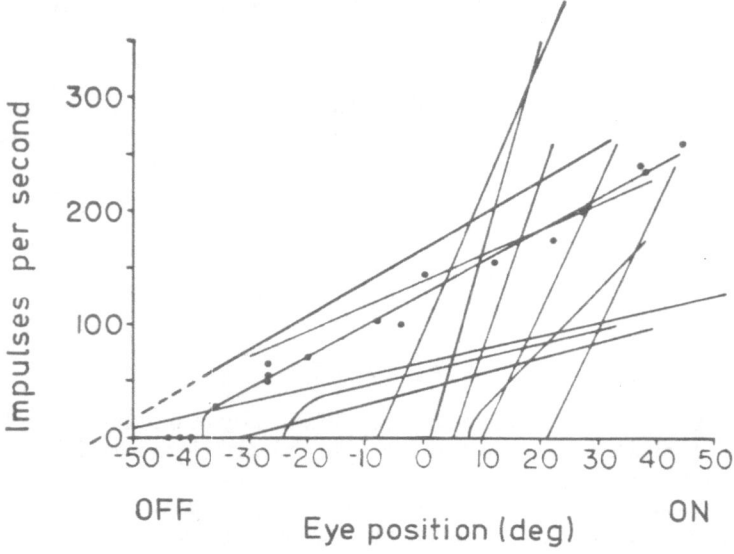

Fig. 1. Relationship between discharge rate and eye position for a selection of motor units. The units which begin to discharge already in off-positions are called low-threshold units. The units which begin to discharge not before on-positions are called high-threshold units. Robinson (1970).

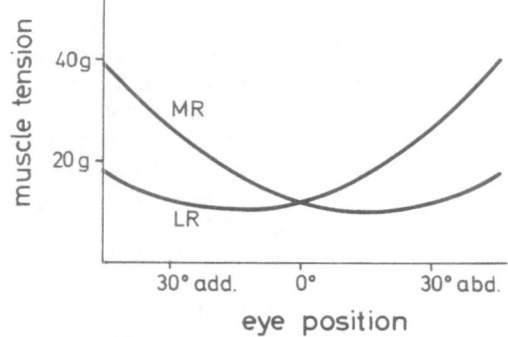

Fig. 2. In situ tendon forces of the lateral rectus (LR) and the medial rectus (MR) of a normal eye. The data are taken from Collins (1975).

produces the well-known paretic incomitance pattern, with a relatively well preserved motility in the nasal field, and a grossly impaired motility in the temporal field. In the case of a partial paresis, a great variation of incomitance patterns occurs. As Virdi (1978) pointed out, the incomitance pattern must depend on the type of motor units which is predominantly affected. A lesion restricted to high-threshold units would leave the eyes parallel up to the mid-position, but abduction would be limited. A lesion restricted to low-threshold

150

units would result in a sizable angle of squint in the midposition, but the paretic eye could reach nearly the extremes of abduction.

Saccades in the presence of muscle palsies

In the case of LR paralysis, abducting saccades are slowed (Metz et al. 1970) because the active pull of the agonist is lacking, and the movement is only due to the sudden relaxation of the MR. This relaxation allows the elastic tissues of the orbit to contract.

Adducting saccades are also abnormal in that they show a twitch. This twitch was observed as early as 1907 by Bielschowsky. We analysed the twitch systematically (Theopold & Kommerell 1974) and found that it can be explained simply by the lack of innervational changes in the LR. The MR receives a completely normal saccadic program. This program consists of a high-frequency pulse of innervation during the saccade, followed by a sustained, lower frequency step of elevated activity after the saccade. This innervational program is reflected exactly in the adducting twitch.

Let us consider an example (Fig. 3). The non-paretic left eye would execute a refixation from 10° to the right to 10° to the left. In the right eye which has a paralytic LR, the saccade begins already in the nasal field, according to the angle of squint at about five degrees adduction. The innervational pulse to the right MR produces a saccade of nearly normal amplitude, and brings the eye to a position of about 20° adduction, but the pulse is unable to hold the eye in the new position: Normally, the LR would relax and thus allow the eye to stay in the new position, but in the case of a paralysis, the LR is extended anyway and cannot relax further. Therefore, the passive elastic forces are relatively strong and pull the globe back to about 15° adduction, as soon as the pulse innervation to the MR is finished.

The relative size of pulse- and step innervations depends on the field of gaze for which the saccade is programmed. In the off-field, the step is relatively small so that the pulse stands out more clearly. If the non-paretic left eye executed the saccade from 40° to the right to 20° to the right, the post-saccadic backdrift of the paretic right eye would be more pronounced than in the example depicted in Fig. 3, and the clinical impression of a twitch would be accentuated.

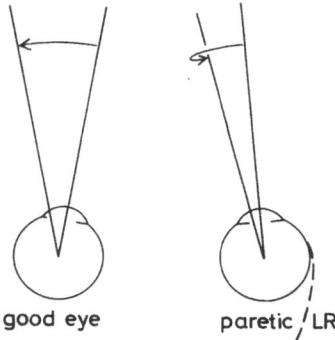

good eye   paretic / LR

Fig. 3. Twitch adducting saccade of the right eye which has a paretic lateral rectus.

The saccadic behaviour can be used in the differential diagnosis between bilateral abducens paralysis and infantile esotropia with crossed fixation. Fig. 4 shows a case of acquired bilateral abducens paralysis. The characteristic pattern of slow abducting saccades and twitch adducting saccades is quite different from the saccadic behaviour of infantile esotropia with crossed fixation. In these non-paretic squints, the abducting saccade is quick, and the adducting saccade is restricted because of the nasal limitation of the eye movement range.

Saccades in myasthenia

In myasthenia, the saccadic abnormalities are often very complicated. The patterns resulting from a LR palsy may interfere with a MR palsy, and the palsies of both muscles may be incomplete in that the first few spikes of the saccadic pulse are still transmitted to the muscle fibers, but not the following spikes. This results in twitches with adducting, as well as with abducting saccades (Schmidt 1975), appearing clinically as 'quiver' movements (Yee et al. 1976).

Saccades in supranuclear versus infranuclear palsies

In infranuclear palsies, the pulse- and step activities are reduced in a fairly constant proportion (although some variation occurs, depending on whether high- or low-threshold neurons are predominantly affected). But in supranuclear lesions, either of these activities may be completely extinguished, and the other may be normal (Kommerell 1975).

An isolated impairment of the pulse activity results in slow saccades with preservation of a full field of gaze. This happens for instance in Huntington's Chorea (Avanzini et al. 1979; Oepen et al. 1981). On the other hand, an isolated impairment of the step activity allows saccades of normal velocity, but eccentric eye positions cannot be held. This results in post-saccadic back-drift and gaze-paretic nystagmus, for instance in cerebellar lesions (Westheimer & Blair 1973).

Internuclear ophthalmoplegia of adduction and prenuclear paresis of

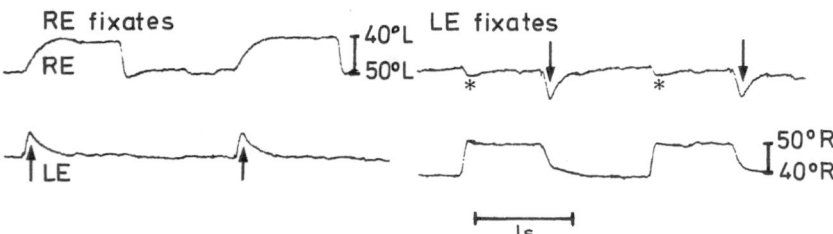

Fig. 4. Slow abducting saccades and twitch adducting saccades in a patient with bilateral traumatic abducens paralysis (StM 190931). The twitch adducting saccades stand out most clearly (arrows) when the innervational program to the medial rectus is such that ten-degree on-saccades, starting from the extreme off-position, are generated. The asterisks * mark artefacts due to electrical cross-talk from the other eye.

152

vertical eye muscles also lead to a pulse-step mismatch (Kommerell 1981; Meienberg et al. 1978). Using the pulse-step mismatch in the differential diagnosis of supranuclear versus infranuclear lesions, it is important to realize that infranuclear lesions also produce slow saccades and post-saccadic backdrift (twitch saccades), and these infranuclear impairments have to be subtracted before a mismatch of pulse- and step activities can be attributed to a supranuclear lesion.

Vestibular and optokinetic nystagmus, and pursuit movements in the presence of eye muscle palsies

All the paretic abnormalities which show up with refixation saccades also disfigure the quick phases of optokinetic and vestibular nystagmus. It is, however, much more difficult to analyse rapid eye movement abnormalities in these more complex supranuclear functions. There are two reasons for this difficulty. The first reason is that the paretic abnormalities of rapid nystagmus phases depend on the field of gaze in which they are executed, just as the paretic abnormalities of refixation saccades do. However, the sector in which the optokinetic and vestibular nystagmus oscillate may change during a record, and is difficult to define. The second reason is that post-saccadic drifts are superimposed on the slow phases of vestibular and optokinetic nystagmus, and therefore cannot be easily recognized.

Tracking responses to a slowly moving target are also very difficult to analyse if a paretic eye is used for fixation. In such a condition, the target image may easily slip off the fovea, and thus may elicit saccades which are superimposed on a smooth pursuit movement. Such a response could be mistaken for a supranuclear abnormality of the pursuit system.

In general, investigations of following movements, optokinetic nystagmus, vestibular nystagmus, and the vestibulo-ocular reflex have their domain in the analysis of supranuclear, and not infranuclear lesions.

SECONDARY CHANGES AFTER EYE MUSCLE PALSY

The paretic muscle: Absence of a stretch reflex in motor units spared from the lesion

A palsy leads to an elongation of the involved muscle. This could theoretically drive the spindle afferents which have been found in the human eye muscle (Manni & Bortolami 1981). It is, however, very unlikely that such afferent signals would increase the discharge of motor units which have escaped the lesion, because a stretch reflex has been refuted in the monkey eye muscle (Keller & Robinson 1971).

Only in 'latent' palsies can the intact motor units compensate for their dropped-out mates. In these cases, it is the retinal disparity, and not a stretch reflex, which drives the residual motor units in the paretic muscle, and inhibits the antagonist, so that binocular fusion can be re-established.

Contracture of the ipsilateral antagonist

There is also no reflex which alters the innervation of the ipsilateral antagonist, as has been shown by electromyography (Björk 1954). The change which does occur in the ipsilateral antagonist, is a structural contracture. It is a general property of muscles and connective tissues to adapt to the range of stretches, which are imposed on them. As a palsy limits stretching of the antagonist, a contracture must ensue. However, the contracture can be overcome when the palsy recovers.

Absence of over- and underactions in the contralateral eye muscles

In the contralateral eye, no innervational changes occur. There is no evidence for a brainstem reflex which could produce an overaction of the contralateral synergist, or an underaction of the contralateral antagonist. The absence of innervational changes in the contralateral eye can be demonstrated by the absence of a head turn with occlusion of the paretic eye. The secondary deviation which occurs when the paretic eye is fixating is not due to a speculative brainstem reflex, but is caused by a change in versional output of the gaze center.

ADAPTIVE REACTIONS OF THE CENTRAL NERVOUS SYSTEM (CNS)

Adaptive correction of refixation saccades

When a paretic eye is habitually used for fixation, and the non-paretic eye is patched or excluded, adaptive changes of several sensory-motor mechanisms can be observed.

In the acute stage, refixation saccades of the paretic eye fall short of the target, because the saccades are still programmed for normally efficient muscles. But in about three days, this hypometria can be corrected (Kommerell et al. 1976; Abel et al. 1978).

Adaptation also alleviates the saccadic abnormalities of a paretic eye which were described above. In a LR palsy, the slowness of abducting saccades is partly compensated by increased pulse activity, and the twitch adduction is partly compensated by increased step activity. These adaptations effect both eyes and thus produce overshoots when the paretic eye is patched, and the patient switches to the use of the non-paretic eye (Kommerell et al. 1976).

Evidence from cerebellar ablations in monkeys has revealed that the cerebellar vermis is essential for the adaptive control of saccadic amplitude (pulse activity), and the flocculi are essential for matching the step activity of the preceding pulse activity, thus preventing post-saccadic drift (Optican & Robinson 1980).

Not only the width, but also the direction of saccades is subject to adaptation. If an eye with a fresh superior oblique palsy attempts a refixation between two targets in the horizontal plane, the adducting saccade runs on an oblique path and terminates above the target. After adaptation to the use of the paretic eye, the saccade will be redirected to the horizontal plane.

We can infer this directional adaptation from experiments in which normal subjects learned to hit a target which was offset upwards whenever the eye took off for a horizontal refixation saccade (Mack et al. 1978).

Adaptive correction of 'incomitant phoria'

In patients who are able to overcome their eye muscle palsy by binocular fusion, i.e. in cases with a latent palsy, the resultant 'incomitant phoria' can be diminished by an adaptive reaction of the CNS.

Henson & Dharamsh (1981) produced an 'incomitant phoria' in normal subjects by means of an optical device, simulating a latent palsy. In a few hours, the latent deviation decreased according to the changing fusional demand in the field of gaze.

In the case of a latent abducens palsy, the fusional demand is small in the off-field and becomes greater in the on-field of the paretic muscle. Applying the evidence from Henson's experiment, one has to assume that the adaptive process in the CNS reduces the latent deviation more in the on-field than in the off-field. Thus, an improvement of incomitance, ascertained with a dissociating technique at the tangent screen, is not necessarily due to a restored conduction of the affected nerve fibers. Only a prolonged occlusion test would isolate the peripheral nerve deficit.

HEALING, AND HEALING DISTURBANCES

Misdirected regeneration

From the severity of a fresh palsy we cannot infer, whether we are dealing with a benign conduction block caused by a localized demyelinisation, or with a complete severance of the neuron. Even a complete paralysis can be due to either of these mechanisms. The distinction can only be made by follow-up. A localized demyelinisation, a so-called neurapraxia, will lead to a complete restitution within three months. In the case of a severance of the neuron, a so-called neurotmesis, healing depends on regeneration from the central stump.

In neurotmesis, a complete recovery cannot be expected, because it is unlikely that all the axons will reach those muscle fibers to which they were originally connected. Thus, misdirected regeneration is the usual outcome. This is especially conspicuous after a lesion of the oculomotor nerve, where for instance neurons which should innervate the MR, reach the levator instead.

It is reasonable to assume that misdirected regeneration also occurs in nerves which serve only one muscle, such as the abducens or the trochlear nerves. Misdirected regeneration in these nerves could become clinically manifest if high-threshold neurons innervated muscle fibers which were originally connected to low-threshold neurons, and vice versa. Such a misdirected regeneration could explain various patterns of residual incomitance, and could also cause secondary concomitance (Kommerell & Mattheus 1981).

Recently, the concept of misdirected regeneration was challenged by Lepore & Glaser (1980), mainly on the basis of an exceptional case in which anomalous synkinesis of the levator and the MR was a transitory phenomenon. These authors suggested two alternative mechanisms. First, an 'ephaptic transmission' of spikes to adjacent axons at the site of the lesion might occur, as has been assumed earlier by D.J. Lyle (1966). Second, the synaptic input of the cells in the nucleus might be altered secondary to an axonal lesion. Experimental support for this latter mechanism is available (Blinzinger & Kreutzberg 1967; Lux & Schubert 1975; Grafstein 1975; Kreutzberg 1979). Although these two mechanisms may indeed play a role in certain cases, the pathology of experimental nerve injuries strongly favours misdirected regeneration. A great number of axonal sprouts have been shown to arise from each severed nerve fiber (Cajal & Ramon 1928; Kreutzberg 1979), and one can hardly imagine that many of these sprouts find their distal correlate through a dense scar.

Whatever the pathophysiological mechanism may be, clinical experience has shown that abnormal synkinesis of muscles after oculomotor nerve lesions tends to be permanent. Correspondingly, surgically transposed muscles retain their original innervation (Metz et al. 1970). These experiences teach a lesson: Obviously, the CNS cannot re-programme false innervations of individual muscles for the sake of binocular vision.

Muscular neurotization

Sprouting of axons also occurs after transection of intramuscular nerve fibers, and such regenerating nerve fibers can cross over to adjacent muscles which lack their own innervation. This so-called muscular neurotization has been seen for instance after resection of malignant parotid tumors. In these cases, nerve fibers from the cut masticatory muscle cross over to denervated facial muscles and produce permanent anomalous synkinesis (Trojaborg et al. 1972). The principle of muscular neurotization has been suggested as a therapy of abducens palsy. Aichmair et al. (1975) used the inferior oblique muscle as the source of regenerating neurons. A success of such a cross-innervation should be detectable from a V-pattern, because the inferior oblique neurons are expected to retain their program as elevators, and would fire the LR with up-gaze.

Duration of reinnervation

The length of time through which the central stump remains capable of regeneration probably lasts much longer than one year, and may even be unlimited (Kreutzberg, personal communication). Obviously, the duration and the success of a reinnervation depends on the amount of scar tissue which has to be penetrated. Another limiting factor is degeneration of the muscle which may become irreversible when the denervation lasts too long.

In clinical eye muscle palsies, most of the healing occurs in the first year, but occasionally, we have seen some improvement as late as two years after the lesion.

Although late recovery cannot be excluded in exceptional cases, it appears practical not to withhold reconstructive surgery longer than one year.

Duane's Syndrome

A lesion of the abducens nerve at a foetal stage, when the muscles acquire their innervation, leads to misdirected innervation of the LR by fibers of the oculomotor nerve. This mechanism was recently confirmed by a superb clinical-pathologic study (Hotchkiss et al. 1980). Branches of the oculomotor nerve were traced to a sector of well developed muscle tissue in the LR, and another sector of the LR which was devoid of innervation showed fibrosis.

The various types of Duane's Syndrome which have been isolated can now be understood as members of a continuous spectrum of innervational disturbances. The clinical appearance of the individual case depends on the proportion of normally innervated, falsely innervated, and non-innervated parts of the LR.

REFERENCES

Abel, L.A., D. Schmidt, L.F. Dell'Osso & R.B. Daroff. Saccadic system plasticity in humans. Ann. Neurol. 4, 313–318 (1978).

Aichmair, H., G. Freilinger, J. Holle, H. Mandl & R. Mayr. Muskuläre Neurotisation bei traumatischer Abduzensparese. Ein neuei Weg der operativen Behandlung. Klin. Mbl. Augenheilk. 167, 580–583 (1975).

Avanzini, G., F. Girotti, T. Caranceni & R. Spreafico. Oculomotor disorders in Huntington's chorea. J. Neurol. Neurosurg. Psychiat. 42, 581–589 (1979).

Bielschowsky, A. Die Motilitätsstörungen der Augen. In: Graefe-Sämisch (eds.). Handbuch der Augenheilkunde, 2. Auflage, Bd. 8, I. Abt., Kap. XI, Nachtrag I, p. 33. Engelmann, Leipzig 1907.

Björk, A. Electromyography studies on the coordination of antagonistic muscles in cases of abducens and facial palsy. Brit. J. Ophthal. 38, 605–615 (1954).

Blinzinger, K. & G. Kreutzberg. Displacement of synaptic terminals from regenerating motoneurons by microglial cells. Zeitschr. f. Zellforschung 85, 145–157 (1968).

Cajal, S. & Y. Ramon. Degeneration and regeneration of the nervous system. Oxford University Press, London 1928.

Collins, C.C. The human oculomotor control system. In: Lennerstrand, G., Bach-y-Rita, P. (eds.). Basic mechanisms of ocular motility and their clinical implications. Pergamon Press, Oxford 1975.

Grafstein, B. The nerve cell body response to axotomy. Exp. Neurol. 48, 32–51 (1975).

Henson, D.B. & B.D. Dharamsh. Binocular adaptation to induced heterophoria and anisometropia. Invest. Ophthal. Vis. Sci. (in print).

Hotchkiss, M.G., N.R. Miller, A.W. Clark & W.R. Green. Bilateral Duane's Retraction Syndrome. A clinical-pathologic case report. Arch. Ophthal. 98, 870–874 (1980).

Keller, E.L. & D.A. Robinson. Absence of a stretch reflex in extraocular muscles of the monkey. J. Neurophysiol. 34, 908–919 (1971).

Kommerell, G. Unilateral internuclear ophthalmoplegia. The lack of inhibitory involvement in medial rectus muscle activity. Invest. Ophthal. and Visual Sciences (in print).

Kommerell, G. Clinical clues for the organization of horizontal quick eye movements and subsequent periods of fixation. In: Lennerstrand, G. Bach-y-Rita, P. (eds.). Basic mechanisms of ocular motility and their clinical implications. Pergamon Press, Oxford 1975.

Kommerell, G. & S. Mattheus. 'Spread of comitance' after palsy: A new explanation based on disproportionate regeneration of motoneuron types. In: J. Mein, S. Moore (eds.) Orthoptics, research and practice. Henry Kimpton, London, 1981.

Kommerell, G., D. Olivier & H. Theopold. Adaptive programming of phasic and tonic components in saccadic eye movements. Investigations in patients with abducens palsy. Invest. Ophthal. 15, 657–660 (1976).

Kreutzberg, G.W. Neurobiological factors influencing regeneration of facial motor neurons. Clinics in Plastic Surgery. 6, 389–395 (1979).

Lepore, F.E. & J.S. Glaser. Misdirection revisited. A critical appraisal of acquired oculomotor nerve synkinesis. Arch. Ophthal. 98, 2206–2209 (1980).

Lux, H.D. & P. Schubert. Some aspects of the electroanatomy of dendrites. Adv. Neurol. 12, 29–44 (1975).

Lyle, D.J. Experimental oculomotor nerve regeneration. Am. J. Ophthal. 61, 1239–1243 (1966).

Mack, A., R. Fendrich & J. Pleune. Adaptation to an altered relation between retinal image displacements and saccadic eye movements. Vision Res. 18, 1321–1327 (1978).

Manni, E. & R. Bortolami. Proprioception in eye muscles. In: Lennerstrand, G. (ed.). Functional basis of ocular motility disorders. Pergamon Press, Oxford 1982.

Meienberg, O., J. Röver & G. Kommerell. Prenuclear paresis of homolateral inferior rectus and contralateral superior oblique eye muscles. Arch. Neurol. 35, 231–233 (1978).

Metz, H.S. & A.B. Scott. Innervational plasticity of the oculomotor system. Arch. Ophthal. 84, 86–91 (1970).

Oepen, G., P. Clarenbach & U. Thoden. Disturbance of eye movements in Huntington's chorea. Arch. Psychiat. Nervenkrankh. 229, 205–213 (1981).

Optican, L.M. & D.A. Robinson, Cerebellar-dependent adaptive control of primate saccadic system. J. Neurophysiol. 44, 1058–1075 (1980).

Robinson, D.A. Oculomotor unit behavior in the monkey. J. Neurophysiol. 33, 393–404 (1970).

Schmidt, D. Diagnostik myasthenischer Augensymptome. Klinische Symptome und elektronystagmographische Befunde sakkadischer Augenbewegungen. Klin. Mbl. Augenheilk. 167, 651–664 (1975).

Trojaborg, W. & S.O. Siemssen. Reinnervation after resection of the facial nerve. Arch. Neurol. 26, 17–24 (1972).

Virdi, P.S. Abduction paralysis and ocular deviation. In: Reinecke, R.D. Strabismus. Grune and Stratton, New York 1978.

Westheimer, G. & S. Blair. Oculomotor defects in cerebellectomized monkeys. Invest. Ophthal. 12, 618–621 (1973).

Yee, D., D.G. Cogan, D.S. Zee, R.W. Baloh & V. Honrubia. Rapid eye movements in myasthenia gravis. Arch. Ophthal. 94, 1465–1472 (1976).

Author's address:
Universitäts-Augenklinik
D-7800 Freiburg, F.R.G.

PRIMARY OVERACTING INFERIOR OBLIQUE MUSCLE
Histopathological and electrophysiological studies

K. MUKUNO, K. FURUNO, H. YOSHIDA & S. ISHIKAWA

(Kanagawa, Japan)

INTRODUCTION

Recently the Primary Overacting Inferior Oblique Muscle (POIOM) is proposed to be secondary to Superior Oblique (SO) palsy by the histopathological study (Spencer & McNeer 1980). In the present study simultaneous observation of histopathological and electrophysiological studies of POIOM was carried out. Morphological alterations in inferior oblique muscle in POIOM and secondary OIOM were observed in conjugation with histochemical fiber types of inferior oblique. Electrophysiological study was carried out intending to disclose the presence of SO palsy in POIOM applying maximum saccadic velocity study by EOG recording.

Fiber types	alkali treated ATPase	acid treated ATPase	SDH	Distributions
1	●	○	○*	global (G)
2a	●	○	⊘	G and orbital (O)
2b	⊘	○	●	G & O
3	○	●	●	G & O
4	○	●	○*	G & O
5	●	●	○*	G
6	⊘	●	●	G & O

Activities: ● : high, ⊘ : intermediate, ○ : negative and ○* : low.

Fig. 1. Classification of fiber types of human extraocular muscle by histochemical technique.

Docum. Ophthal. Proc. Series, Vol. 32, ed. by A.Th.M. van Balen & W.A. Houtman 159
© *1982, Dr W. Junk Publishers, The Hague. ISBN 90 6193 728 0*

RESULTS AND COMMENTS

Histochemical study of fiber types of normal human inferior oblique (IO) was carried out (Furuno & Mukuno 1979). The fiber types disclosed were classified into six types (Fig. 1). The classification was very reasonable compared with that of previous reports on sheep and cat extraocular muscles except few reports (Table 1) on human extraocular muscles. POIOM and secondary OIOM were observed histochemically. The 'cored fiber',

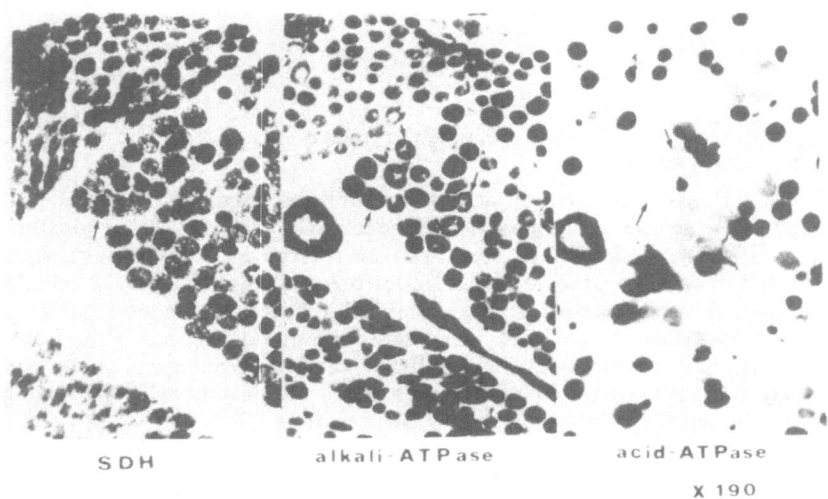

SDH   alkali-ATPase   acid-ATPase

X 190

core lesion   T. I. 5Y (F)

(a)

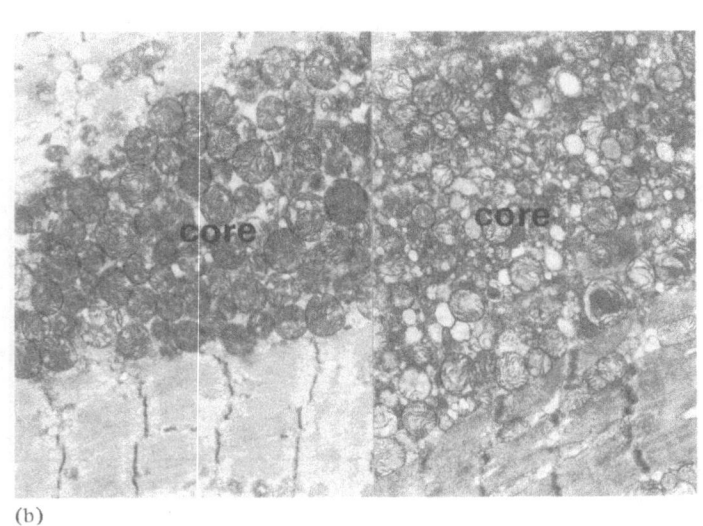

(b)

Fig. 2.

160

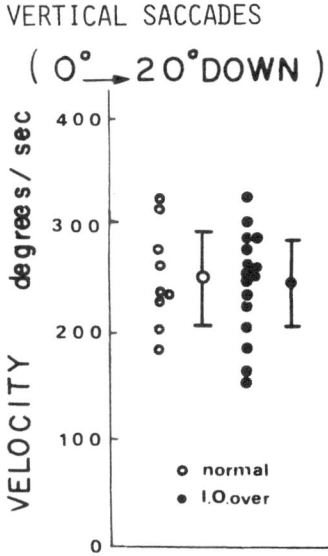

VERTICAL SACCADES

(0°→20°DOWN)

Fig. 3.

Table 1. Comparison of fiber types in the human EOM, mammalian EOM and mammalian limb muscle.

	Author	Harker (1972)	Ringel (1978)	Alvarado (1975)	Brooke (1971)	
Materials	Human inferior oblique	Sheep sup. rect. Levator palp.	Human all EOM	Cat inferior oblique	Cat gastro-cnemius	Inner-vation
techniques	Histo-chemical[a]	Histo-chemical & electron microscopic	Histo-chemical	Electron micro-scopic	Histo-chemical & physiological[c]	
Classifi-cation of fiber types	1 (G)	A fiber	granular	1	type IIB (FF)	single
	2a (G & O)	C fiber				single
	2b (G & O)	C' fiber	coarse (multiple?)	2	type IIA (FR)	single
	3 (G & O)	B fiber (levator only)	_b	3	type I (SR)	single
	4 (G & O)	G fiber	fine	4	—	multiple
	5 (G)	_b	_b	_b	—	?
	6 (O)	_b	_b	5	—	multiple?

[a]Distribution of fibers: G = global layer; O = orbital layer.
[b]Fibers not found.
[c]FF = fast contracting, fast fatigue; FR = fast contracting, fatigue resistant; SR = slow contracting, fatigue resistant.

161

accumulation of mitochondria in the center of the fiber, (Mukuno et al. 1976) is also reconfirmed to be characteristic changes in both POIOM and secondary OIOM in the present observation (Fig. 2). According to the classification the cored fibers were identified to be type 2a and 2b fibers and seem to correspond to type IIA fibers of skeletal muscles, i.e. fast contracting, fatigue resistant fiber. These morphological alterations found in both POIOM and secondary OIOM suggested to be secondary to overaction of IO associated with primary SO palsy or primary overaction of specific motor neurons according to supranuclear anomalous innervation suggested in A-V syndrome (Ghi 1969) and exotropia (Mitsui et al. 1979).

To elucidate the presence of SO palsy in POIOM vertical maximum saccadic velocity study was performed following Rosenbaum's method (Rosenbaum et al. 1977). According to comparative study to normal subjects velocity of 20 degrees downwards gaze in 20° adducted position was not decreased in the POIOM (Fig. 3). Therefore, the presence of SO palsy in POIOM seems to be unlikely.

Based on these morphological and electrophysiological data, POIOM (primary overacting inferior oblique muscle) may have lesions at the supranuclear portion as have been suggested in ordinary exodeviation (Mitsui et al. 1979; Mukuno et al. 1980) and A-V syndrome (Ghi 1969).

REFERENCES

Furuno, K. & K. Mukuno. Histochemical classification of the fiber types in human extraocular muscles, and further histochemical study of the overacted inferior oblique muscles (in Japanese with English abstract) Jpn. Rev. Clin. Ophthalmol. 73, 947–953 (1979).

Ghi, S. Study of the A-V patterns in horizontal strabismus (in Japanese with English abstract) Acta Soc. Ophthalmol. Jap. 73, 886–897 (1969).

Mitsui, T., K. Hirai, K. Akazawa & K. Masuda. The sensorimotor reflex and strabismus Jpn. J. Ophthalmol. 23, 227–256 (1979).

Mukuno, K., S. Ishikawa, T. Togo & Y. Minei. Histopathological study on the overacted inferior oblique muscles with special reference to 'central core' within the muscle fibers. Jpn. J. Ophthalmol. 20, 166–176 (1976).

Mukuno, K., S. Aoki & S. Ishikawa. Innervational anomalies in exodeviation (in Japanese with English abstract and Table) Jpn. Rev. Clin. Ophthalmol. 74, 794–797 (1980).

Rosenbaum, A.L., M.R. Carlson & R. Gaffney. Vertical saccadic velocity determination in superior oblique palsy Arch. Ophthalmol. 95, 821–823 (1977).

Spencer, R.F. & K.W. McNeer. Structural alterations in overacting inferior oblique muscles Arch. Ophthalmol. 98, 128–133 (1980).

Authors' address:
Department of Ophthalmology
School of Medicine, Kitasato University
Sagamihara
Kanagawa, Japan 228

ELECTROOCULOGRAPHIC EXAMINATIONS IN COMITANT AND INCOMITANT STRABISMUS

V. DORN & M. ČELIĆ

(*Zagreb, Yugoslavia*)

SUMMARY

Besides sensoric disturbances in strabismus it is also possible, by means of electrooculography, to analyse as well the kinetic disturbances in harmonic motility of both eyes (or conjugate eye movements) as in disjunctive movements. We performed our electrooculographic examinations in patients with acute convergent strabismus, chronic progressive external ophthalmoplegia (von Graefe) and in typical and atypical Duane's syndrome. The saccades, smooth-pursuit movements and optokinetic nystagmus in horizontal eye movements are analysed revealing the different electrooculographic dyssynergies. In the Duane's syndrome we noted the reduction of movement in the affected eye always in both horizontal directions (abduction and adduction). The purpose of examinations was to ascertain the more exact diagnosis and to point the indication for operative treatment.

Kinetic disturbances in different forms of comitant as well as incomitant squint can be objectively recorded by means of electrooculography (EOG) and analysed (Quéré 1978; Quéré et al. 1981).

METHOD

For EOG examinations we used an AC amplifier, a commercial electro-encephalograph (EEG) instrument (T.C. 0.1–1.0 s) with linear ink writers. Horizontal and vertical saccades were tested on the tangent scale. (Mackensen & Harder 1954). Light fixation targets were viewed from the midline to the lateral side at a visual angle of 20°. To test the smooth-pursuit eye movements, the harmonic swinging of a simple pendulum in the frequency of 0.35 Hz was to be used. (Hülse & Partsch 1973). The saccades of optokinetic nystagmus in both directions were elicited by a black and white striped rotating drum. (Mackensen 1954; Mackensen & Schumacher 1960). The speed of rotation was usually about 140°/second (96–144°).

Ocular saccades of each eye were recorded and analysed in four movements. The patient was asked to fixate: 1) centre to right (centrifugal movement in relation to midline straight ahead – CF), right eye (RE) movement – abduction (Abd), left eye (LE) movement – adduction (Add); 2) right to centre (centripetal movement (CP) − RE CP Add, LE CP Abd; 3) centre to left − RE CF Add, LE CF Abd; and 4) left to centre − RE CP Abd, LE CP Add (Bird & Leech 1976; Nóbrega et al. 1976). Readings for peak and angular saccadic velocities were taken directly in millimeters as shown by Nóbrega et al. (1976). Saccades of optokinetic nystagmus − angular velocities of the rapid nystagmus phase (Metz et al. 1971) − were calculated according to Mackensen (1954).

CASE REPORTS AND RESULTS

Case 1

An 8-year-old boy with sudden onset of convergent squint. An acute eso-tropia of about 35° occurred after the interruption of binocular vision by temporary occlusion of one eye caused by trivial superficial eye injury. Clinically, abduction of the left was limited, diplopia was not noted. Electro-

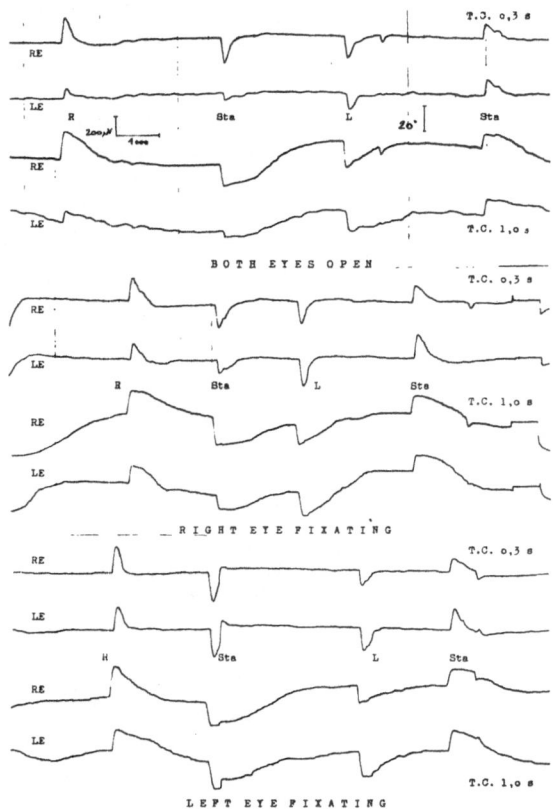

Fig. 1. Acute convergent strabismus. Reduction of the LE centripetal abduction (RE = right eye; LE = left eye) R = right gaze, Sta = Straight ahead gaze, L = left gaze.

oculographically the peak angular saccadic velocity of LE was commonly reduced, especially centripetal abduction (Fig. 1). The angular velocity of the rapid nystagmus phase on the LE was decreased in both directions, and markedly to the left side (Table 1).

Case 2

.A 20-year-old young man since 15th year with bilateral ptosis. He presented a narrowed palpebral fissure, slight exotropia, a decrease of eye motility especially of elevation, and head-tilt keeping the chin elevated. (Čelić et al. 1980).

Electroretinography (ERG) and EOG Arden's quotient were normal. Electromyography (EMG) of the sceletal muscles revealed a physiological pattern. EMG of the levator muscle revealed normal electrical activity which was opposite to failure motion effect (Huber & Mayer 1976). EOG tracings showed slowing of the peak angular saccadic velocity in all directions (Metz & Meshel 1974; Metz 1976a, 1976b) particularly in centrifugal abduction (Table 2).

This finding was also confirmed by poor optokinetic response and with slow angular velocities of the quick nystagmus phase (Fig. 2).

Case 3

A 9-year-old girl with a bilateral Duane's syndrome and orthophoria in primary position, but with severe motility disturbance and retraction phenomena (Fig. 3). Limitation of abduction as well as adduction was bilaterally present (Fig. 4). Peak angular saccadic velocities are considerably slowed in abduction in the both eyes but abduction saccadic speed of the left eye is significantly slow (Table 3).

Case 4

A girl age 16 with strabism from birth and unequally pronounced bilateral involvement. While the RE adduction was markedly reduced, LE showed an inability of abduction. Torticollis was very marked. This unique case has in the RE Duane's syndrome of type II and in the LE a Duane's syndrome of

Table 1. Acute convergent strabismus. Decrease of the angular velocities of the rapid nystagmus phase on the LE (degree/s).

SACCADES OF OPTOKINETIC NYSTAGMUS				
	▌▌▌▌ ← Drum rotated right to left		→ ▌▌▌▌ Drum rotated left to right	
	RE	LE	RE	LE
Both eyes open	340	241	362	175
Right eye fixating	350	219	350	263
Left eye fixating	306	263	197	296

Table 2. Case 2. Chronic progressive external ophthalmoplegia. Slowing of the peak angular saccadic velocity in all directions, especially CF Abd (in mm).

| | Right gaze 20° | | | | Left gaze 20° | | | |
| | Left to straight ahead | | Straight ahead to right | | Right to straight ahead | | Straight ahead to left | |
	RE CP Abd.	LE CP Add.	RE CF Abd.	LE CF Add.	RE CP Add.	LE CP Abd.	RE CF Add.	LE CF Abd.
Both eyes open	4,5	4,5	3,25	4,25	5,0	4,5	3,5	2,0
Right eye fixating	4,5	5,0	3,0	4,75	5,5	5,5	3,0	1,75
Left eye fixating	5,0	5,0	3,0	3,0	4,5	3,5	3,75	3,0

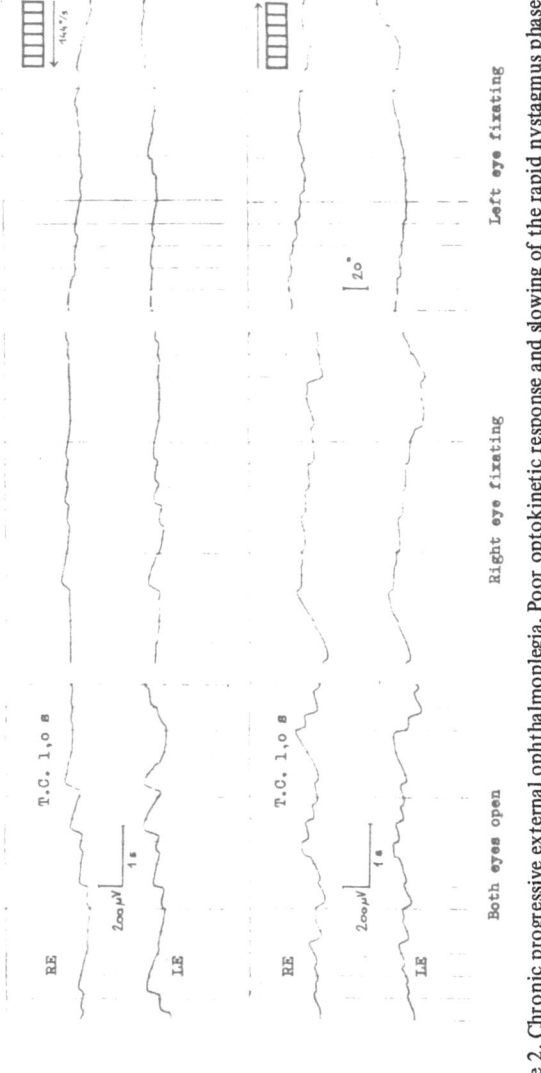

Fig. 2. Case 2. Chronic progressive external ophthalmoplegia. Poor optokinetic response and slowing of the rapid nystagmus phase.

167

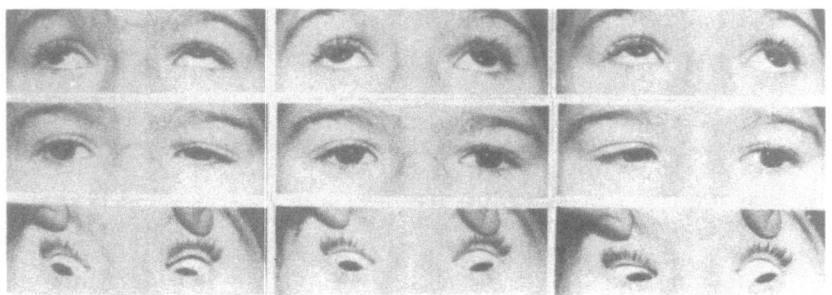

Fig. 3. Case 3. Bilateral Duane's syndrome with orthophoria in primary position. Clinical aspect.

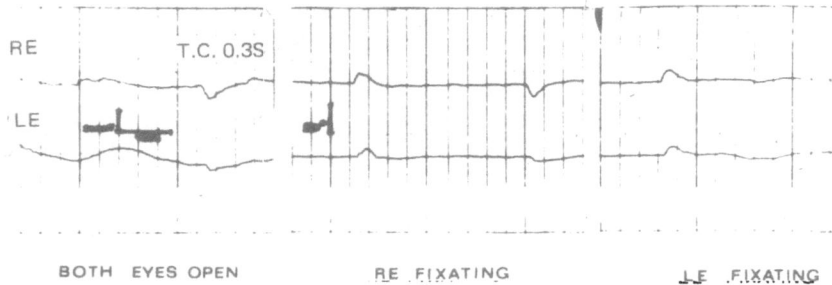

BOTH EYES OPEN   RE FIXATING   LE FIXATING

Fig. 4. Case 3. Bilateral Duane's syndrome. Limitation of motility in both abduction and adduction of both eyes.

Table 3. Case 3. Bilateral retraction Duane's syndrome. Slowing of the peak angular saccadic velocities (in mm).

| | Right gaze 20° | | Left gaze 20° | |
| | Straight ahead to right | | Straight ahead to left | |
	RE CF Abd.	LE CF Add.	RE CF Add.	LE CF Abd.
Both eyes open	3,0	4,0	4,5	2,0
Right eye fixating	3,5	3,0	4,25	1,5
Left eye fixating	4,0	3,0	5,0	1,75

type I, according to Malbran's classification (Fig. 5). The objective angle of squint in $-9°$, LE/RE. EOG of horizontal saccadic eye movements (Fig. 6) revealed a reduction of motility in both eyes but more considerably in the RE. There was no abduction saccade in the LE (Table 4). Simultaneously the RE saccadic velocity is reduced. (Metz et al. 1975; Nóbrega et al. 1976; Rosenbaum 1976). The horizontal pursuit movements in both eyes are not 'smooth' and show the low amplitudes, especially the left eye.

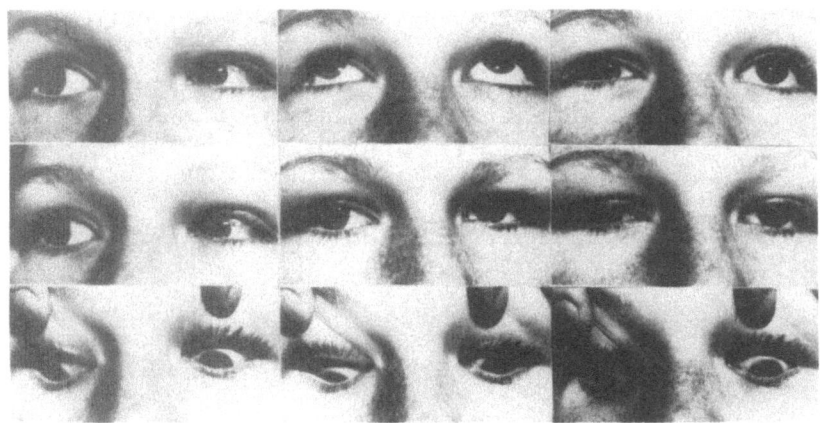

Fig. 5. Case 4. Bilateral Duane's syndrome with exodeviation in primary position. Clinical aspect.

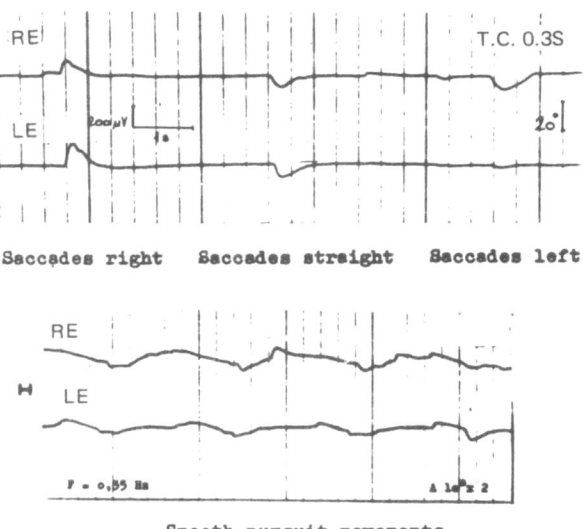

Fig. 6. Case 4. EOG of horizontal saccadic (upper tracings) and smooth-pursuit eye movements (lower tracings).

Table 4. Case 4. Duane's syndrome II in the RE and Duane's syndrome I in the LE. Reduction of motility in both abduction and adduction. Peak angular saccadic velocity (in mm).

	Right gaze 20°		Left gaze 20°			
	Straight ahead to right		Right to straight ahead		Straight ahead to left	
	RE CF Abd.	LE CF Add.	RE CP Add.	LE CP Abd.	RE CF Add.	LE CF Abd.
Both eyes open	4,0	6,5	3,25	4,0	4,0	0,75

CONCLUSIONS

EOG analysis of eye motility in exposed clinical examples revealed:

In acute esotropia a decrease of velocity is noted in the deviating eye. Velocity of the deviated eye is faster when eye is fixating.

Among the myopathies in progressive external ophthalmoplegia a general slowing of saccades was recorded.

Unilateral and bilateral typical and atypical Duane's syndrome showed a dyssynergy of eye movements. The patient with orthophoria in primary position presented the limitation of abduction and adduction bilaterally, but also the patient with strabism, as our case with bilateral atypical retraction Duane's syndrome, which had more reduced adduction in the RE and abduction in the LE.

The degree of the reduction in movement (adduction and abduction) varies individually so no classification seems to be acceptable.

EOG presents a useful and valuable aid in the clinical examination of the ocular motility.

REFERENCES

Bird, A.C. & J. Leech. Internuclear ophthalmoplegia. An electro-oculographic study of peak angular saccadic velocities. Brit. J. Ophthalmol. 60, 645–651 (1976).
Čelić, M., V. Dorn, P. Žeškov & N. Raić. Ophthalmoplegia externa chronica progressiva mit atypischer Netzhautpigmentdystrophie. Klin. Mbl. Augenheilk. 177, 677–683 (1980).
Huber, A. & M. Meyer. Die elektrookulographisch-elektromyographische Analyse periferer und zentraler Störungen der Augenmotorik. Ophthalmologica 172, 194–204 (1976).
Hülse, M. & C.J. Partsch. A Short Introduction to Nystagmography. (Edit. Dr. -Ing. J.F. Tönnies Erben KG), pp. 37–38. Freiburg i. Br. (1971).
Mackensen, G. Untersuchungen zur Physiologie des optokinetischen Nystagmus. Albrecht von Graefes Arch. klin. Exp. Ophthalmol. 155, 284–313 (1954).
Mackensen, G. & S. Harder. Untersuchungen zur elektrischen Aufzeichnung von Augenbewegungen. Albrecht von Graefes Arch. klin. exp. Ophthalmol. 155, 397–412 (1954).

Mackensen, G. & J. Schumacher. Die Geschwindigkeit der raschen Phase des optokineti-schen Nystagmus. Albrecht von Graefes Arch. klin. exp. Ophthalmol. 162, 400–415 (1960).

Metz, H.S. Saccadic velocity measurements in internuclear ophthalmoplegia. Am. J. Ophthalmol. 81, 296–299 (1976a).

Metz, H.S. Saccadic velocity tests in various neurological diseases. In: Smith-Kettlewell Symposium on Basic Sciences in Strabismus, (Edit. C. Souza-Dias), Oct. 16th–17th, Guarujá – Brasil, pp. 50–59 (1976b).

Metz, H.S. & L. Meshel. Ocular saccades in progressive external ophthalmoplegia. Ann. Ophthal. 6, 623–628 (1974).

Metz, H.S., A.B. Scott & D. O'Meara. Saccadic velocities in infants and children. Am. J. Ophthalmol. 72, 1130–1135 (1971).

Metz, H.S., A.B. Scott & W.E. Scott. Horizontal saccadic velocities in Duane's syndrome. Am. J. Ophthalmol. 80, 901–906 (1975).

Quéré, M.A. Elektro-Okulographie bei Blockierungssyndromen. Beiheft Klin. Mbl. Augenheilk. 72, 32–47 (1978).

Quéré, M.A. Kinetic Electro-Oculography: Aims – Disadvantages and Limitations. Ophthalmologica 182, 73–80 (1981).

Nóbrega, J.F.C., H.E.A. Bicas & S.J. Faria e Souza. Saccadic movements in normal and strabismic patients. In: Smith-Kettlewell Symposium on Basic Sciences in Strabismus (Edit. C. Souza-Dias) Oct. 16th–17th 1976, Guarujá – Brasil, pp. 128–150 (1976).

Rosenbaum, A. The clinical application of saccadic velocity testing. In: Smith-Kettlewell Symposium on Basic Sciences in Strabismus (Edit. C. Souza-Dias) Oct. 16th–17th 1976, Guarujá – Brasil, pp. 42–49 (1976).

Authors' address:
Department of Ophthalmology
Faculty of Medicine, University of Zagreb
Kišpatićeva 12
YU-41000 Zagreb, Yugoslavia

171

ELECTROPHYSIOLOGICAL DIAGNOSIS IN NON-COMITANT STRABISMUS

R. FROSINI, M.C. BOSCHI & D. BARONCELLI

(Firenze, Italy)

INTRODUCTION

Electrophysiological studies of ocular kinetics are made possible by the existence of the antero-posterior eye potential.

These techniques have greatly advanced in the last few years and electro-oculograms (EOG) have largely contributed to the understanding of some alterations of eye motility.

In particular, it has been possible to evidence, in the so-called concomitant strabismus, those kinetic alterations which are referred to as dissynergy, amblyopic kinetic anarchy, ataxia.

A typical behaviour is shown by the tracings of paralitic strabismus (i.e. paralitic dissynergy) which make it possible to recognize this form of strabismus even many years after the onset.

These techniques, however, are somewhat limited. To start with, the analysis can be carried out only on the horizontal plane and consequently it yields little information.

Data on the positions of the eyes, both relative and absolute, is also scanty.

In order to obtain more data on these very important features of eye kinetics, particularly in non-comitant strabismus, a more sophisticated stimulation and recording system is now being worked out in our department.

We report here the preliminary data and a description of the device we used.

MATERIAL AND METHODS

The recording system (Fig. 1) consists of four DC amplifiers which collect and amplify the potentials received by eight electrodes — four for each eye. These electrodes are placed on the skin at the internal and external corners as well as above and below the eye.

Through a digital-analog converter, the signal reaches the central processing unit which controls the automatic elimination of the offset. It also stores the signals on eight memories and operates the stimulation. It is equipped with a CRT display, with an x-y plotter and a serial output for possible further processing.

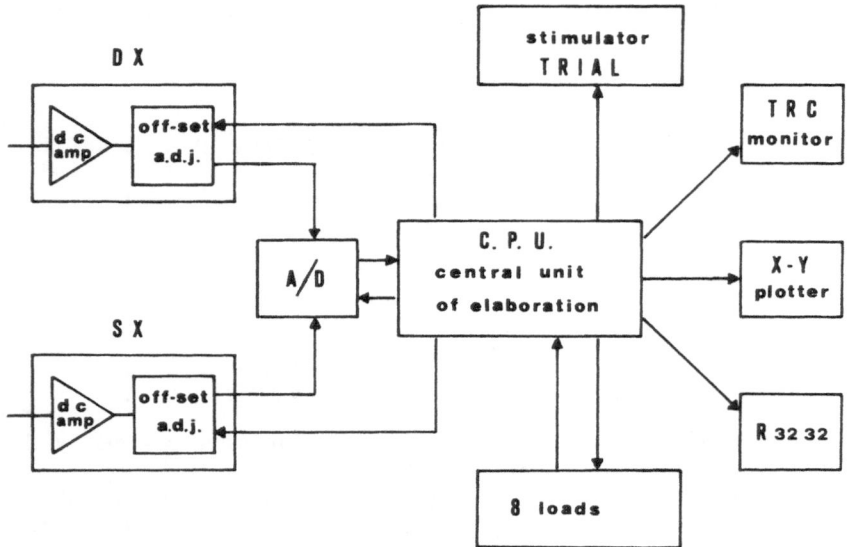

Fig. 1.

The stimulator consists of a black tangent screen placed at 1.5 m in front of the patient. On the screen there are 128 red LEDs of which 72, with a 5° distance between them, form a 30° radius circumference, and one is in the centre. The remaining 55 were not employed in this experience.

So far we have done only circular stimulation consisting of sequence ignition along the LED circumference in a total time of 5 seconds.

The patient is asked to look at the central target while the device is automatically set at Zero on the centre of the CRT screen. When the centre appears stable, the patient is asked to look up fixedly at the higher LED of the circumference. At that point there starts the sequence of ignitions that the patient has to follow.

At the end of each circular run the tracings are stored; then they are recorded on paper and compared.

RESULTS

We have not been using this device long enough to obtain statistically significant data. We therefore report only some examples of those tracings we were able to observe using the circular stimulation only.

In Fig. 2 we can see the tracing of the right eye and of the left eye of a normal individual. It can be noted that the tracing of the eye movement is practically circular and concentric to the primary position indicated by the centre.

In Figs. 3 and 4 is shown the tracing relating to a patient affected by recent paresis of the left eye lateral rectus.

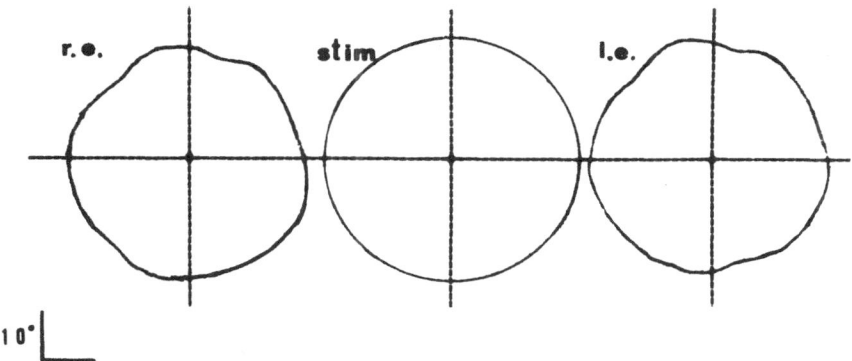

normal

Fig. 2.

Some of the more evident features are clearly visible. When the subject fixated with his unaffected eye, the tracing of this eye was practically circular like that in the normal individual; in the affected eye there was a sharp reduction in the left portion of the tracing, indicating motor failure in that direction.

When the patient looked with his affected left eye, this eye succeeded in overcoming the medial line, but a kind of 'hump' indicating the secondary deviation appeared in the left portion of the tracing of the right eye.

Finally, Figs. 5 and 6 show the picture of a child affected by Stilling-Türk-Duane syndrome bilaterally.

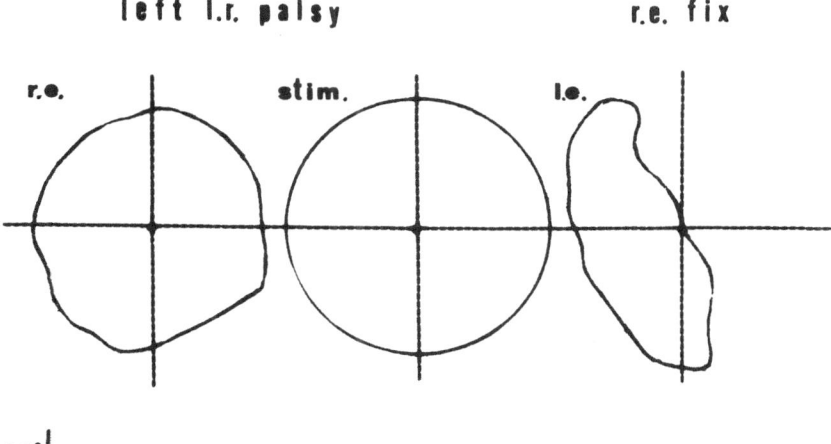

left l.r. palsy   **r.e. fix**

Fig. 3.

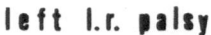
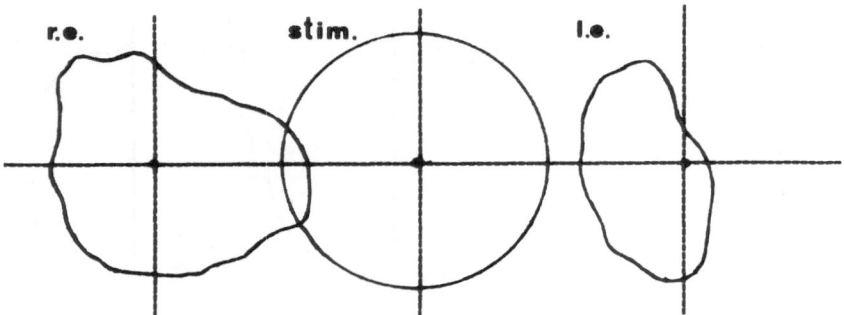

left l.r. palsy   **l.e. fix**

r.e.   stim.   l.e.

1 0°

Fig. 4.

There is a clear reduction in the lateral portions of the field of gaze in either fixing eye. No increase seems to be revealed in the nasal portions of the fields of gaze which might indicate the presence of a secondary deviation.

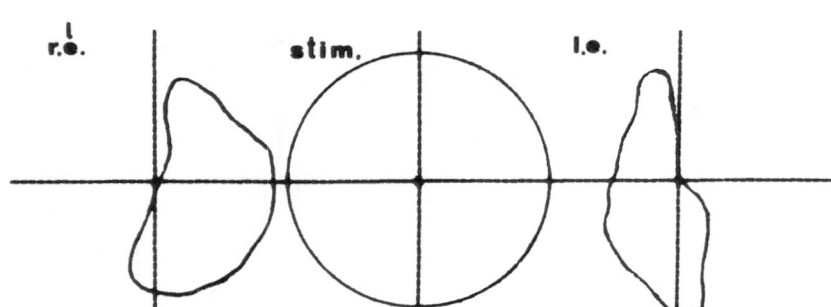

Stilling Türck Duane S.   **r.e. fix**

r.e.   stim.   l.e.

1 0°

Fig. 5.

176

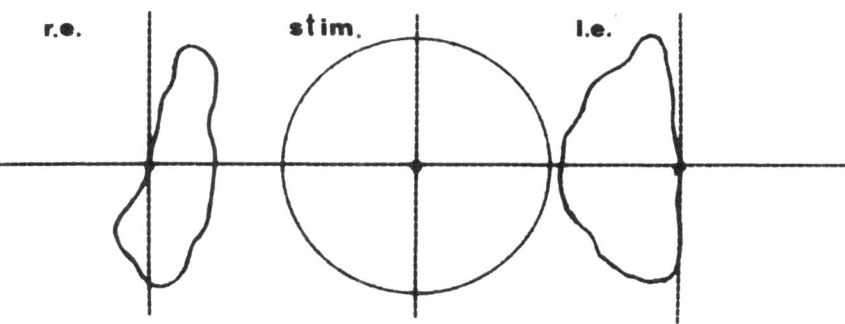

Stilling Türck Duane S. **l.e. fix**

r.e.   stim.   l.e.

1 0°

Fig. 6.

CONCLUSION

The first results supplied by our device for recording eye movements seem to be satisfactory.

In particular, it has made it possible to visualize the positions of the eyes not only horizontally, but also vertically and obliquely.

It has also enabled us to compare directly the positions reached by the eyes, in a way similar to Hess's screen, but with the advantages of not being subjective and of identifying the position of the eye even when it is occluded. This way it is possible to continually check the fixing eye.

We believe that the setting-up of more suitable stimulation modes and of more sophisticated data processing programmes will allow useful applications of this technique in many alterations of eye movements.

REFERENCES

Frosini, R., F. Galassi & D. Baroncelli. Dispositivo per la generazione di uno stimolo induttore nella tecnica elettrooculografica. Boll. Ocul. 58, 709–715 (1979).

Huber, A. & E. Meyer. A new method oculography. In Strabismus Robert, D., Reineke, M.D. Ed. New York (1978).

Quéré, M.A., C. Frettay, R. Le Borgne, M.P. Delplace & S. Devlamynck. Etude electro-oculographique des mouvements de porsuite. 1) L'explorateur multiparametrique de la cinetique oculaire. Ann. Ocul. Paris 205, 1307–1320 (1972).

Suarez, H.E., I. Macadaro & D. Cibilis. Analyse dynamique de la porsuite oculaire et son applications clinique. Rev. Otoneuroophtal. 52, 143–146 (1980).

Weiss, J.B. Differential electro-oculography. In Strabismus Robert, D., Reineke, M.D. Ed. New York (1978).

Yuzawa, H. & G. Matsui. Studies on clinical application of electrooculography – part 1; An improved method for measuring electrooculography. Dept. Acta Soc. Ophthal. JPN 82, 10 (1978).

Authors' address:
Istituto di Clinica Oculistica
Cattedra di Ottica fisiopatologica
Università degli Studi di Firenze
Firenze, Italy

178

THE BIELSCHOWSKY HEAD TILT TEST AND OCULAR COUNTER-ROLLING

J. VAN DER MEER

(Amsterdam, The Netherlands)

SUMMARY

Ocular counter-rolling was measured in 16 normal subjects and 11 patients with superior oblique palsy by means of photographic recording. We did not find a correlation between the degree of counter-rolling and the effect of the Bielschowsky head tilt test.

In the study of incomitant strabismus the Bielschowsky head tilt test (BHTT) is one of the important methods of examination. The diagnosis may depend on the result of this test: a palsy of an oblique or a rectus muscle, or, perhaps, neither of the two.

Since the work of Hofmann & Bielschowsky (1900) it is generally assumed that the head tilt test is based on vestibular counter-rolling of the eyes. Although the existence of a static otolith response has recently been challenged by Jampel (1981), the evidence for counter-rolling is very strong (vide inter al. Miller 1962; Scott 1967).

The mechanism of the Bielschowsky test is easy to understand. Head tilting to the right causes compensatory eye torsion to the left by contraction in the right eye of the superior oblique and, to a lesser degree, of the superior rectus; in the left eye, by contraction of the inferior oblique and, to a lesser degree, of the inferior rectus. If there is a paretic right hypertropia, strongest during laevoversion, the cause may either be a paralysis of the right superior oblique or of the left superior rectus. In the first case the hypertropia will become larger during head tilt to the right shoulder, in the second case the hypertropia will decrease.

Although there can be little doubt on the mechanism of the Bielschowsky test many questions remain to be answered. How to explain that the amplitude of the Bielschowsky phenomenon is only $5°$ in one case of trochlear palsy and $25°$ in another? Do differences of counter-rolling lie at the root of this? Or is there a relation with anatomical peculiarities, in so far as obliques which run a more sagittal course, have a larger vertical component? Or is there more passive resistance against torsion in one patient than in another? We still know very little about these problems.

In the individual case of incomitant squint we do not know the amplitude of counter-rolling, neither the anatomy of the ocular muscles, nor the active and passive forces in the muscles and other tissues concerned.

The aim of this preliminary study is the measurement of counter-rotation, in a number of normal subjects and in patients with superior oblique palsy. We employ a tilting chair as illustrated in Fig. 1. The fixating eye is photographed in its primary position, while it looks at a small red fixating light. The other eye is occluded. The room is darkened so that there are no visual cues for vertical orientation. The camera is fixed to the skull by means of a bite board with dental impression. The accuracy of the measurement depends on the accuracy in which the bite board is held by the subject. Measurements are not possible in subjects with a bad set of teeth.

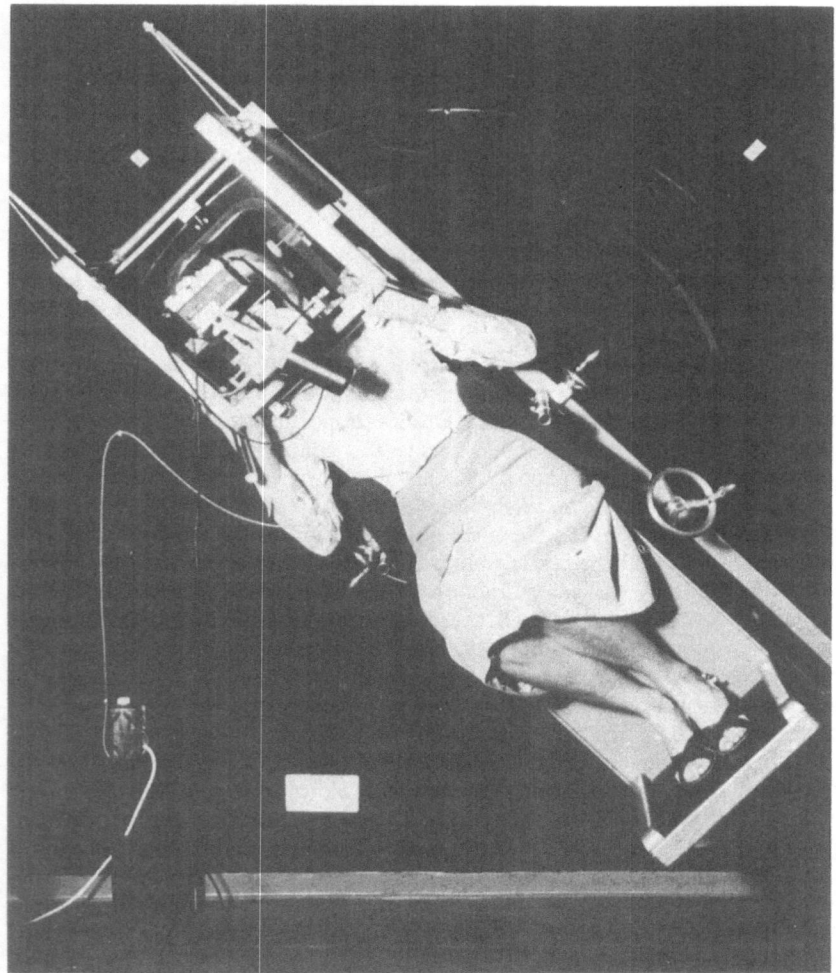

Fig. 1. Tilting chair for the photographical recording of ocular counter-rolling.

Counter-rotations of 16 normal subjects

In two subjects the torsional eye position was measured after every 5° of head and body tilt (Fig. 2). In the remaining cases we measured as a routine only the counter-rolling in 45° tilt, because we are used to perform the Bielschowsky head tilt also with 45° tilt. The total counter-rolling of all normal subjects is arranged in Fig. 3 in order of increasing amplitude of the right eye torsion. The subsequently measured torsions of the left eye are not exactly identical to those of the right eye. Whether this discrepancy is caused by experimental errors or by differences of counter-rolling is impossible to decide.

Counter-rotation in 11 patients with superior oblique palsy

As could be expected we found a decreased counter-rolling on the affected side. Usually, but not invariably, the intorsion was most limited. Fig. 4 depicts a rather typical case of acquired superior oblique palsy, in which the effect of head tilt on counter-rolling and on the hypertropia has been measured. We hoped to find a correlation between the amplitudes of counter-rolling and the Bielschowsky test, because they should be strongly inter-related, according to the classical theory of Hofmann and Bielschowsky. We did indeed find cases in which a strong counter-rolling was accompanied

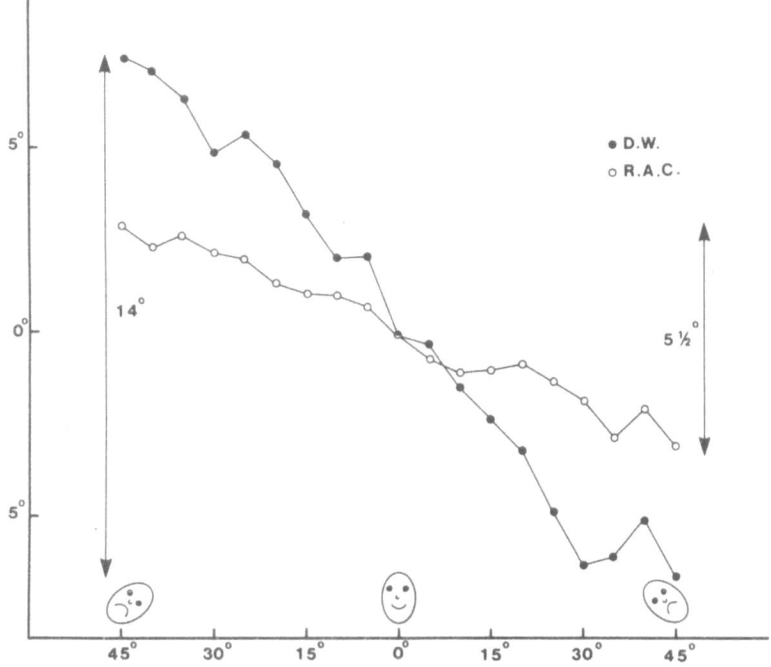

Fig. 2. Counter-rolling in 2 normal subjects.

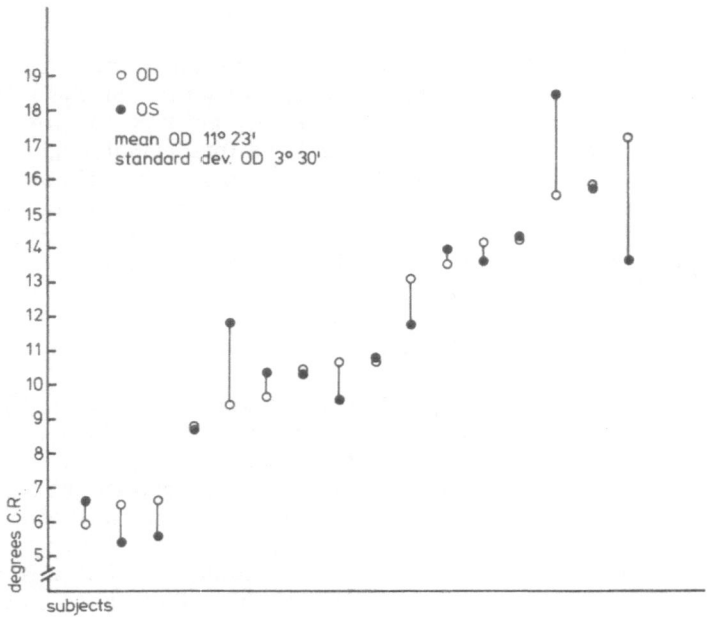

Fig. 3. Total counter-rolling in 16 normal subjects arranged in order of magnitude of right eye torsion.

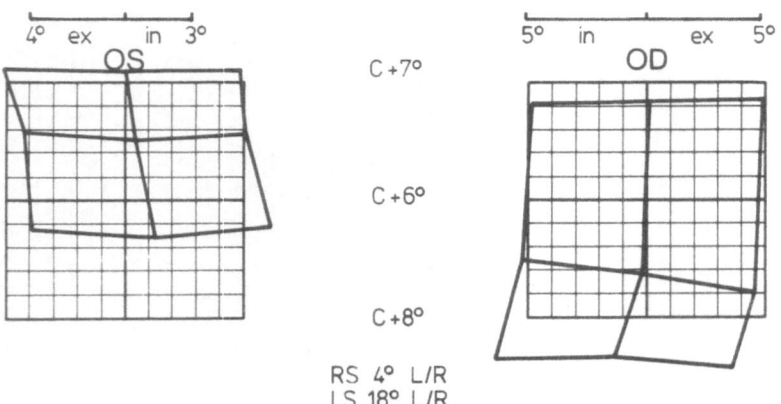

Fig. 4. Acquired left superior oblique palsy. Each small square is 5 × 5 degrees. Above the motility diagram: counter-rolling of each eye C: cyclotropia in primary direction of gaze and during 25° upward and downward gaze. RS, LS: 45° head tilt towards R, L shoulder.

182

by a strongly positive Bielschowsky test, as, for instance, the case of Fig. 5. Disappointingly, however, in our 11 cases we did not find the presumed correlation (Fig. 6). Probably in the study of the BHTT the degree of palsy has to be taken into account, and torsional forces, both active and passive, will have to be measured.

Certainly information on torsional forces will be necessary for a better understanding of the case of Fig. 7, a traumatic superior oblique palsy in a young person. Both inferior oblique had generous recessions so that the function of all 4 obliques must be minimal. In accordance with this the measured counter-rolling is very slight. The more impressive is the large amplitude of the Bielschowsky test. If the patient does not keep her head exactly straight, she has double vision. One wonders how the balance of forces is in the extraocular muscles, and why the same phenomenon is absent in most other comparable cases.

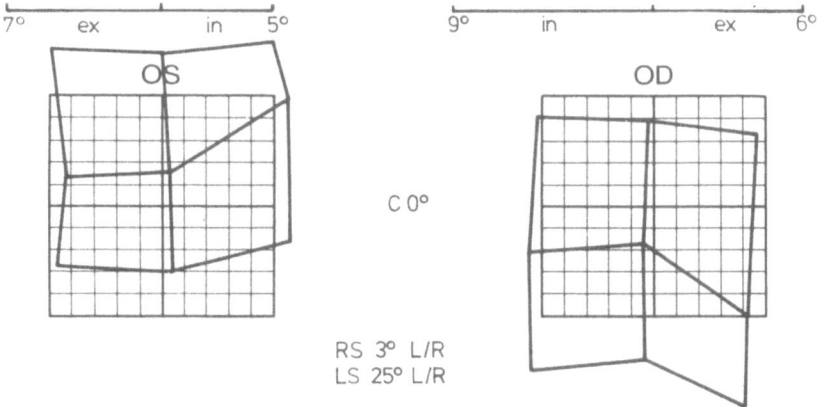

Fig. 5. Congenital left superior oblique palsy. Large effect of tilt on torsion and hypertropia.

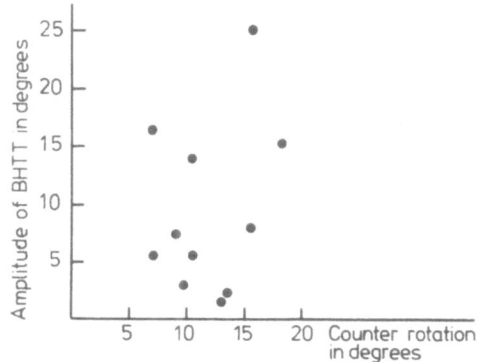

Fig. 6. Relation between counter-rolling and amplitude of Bielschowsky test.

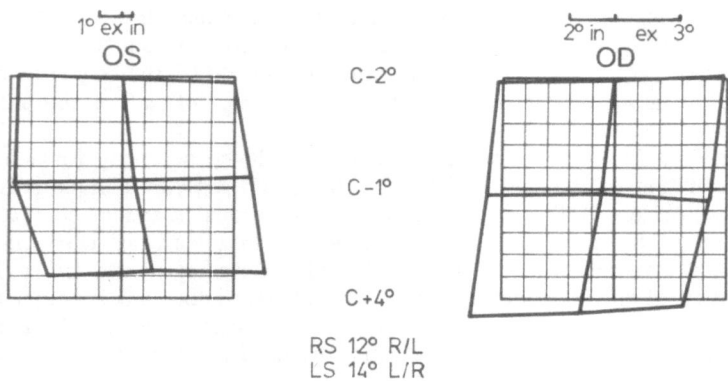

Fig. 7. Bilateral traumatic superior oblique palsy, after bilateral inferior oblique recession. Small effect of tilt on compensatory torsion, very large effect on hypertropia.

REFERENCES

Hofmann, F.B. & A. Bielschowsky. Die Verwertung der Kopfneigung zur Diagnostik von Augenmuskellähmungen aus der Heber- und Senkergruppe. Albrecht v. Graefes Arch. Ophthal. 51, 174–185 (1900).

Jampel, R.S. Ocular torsion and the primary retinal meridians. Am. J. Ophthalmol. 91, 14–24 (1981).

Miller, E.F. Counterrolling of the human eyes produced by head tilt with respect to gravity. Acta otolaryng. (Stockh.) 54, 479–501 (1962).

Scott, A.B. Extraocular muscles and head tilting. EMG measurements of activity of individual muscles. Arch. Ophthal. 78, 397–399 (1967).

Author's address:
Oogheelkundige Kliniek
Academisch Ziekenhuis bij de
Universiteit van Amsterdam
le Helmersstraat 104
1054 EG Amsterdam, The Netherlands

L'ELECTRO-OCULOGRAPHIE DES PARALYSIES OCULO-MOTRICES HORIZONTALES INTERET PHYSIO-PATHOLOGIQUE, DIAGNOSTIQUE ET THERAPEUTIQUE

M.A. QUÉRÉ, A. PECHEREAU & F. LAVENANT

(*Nantes, France*)

RESUME

L'étude des tracés électro-oculographiques pré et post-opératoires de 150 cas de paralysie oculo-motrice horizontale traités chirurgicalement prouve que cette exploration fonctionelle est indispensable pour révéler leurs troubles cinétiques.

A la phase initiale la dyssynergie paralytique est constamment retrouvée alors qu'elle est notée dans moins de 5% des strabismes infantiles.

l'analyse des enregistrements montre que l'induction opto-motrice est assurée par l'ensemble de la rétine et non seulement par la fovéa. Par ailleurs, il apparaît que l'inhibition motrice joue un rôle essentiel dans la conservation de la phase lente du N.O.C.

En pratique journalière l'électro-oculographie cinétique est indispensable pour poser un diagnostic exact dans les paralysies anciennes, suivre objectivement l'évolution, enfin, pour déterminer un plan opératoire correct.

SUMMARY

The study of pre and post-operative electro-oculographic recordings in 150 cases of horizontal palsies surgically treated prove that functional investigation is absolutely necessary to reveal the kinetic troubles.

At the early stage the paralytic dyssynergy is ever noticed, whereas less than 5% of children squints have such a symptom.

The recording analysis demonstrates the opto-motor induction is related with the retina as a whole and not only with the fovea. On the other hand the motor inhibition appears to play at utmost part in the slow phasis of opto-kinetic nystagmus.

In daily practice, kinetic electro-oculography is the best way to set an accurate diagnosis in long standing palsies, to get an objective follow-up, and to settle a correct surgical plan.

Docum. Ophthal. Proc. Series, Vol. 32, ed. by A.Th.M. van Balen & W.A. Houtman 185
© *1982, Dr W. Junk Publishers, The Hague. ISBN 90 6193 728 0*

INTRODUCTION

Tous les tests cliniques usuels d'examen de l'oculomotricité sont, sans exception, basés uniquement sur l'étude de la statique oculaire. Or, si l'on veut parler valablement de la motilité oculaire, il est évident que l'étude de la cinétique des divers types de mouvements de version et de vergence est indispensable. Celle-ci exige impérativement une méthode d'enregistrement.

Pour diverses raisons que nous avons à nouveau récemment exposées dans Ophthalmologica (Quéré & Péchereau 1981), la méthode électro-oculographique reste pour le moment la seule technique commode permettant de faire face à nos besoins cliniques. Malheureusement, elle comporte de sérieux aléas et d'étroites limites. En particulier, avec Mme Devlamynck en 1972 et Coat en 1976, nous avons montré que les particularités de la constitution anatomique orbitaire en général et celle de chaque individu en particulier entraînent une transmission non uniforme des potentiels oculographiques vers les divers secteurs du pourtour orbitaire où ils sont captés.

L'analyse statistique d'un très grand nombre de cas a prouvé que sur les axes obliques de déplacement les corrélations cinétiques électriques ne sont pas significatives. En revanche, elles sont excellentes sur l'axe horizontal, et satisfaisantes sur l'axe vertical.

Aussi, nous ne parlerons que des P.O.M. horizontales, et, à cause de leur fréquence, plus particulièrement des paralysies de la VIème paire.

Pour nos enregistrements standard, nous utilisons un amplificateur E.C.E.M. à 8 pistes on courant alternatif. Le déplacement du potentiel de repos de

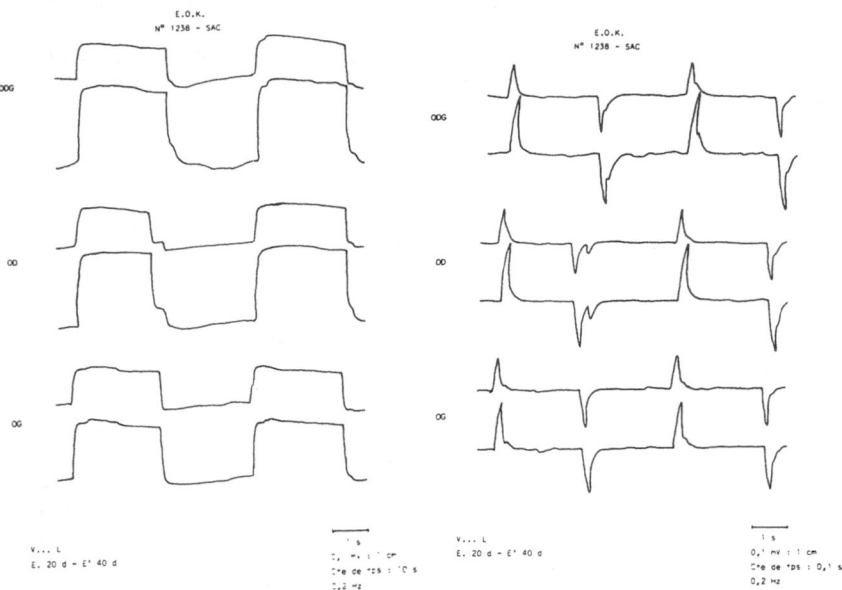

Fig. 1. Paralysie du VI droit. a: saccades – constante de temps 10 secondes. (altération de l'amplitude du mouvement) b: saccades – constante de temps 0,1 seconde. (altération de la vitesse du mouvement).

chaque oeil entre le même couple d'électrodes est simultanément analysé sur deux pistes (Figs. 1a et b).

— l'une en constante de temps longue de 10 secondes dont le tracé est avant tout l'expression de l'amplitude du mouvement,

— l'autre en constante de temps courte de 0,1 seconde qui donne un tracé avant tout du reflet de la vitesse du mouvement.

LA SEMEIOLOGIE CINETIQUE DES PARALYSIES HORIZONTALES

Le symptôme cinétique majeur, constant et stéréotype est la dyssynergie paralytique qui représente l'expression spécifique de l'atteinte du neurone moteur périphérique et de ses effecteurs musculaires (Fig. 2).

Elle est en effet observée dans 100% des paralysiés avérées et des syndromes de rétraction. Elle se traduit par une diminution de l'amplitude et de la vitesse du tracé de l'oeil impotent par rapport à celles du tracé de l'oeil sain. La dyssynergie paralytique altère les trois types fondamentaux de version: poursuite, saccades et N.O.C. L'impotence cinétique de l'oeil atteint est permanente; elle est évidente quelles que soient lest modalités de fixation: binoculaire, monoculaires droite ou gauche.

Enfin, son intensité est proportionnelle au degré de l'impotence. Elle est présente tant que l'impotence persiste. La dyssynergie paralytique est par conséquent parfaitement logique et apparemment sans aucun mystère.

Néanmoins, l'étude analytique de ses caractères sur les enregistrements pré et post-opératoires de 150 cas de P.O.M. horizontales opérés ces dernières

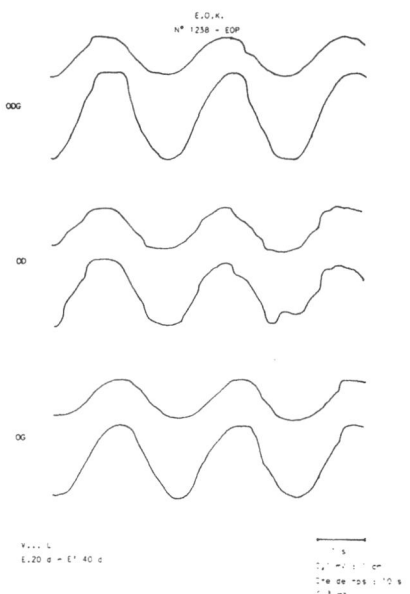

Fig. 2. Paralysie du VI droit. Poursuite — Dyssynergie paralytique OD.

années nous a permis de dégager un certain nombre de faits d'un intérêt majeur du point de vue physio-pathologique, diagnostique et thérapeutique.

INTÉRÊT PHYSIO-PATHOLOGIQUE

P.O.M. horizontales et strabismes infantiles

Nos séries successives portant sur près de 2000 cas de strabismes infantiles ont prouvé que moins de 5% ont une dyssynergie paralytique. La généralisation de la théorie paralytique à leur étiologie est donc erronée. (Fig. 3).

70 à 80% des ésotropies présentent une dyssynergie mais dont la morphologie est totalement différente; en fonction des modalités de la fixation inductrice, elle change totalement de côté ou disparaît. Il n'y a pas d'impotence des ductions, il s'agit exclusivement d'un trouble innervationnel caractérisé par une perturbation de la correspondance motrice des versions. Le mouvement de l'oeil découvert a une amplitude et une vitesse normale et seul le tracé de l'oeil occlu est altéré.

En effet, on constate soit une dyssynergie alternante soit une dyssynergie monolatérale; elles révèlent un dérèglement du système opto-tonique qui assure l'équilibre stato-cinétique réciproque des globes. De nombreux arguments donnent à penser que les réseaux oculogyres occipitaux et de la jonction visuomotrice sont en cause.

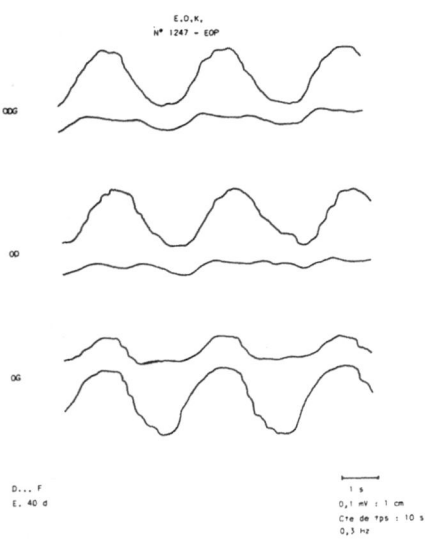

Fig. 3. Poursuite – Dyssynergie alternante dissociée dans un strabisme fonctionnel.

Angle de déviation et dyssynergie

Que le trouble moteur originel soit périphérique ou supra-nucléaire, fort logiquement plus il est important, plus la déviation est marquée.

Récemment certains auteurs (Weiss 1979; Bérard 1980) ont pu dire que la dyssynergie oculographique est seulement l'expression de cette déviation, c'est-à-dire de la position de l'oeil dévié par rapport aux électrodes; ce serait un simple artéfact sans aucune réalité cinétique; bien entendu, cette opinion ôte toute signification à la dyssynergie dissociée.

Mais l'existence même de la dyssynergie paralytique prouve de façon éclatante le contraire. Ce facteur existe, mais il n'intervient que pour les angles au-dessus de 30 degrés et il est minime en regard des perversions cinétiques considérables par ailleurs constatées. (Figs. 1a et b).

Les modalités de l'induction opto-motrice

Un rôle sinon exclusif, du moins essentiel a depuis toujours été attribué à la fovéa dans l'induction des saccades et surtout de la poursuite.

Les tracés de sujets atteints d'ophtalmoplégie complète prouvent que cette conception est inexacte. En effet, chez un sujet coopérant, quand on masque l'oeil sain et qu'on lui demande d'essayer de suivre le mobile inducteur avec l'oeil paralysé, ce qu'il est évidemment incapable de faire, on voit apparaître sur l'oeil sain occlu un mouvement parfaitement harmonieux. (Fig. 4).

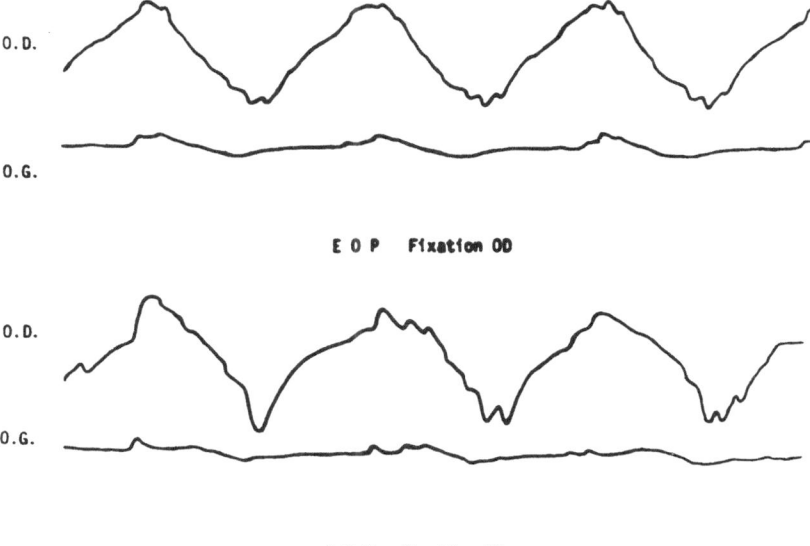

Fig. 4. Poursuite — Paralysie complète du VI gauche. Poursuite harmonieuse de l'oeil droit occlu. Même phénomène pour les saccades sur la figure 1a.

189

Nous avons prouvé que la poursuite volontaire sans support visuel est impossible. On doit donc conclure que le mouvement harmonieux de l'oeil sain masqué est assuré par le balayage rétinien de l'oeil paralysé; par conséquent, l'induction motrice est déterminée par l'ensemble de la hiérarchie spatiale des diverses zones rétiniennes, et dans cette fonction le rôle de la fovéa est d'être seulement le centre de cette organisation. (Fig. 5).

Les preuves corollaires sont apportées par la conservation de l'induction motrice dans les scotomes centraux organiques et au contraire sa complète désorganisation dans les amblyopies par inhibition (anarchie cinétique amblyopique). (Figs. 6, 7).

Le rôle de l'inhibition

Dans les paralysies récentes et complètes du VI on constate toujours une abolition du N.O.C. – c'est-à-dire de la phase rapide – qui bat vers le droit externe impotent, et, au contraire, sa conservation quand il bat vers le droit interne antagoniste homolatéral. C'est ce que nous avons appelé avec Larmande 'les paralysies du type 1'. (Fig. 8).

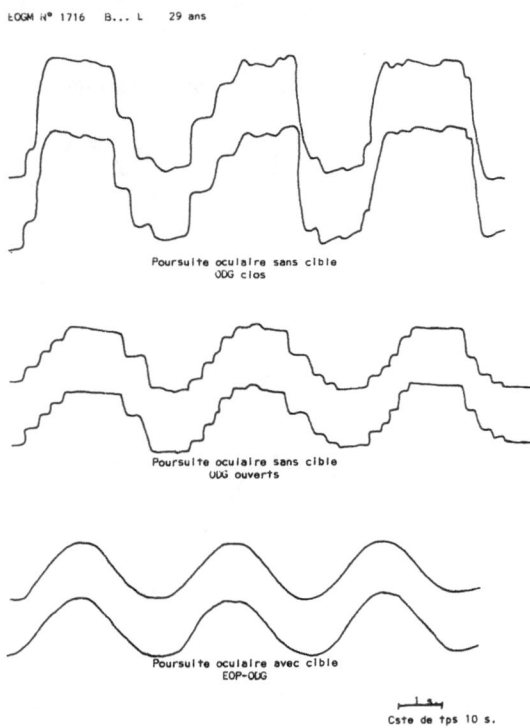

Fig. 5. Poursuite chez un sujet normal. – en haut: poursuite volontaire les yeux cachés. – au mileu: poursuite volontaire les yeux ouverts sans cible mobile. – en bas: poursuite avec cible mobile.

190

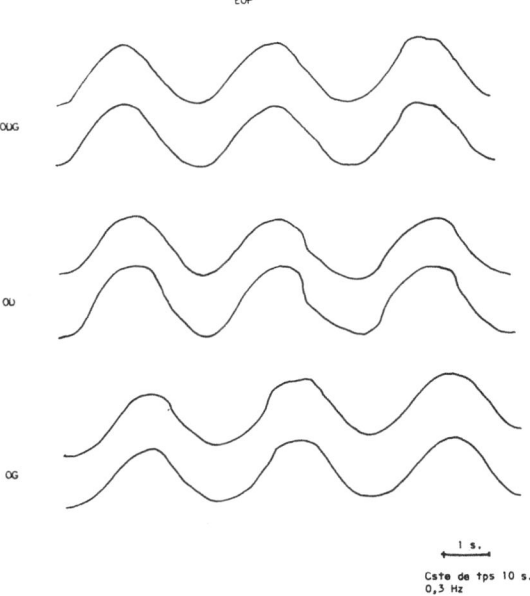

LOP

OUG

OU

OG

1 s.

Cste de tps 10 s.
0,3 Hz

Fig. 6. Poursuite – amblyopie organique. VOG 1/50. Poursuite excellente en fixation OG.

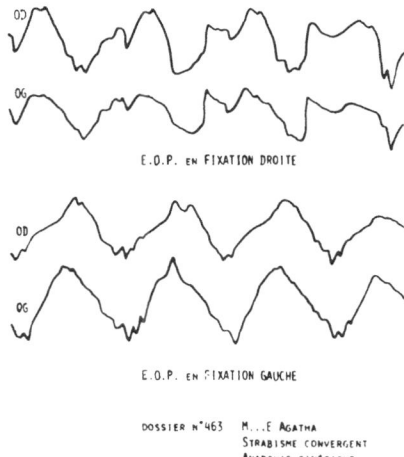

OD

OG

E.O.P. EN FIXATION DROITE

OD

OG

E.O.P. EN FIXATION GAUCHE

DOSSIER N°463   M...E AGATHA
STRABISME CONVERGENT
ANARCHIE CINÉTIQUE

Fig. 7. Poursuite amblyopie fonctionnelle strabique – OD 3/10. Anarchie cinétique en fixation droite.

191

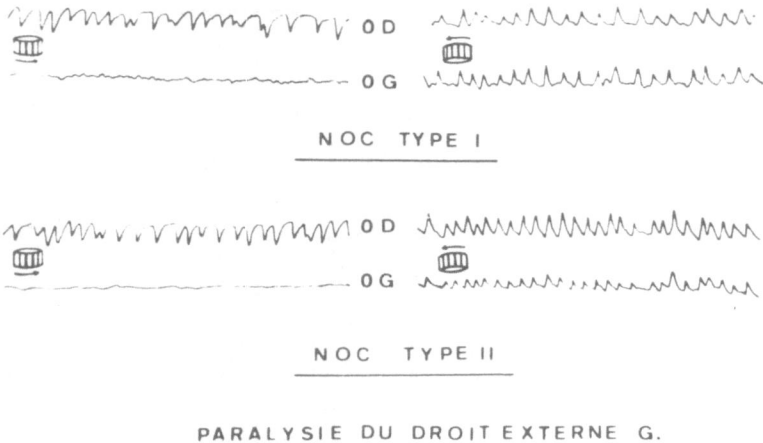

NOC TYPE I

NOC TYPE II

PARALYSIE DU DROIT EXTERNE G.

Fig. 8. N.O.C. – Paralysie du VI gauche. – en haut: paralysie type 1 – en bas: paralysie type II.

Cette conservation a une importance capitale. La phase rapide normale signifie en effet qu'elle a été précédée d'une phase lente; or, celle-ci ne peut être que le résultat de l'inhibition active du droit interne. On arrive donc à la conclusion qu'l'inhibition peut compenser une phase lente, mais jamais une phase rapide.

La compensation d'une phase rapide ne se voit que dans les vraies paralysies congénitales du VI.

Le plus souvent après un certain temps d'évolution, un spasme réactionnel de ce droit interne antagoniste gene à des degrés divers cette compensation. Ce sont les paralysies du type II.

La compensation de la phase lente mais pas de la phase rapide semble une règle de l'ensemble du système oculogyre. En effet, on constate exactement le même phénomène à l'autre extrême des voies oculogyres dans les lésions pariéto-occipitales responsables du syndrome de Barany.

INTÉRÊT DIAGNOSTIQUE

Dans les paralysies anciennes

On sait que le passage à la concomitance rend souvent le diagnostic exact de l'impotence séquellaire difficile et parfois même impossible. Au contraire, le simple enregistrement électro-oculographique le révèle sans aucune ambiguité. (Fig. 9).

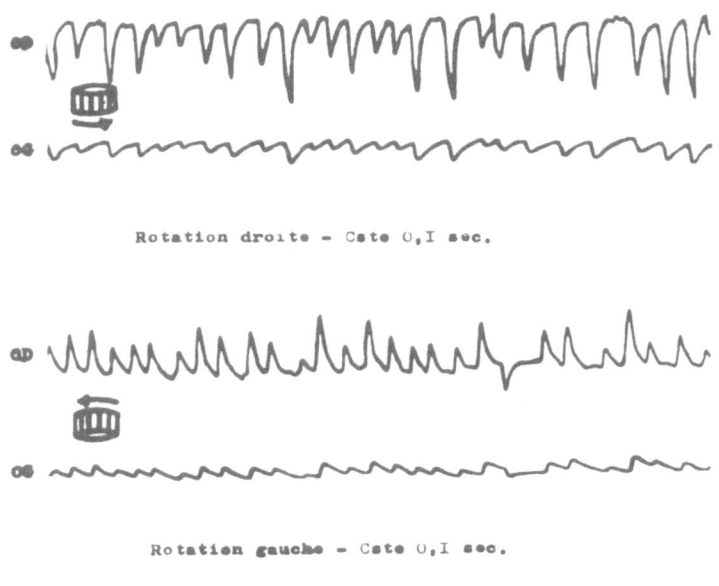

Rotation droite - Cste 0,I sec.

Rotation gauche - Cste 0,I sec.

V....E Romaine N° 10

Fig. 9. N.O.C. – Esotropie post-traumatique concomitante vieille de 10 ans. La paralysie de type II à gauche est évidente sur les tracés. Diagnostic clinique impossible.

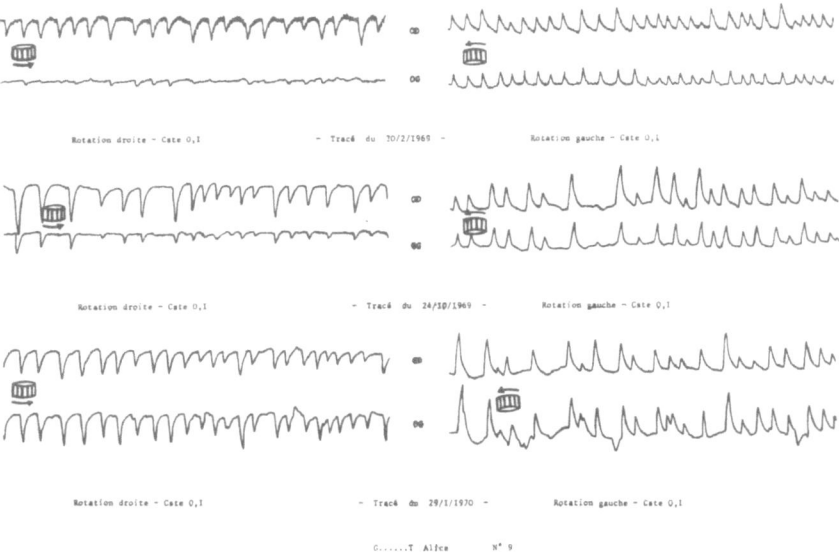

Fig. 10. N.O.C. – Paralysie du VI gauche. Evolution objective sur 11 mois.

Elle est évidente sur les enregistrements successifs et l'on peut ainsi suivre de façon parfaite la régression ou au contraire la persistance de l'impotence primitive. (Fig. 10).

On conçoit les avantages de la méthode pour décider le moment opportun de l'intervention.

INTÉRÊT THÉRAPEUTIQUE

Quand le trouble moteur se stabilise et que la chirurgie se révèle indispensable, l'examen des tracés révèle clairement le degré de l'impotence résiduelle, des hyperactions de l'antagoniste homolatéral et du synergiste contro-latéral, donc les points d'impacts de la chirurgie.

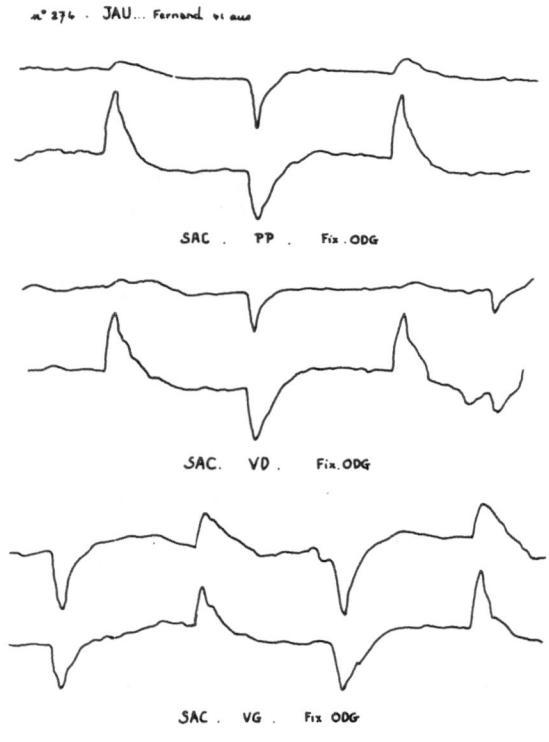

Fig. 11. Saccades – Constante de temps 0,3 sec. Paralysie du VI droit. La dyssynergie diminue dans la version gauche.

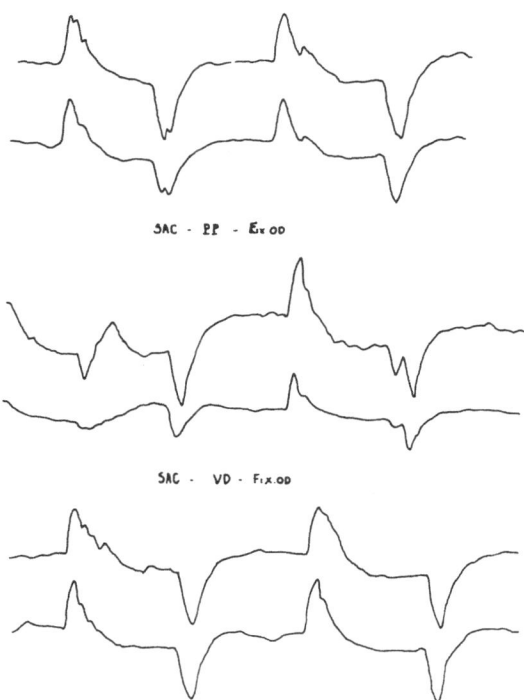

3AC - P.P - Ex OD

SAC - VD - Fix.OD

Fig. 12. Saccades – Constante de temps 0,3 sec. Paralysie du VI gauche. La dyssynergie diminue de façon paradoxale en version gauche (en bas) et augmente en version droite (au milieu).

Le rôle des hyperactions

Sur les enregistrements il est fréquent de constater la disparition de l'impotence initiale et que seules persistent les hyperactions secondaires; or, elles sont responsables de déviations séquellaires parfois considérables.

L'aspect le plus typique est marqué par une dyssynergie qui diminue dans la version vers le droit externe primitivement atteint et augmente dans le sens opposé. Dans ces cas le traitement prismatique appliqué précocément peut, à lui seul, donner la guérison; mais s'il est inopérant le résultat chirurgical est toujours excellent. (Figs. 11, 12).

Parésies séquellaires et efficacité des opérations de suppléance

Quand un degré plus ou moins marqué de paralysie persiste, les interventions ont toujours un résultat beaucoup plus modeste. De la même façon, il faut naturellement doser les actions opératoires en fonction de l'impotence résidu-

195

elle et des hyperactions secondaires. Mais l'électro-oculographie nous a montré que les opérations de suppléance type O'Connor sont totalement incapables de réanimer une fonction de duction altérée du fait d'une parésie persistante.

Chaque fois que par ces procédés nous avons supprimé la déviation dans toutes les positions du regard, et par conséquent rétabli la duction de l'oeil primitivement parésié, l'examen des tracés pré-opératoires a montré que le trouble moteur séquellaire était uniquement dû aux hyperactions secondaires, et plus particulièrement à celle de l'antagoniste homolatéral.

A notre avis, l'opération d'O'Connor n'apporte jamais de vraie suppléance motrice dynamique; elle a un effet purement mécanique, et l'on peut obtenir un tel résultat avec des actions opératoires beaucoup moins mutilantes; c'est pourquoi nous avons abandonné cette technique depuis plusieurs années.

BIBLIOGRAPHIE

Berard, P.V., A. Tassy, J.C. Deransart-Ferrero & N. Mouillac-Gambarelli. Valeur séméiologique de l'électro-oculographie motrice de poursuite dans les ésotropies de l'amblyopie strabique. J. fr. Ophtal. 3, 719–730 (1980).

Coat, A. Etude expérimentale et analyse statistique des potentiels électro-oculographiques, physiologiques dans les mouvements oculaires saccadiques et de poursuite. Thèse, Nantes, p. 60, (1976).

Devlamynck, S. L'électro-oculographie pendulaire (poursuite de type sinusoïdal). Physiologie et enregistrement. Thèse, Tours, p. 98 Ronéo (101 réf.), (1972).

Larmande, A.M., M.A. Quéré & M.P. Delplace. Le nystagmus opto-cinétique dans les paralysies de la VIème paire. Bull. Mem. Soc. Franç. Ophtal. 123, 218–489 (1970).

Quéré, M.A., S. Devlamynck, M.P. Delplace & R. Le Borgne. Etude électro-oculographique des mouvements de poursuite. II – Aspects physiologiques de la poursuite sinusoïdale (épreuve pendulaire). Ann. Oculist. 205, 1321–1338 (1972).

Quéré, M.A. Abnormal ocular movements in amblyopia. Trans. Ophthal. Soc. U.K. 99, 401–406 (1979).

Quéré, M.A., A. Péchereau & F. Lavenant. Les troubles oculogyres des traumatisés crâniens. Rev. oto. neuro. Ophtal. 52, 392–399 (1980).

Quéré, M.A., A. Péchereau & F. Lavenant. Kinectic-electro-oculography. Aims – Disadvantages and limitations. Ophthalmologica, 182, 73–80 (1981).

Weiss, J.B. Le blocage existe-t-il? J. fr. Ophtal. 2, 715–722 (1979).

Authors' address:
Clinique Ophtalmologique Universitaire de Nantes
Hôtel Dieu
44035 Nantes, France

THE TREATMENT OF NON-COMITANT STRABISMUS

P. FELLS
(*London, U.K.*)

INTRODUCTION

I want to make it clear that this paper deals with some forms of squint where certain movements are limited but not because of any ocular muscle paralysis. I have been asked to include specifically dysthyroid ophthalmopathy in this paper and not all ophthalmologists would include such cases under the term 'paralytic' strabismus. Reduced ocular rotation may result from decreased innervation input to a muscle or failure of its antagonist to relax and extend normally. Furthermore, changes in orbital connective tissue may prevent normal movement of the eye despite the muscles contracting powerfully.

METHODS

Certain points in the management of non-comitant strabismus should be emphasised since they must be considered in every case. In the adult diplopia is a distressing symptom which forces most patients to seek urgent medical advice. Every attempt should be made to try to establish the diagnosis once recent head trauma has been eliminated which is an obvious and common cause in many patients. The excellent work by Heinze (Heinze 1969) has shown that head trauma producing avulsion of the nerve rootlets as they leave the brain stem is the most common cause of third, fourth and sixth nerve pareses but that there is rarely total avulsion and some nerve rootlets remain. Birth trauma is much more difficult to evaluate in this connection. Neoplasms are a frequent cause of abducent palsy in all ages with metastatic tumours being found much more often in adults. Infection of the brain and meninges is much commoner in children, but diabetes, vascular disease and aneurysms belong to the adult group. Altered thyroid function must always be considered in adults since diplopia can be the presenting symptom without any preceding proptosis or phase of ocular muscle swelling. Appropriate treatment of the underlying conditions must be instituted. Last, but by no means least, is the eternal question – is this due to decompensation of a congenital or long-standing strabismus? The study of old photographs in these cases can prove invaluable in that a compensatory head posture may be seen to have been present for many years.

Docum. Ophthal. Proc. Series, Vol. 32, ed. by A.Th.M. van Balen & W.A. Houtman 197
© *1982, Dr W. Junk Publishers, The Hague. ISBN 90 6193 728 0*

It is necessary to look for associated changes that may influence the outcome. Trauma is the most important factor here since severe head injury can cause loss of fusion which is usually permanent. A very few proven cases of normal fusion before the accident, followed by loss of fusion for eighteen months to two years, and subsequent fusional recovery are known. (Hart 1969; Stanworth 1974.) This will be referred to later. Traumatic visual field loss, such as occurred in a pilot who crashed and suffered a right homonymous hemianopia plus a right sixth nerve palsy of his dominant eye, caused severe handicap as the usable visual field of the esotropic right eye was almost zero. Furthermore, when the visual fields are reduced the total area of visual field common to each eye may be very small and inadequate for fusional purposes even when the eyes have been rendered as straight as possible. Trauma can also have widespread effects on both the vestibular and cerebellar systems so that even if the eyes can be anatomically aligned in due course there is great functional deficiency because the ability to adjust the gain in the vestibulo-ocular reflex has been altered.

A simple clinical test has recently been shown by Dichgans (Dichgans et al. 1978) to be an excellent indicator of cerebellar pathology. The patient stands, holding his hands together, elbows firmly against his side, and he fixates his extended thumbs. The doctor rotates the patient by his shoulders from side to side whilst watching the patient's eyes. Patients with inadequate suppression of their vestibulo-ocular reflex show nystagmus due to flocculus involvement. Normal subjects can keep their eyes steady.

When trying to assess the local, ocular causes of acquired incomitant squint it is important to differentiate restrictive from paralytical causes. Simple clinical tests include inspecting the affected eye from the side to see if powerfully attempted up gaze causes retraction of the globe into the orbit. This is often positive in dysthyroid patients with inferior rectus tethering, and in orbital floor fractures. More subtle forms of restricted movement may be elicited by the applanation test which shows a rise of more than 4 mm Hg. on trying to look into the field of restricted movement. The patient has to be positioned at the slit-lamp carefully to give reliable results.

The standard traction test using local anaesthesia does not always give easily interpreted results, particularly when slight restrictions are being tested for. Increase in muscle stiffness due to contracture is said to feel different to the connective tissue shortening that causes an abrupt increase in resistance — the so-called 'leash' effect. I find the traction test is only useful with the patient under general anaesthetic. Scott (Scott 1971) has elaborated the test under local anaesthetic to assess the active force that can be generated by the muscle under consideration. Here the surgeon grasps the muscle tendon and tries to hold the eye still against the direction of attempted eye movement. Generated force may be estimated indirectly by comparing saccadic velocities towards and away from the direction of action of the suspect muscle. Electro-oculographic measurements are best for this purpose. These tests not only distinguish restrictive from paralytic causes but also indicate the severity of the paresis and when recovery begins.

Knowledge of the natural history of the various conditions involving the eye movements is essential in planning treatment. Dysthyroid patients who are having treatment for hyperthyroidism have a better chance of a successful result from ocular muscle surgery if they are biochemically euthyroid at the time of operation. (Fells & Waddell 1979). The results are better still if they are euthyroid without the need for anti-thyroid medication. Following orbital blow-out fractures the majority of patients show spontaneous improvement of their ocular rotations over the ensuing weeks and months. Planned surgical intervention within the first two weeks is still indicated if there is gross tethering of the globe inferiorly, or more than 3 mm of enophthalmos, or the ocular rotations are not beginning to show any improvement. The enigma of Brown's syndrome of absent elevation in adduction has been largely solved by studying its natural history. (Waddell) Recalling patients who presented with the condition up to fifteen years ago showed that improvement began around seven years of age, regardless of any surgical treatment, and was complete by twelve to fifteen years of age. Adult patients with the signs of Brown's syndrome are virtually all of the acquired form, mostly traumatic but occasionally iatrogenic trauma from frontal sinus operations.

It is indeed fortunate that many adult neurogenic ocular palsies of whatever cause will improve with time. Most ophthalmologists will wait for six months for such improvement and only consider surgery after that time. During this time the patient must be helped by being encouraged to use a compensatory head posture if this permits a useful area of binocular vision with or without the aid of Fresnel prisms. Partial occlusion of one spectacle lens may be required in some patients and occasionally total occlusion is necessary. Total occlusion should be alternated with the affected eye being left uncovered when the patient is at home in familiar surroundings.

Sixth nerve palsies may be helped surgically in five ways if symptoms persist after six months. Where the affected eye can abduct at least $10°$ beyond the mid-position and saccadic velocity for this appears clinically adequate, then medial rectus recession plus lateral resection of the affected eye should suffice. If the eye cannot abduct to the midline and the traction test at the time of surgery shows no restriction then muscle transfer procedures may be used in young patients, i.e. under twenty years of age (Fells 1971). Recession of the medial conjunctiva may also be necessary at the end of this operation in which the medial rectus is recessed and then the whole of the superior and inferior recti are moved temporally to give a combined vecter force of abduction. Older patients should have Jensen's operation (Jensen 1964) carried out where adjacent halves of the split vertical recti and lateral rectus are sutured together at the level of the equator, plus medial rectus recession. This leaves the anterior ciliary artery over the medial half of each vertical rectus intact to maintain the blood flow to the anterior segment. The following case indicates the importance of considering the anterior blood supply to the eye (Fells 1980).

A twenty-two-year old male suffered a left partial third nerve palsy and left zygomatic triple fracture, together with right seventh and eighth nerve damage plus total failure of right abduction. The fractured right ethmoidal bones were thought· to be responsible for medial tethering and failure of abduction. At operation the traction test was quite normal, indicating total sixth nerve palsy with no recovery in five months. Because of his age, only twenty-two, and no evidence of deficient carotid circulation it was decided to do whole muscle temporal transfers of both vertical recti plus the medial rectus recession. Surprisingly at forty-eight hours there were unequivocal signs of anterior segment ischaemia with wrinkles in Descemet's membrane and an irregularly dilated pupil. Local and systemic steroids were given and the cornea and aqueous cleared over the next few days but not before fine, anterior subcapsular lenticular opacities had been noted at seventy-two hours. These lens changes were identical with those described in acute glaucoma, yet daily measurements of the intra-ocular pressure had never been higher than 14 mm Hg. This case suggests that not only are iris atrophy and spiralling in acute glaucoma due to ischaemia, but also the 'Glaukomflecken'. The second conclusion to be drawn is that the arbitrary rule that I proposed in 1972 that after twenty years of age a Jensen type of operation leaving at least two anterior ciliary arteries should be used is not to be broken with impunity.

A fourth operation that introduces the use of adjustable sutures in lateral rectus palsy has recently been described by Carlson & Jampolsky (1979). Here the temporal halves of the superior and inferior recti are detached and their tendons sutured together deep to the lateral rectus making an adjustable bridle. The medial rectus is recessed, also on an adjustable suture, and then the horizontal forces can be balanced to give optimal position and movements of the eyes. After any of these methods have been used and there is still diplopia on full lateral gaze because of incomplete restoration of abduction, a weakening procedure of recession, or Fadenoperation, or both may be made on the yoke medial rectus. If there is no deviation in the primary position the proponents of the Fadenoperation would claim this as the best manoeuvre since it would reduce innervational factors alone. In practice the recession operation may be equally effective and simpler to do.

Unilateral fourth nerve palsies needing surgery have had a bad reputation because initial accurate alignment or even undercorrection by recession of the yoke inferior rectus may sometimes be followed by an overcorrection despite good fusion pre-operatively. Recession of the direct antagonist, the ipsilateral inferior oblique, by itself often leaves an undercorrection, necessitating a second operation. Combining these two procedures, with the inferior rectus being placed on an adjustable suture gives the best chance of a good result from one operation.

Bilateral fourth nerve palsies, typically traumatic in origin, cause disproportionate disability because of the torsional diplopia, particularly on down gaze, that results. I have long advocated (Fells 1972) and used with success the re-alignment of the anterior half of each superior oblique muscle to produce more intorsion without affecting vertical movements. Although this procedure usually gives excellent relief of symptoms there is often some residual underaction. Rarely, however, it may produce overaction with excessive intorsion on down gaze. Metz (1981) has recently adapted the adjustable technique to this anterior half advancement of the superior oblique with good effect.

I now propose to describe the adjustable suture technique that I use in sufficient detail to allow its proper use. First it is apparent that the procedure may be performed in one or two stages. It is possible that the whole operation and adjustment could be done using local anaesthesia. However, in practice I first used the two stage method of surgery under general anaesthesia followed the next morning by adjustment with local anaesthesia. I prefer to adjust recessed muscles and aim to maintain full insertional width. The option of further recessing the muscle and not only being able to pull the recessed muscle forwards should be available. At the end of the operation the Dexon suture should be fully covered by conjunctiva.

Initially I limited myself to working on rectus muscles and having only one adjustable suture per eye. This latter rule may be broken as soon as familiarity with the technique is gained. 6-0 double-armed Dexon with spatulate needles is attached securely to the muscle via a conjunctival opening over the normal insertion of the muscle. The muscle is disinserted and each suture end is passed through the original scleral insertion twice to maintain full muscle width. The suture is tied over a squint hook with a single throw and temporarily completed with half of a bow leaving a loop (Fig. 1). If this knot is

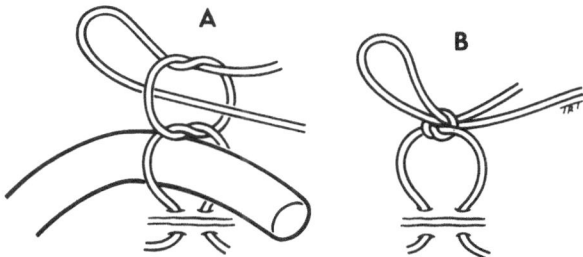

Fig. 1. A. Showing the adjustable suture being tied over the end of a strabismus hook. B. When the second throw with the loop is pulled tight the knot holds securely but can be readily undone at adjustment because it has been prevented from embedding itself in the sclera.

pulled tight against the sclera it is difficult to loosen the suture during adjustment. I instill one drop of prednisolone before suturing the lateral ends of the conjunctival incision but leave a central access gap. Only chloramphenicol drops are used at the end of the operation, not ointment, which would make the sutures slippery.

Next morning the patient must be fully alert for the adjustment and to this end special premedication before the original operation is used. I give pethidine and perphenazine pre-operatively, and my anaesthetist uses nitrous oxide gas induction and so avoids intravenous thiopentone. For the adjustment the patient is seated and 1% amethocaine drops instilled. The ocular movements are checked subjectively and objectively for both near and far using either the cover test or the Maddox rod. If the eyes are satisfactory the loop is pulled through, completing the knot, the ends trimmed and buried beneath the conjunctiva. I wear telescopic glasses with a headlight and use Max Fine corneal forceps whilst my assistant holds the lids apart with cotton bud sticks. If the muscle is too far back the suture is pulled forwards in two stages, tied temporarily with the half bow and the ocular position re-checked (Fig. 2). It is possible to further recess the muscle by slackening the sutures and then making the patient contract the muscle briskly whilst I hold the globe

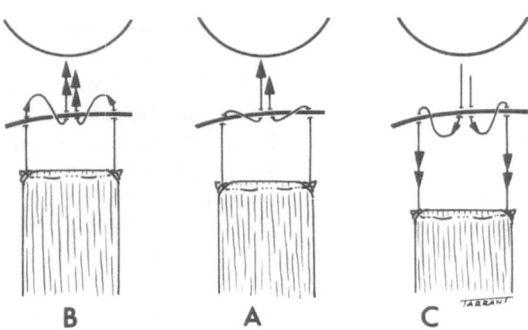

Fig. 2. A. Shows position of recessed muscle when the suture has been untied and is ready for adjustment. B. To bring the muscle forwards, i.e. to *decrease* the recession, a loop is pulled forwards as shown by the single arrow each side, the double arrows show second part of drawing the suture forwards. C. To *increase* the recession the sutures are pulled through in 2 stages as indicated by the single and double arrows. See main text.

firmly by the sclera so that the muscle moves further back. These manoeuvres are repeated as necessary to produce the required position of the eyes.

Although good results were obtained with seven out of eight unilateral fourth nerve palsies so treated there was an interesting complication in one patient. This twenty-three year old man had been unconscious for six days following a severe road traffic accident which left him with constant diplopia and no demonstrable fusion due to a right superior oblique palsy. He accepted the risk that surgery might make his diplopia worse by merely bringing the two images closer. At operation under general anaesthetic the right medial and left inferior recti were recessed on adjustable sutures. Next morning the patient was suppressing and adjustment had to be carried out using objective assessment alone. This was easy for the height but he was left esotropic in the distance. Four hours later his diplopia had returned and with base out prisms he could fuse. Over the next five months the esotropia has decreased and he now has a full field of binocular single vision without prisms.

Dysthyroid ophthalmopathy is particularly suitable for the adjustable suture technique because the results of conventional strabismus therapy where the tight rectus muscle are recessed are peculiarly unpredictable. Often a greater than standard recession of the tethered medial and inferior recti is needed. Some patients require recession of both medial and both inferior recti. In these circumstances I do a maximal recession of the medial rectus on one side and of the inferior rectus on the other. The inferior rectus of the first side and the medial rectus of the other are placed on adjustable sutures, keeping to one adjustable per eye. Next day the height is corrected first using the inferior rectus and the horizontal diplopia corrected at near and far using the medial rectus. When the superior rectus is too tight this may be recessed using a sliding suture but at adjustment next day is not quite so accessible.

Although at operation I try to place the muscle in the position that I judge to be correct in practice only seven patients out of thirty-five needed no adjustment. This means that by conventional assessment of muscle placement I was getting it right in only 20% of cases. After adjustment twenty-six out of thirty-five, i.e. over 77%, had good to excellent results.

A number of factors led me to consider carrying out the whole procedure with local anaesthetic so that surgery and adjustment took place in one operation. One patient needing diplopia correction had already had a large number of general anaesthetics for orthopaedic operations and I wished to avoid additional anaesthetics. Another patient had suffered massive, near-fatal pulmonary embolism after his last general anaesthetic for some non-ocular condition and I was not prepared to give him another general anaesthetic. Where both eyes need surgery, or the eye cannot be voluntarily moved to a position that would allow surgical access, the two stage method must be used.

In the one stage procedure a different pre-medication of propranolol (Inderal) 40 mg orally was used. Local anaesthetic drops of G. Adrenaline 0.01% and G. Cocaine 4% are given and *no* anaesthetic is injected into the muscle sheath. This is to ensure that as far as possible normal muscle innervation is maintained. All movements by the surgeon are as gentle as possible, in particular the use of the squint hook, and stretching of tissues kept to a minimum. It is possible using local anaesthetic drops alone to operate on any of the four recti and even to recess the inferior oblique. If a recession/resection operation is required then the muscle is recessed and left on an adjustable suture and then the second muscle resected. Adjustment is carried out using a Maddox rod but it is not so easy to check the distance position. At the end of the operation the conjunctiva can be closed completely so that no irritable Dexon remains on the surface. The time taken for this one stage procedure is often less than the total time for the two stage method.

Patients whose affected eye is centrally positioned but with generally restricted movements and a very small field of binocular fixation may be helped by surgery to the fellow eye. This boy still had considerable vertical diplopia after orbital floor surgery so the next operation was simultaneous recession of both the superior and inferior recti of the unaffected eye with a great improvement in his binocular field. It appears this is not a widely used method although it is merely the logical extension of the long-established practice of weakening the overacting yoke muscle (Fig. 3).

When this same principle is applied to third nerve palsies the results are usually far from satisfactory. The reason is that the orbital fracture patient has intact cranial nerves and normal vestibulo-ocular reflexes. The misdirection-regeneration after third nerve palsies means that the opportunities for normal binocular control of movements have usually been irretrievably lost. A reasonable, static, primary position is the best that can be hoped for. Two recent operations may help to achieve this. Scott's transposition of the still acting superior oblique insertion to in front of the medial end of superior rectus insertion without releasing its tendon from the trochlea reduces the hypotropia while preserving intorsion (Scott 1977). Where re-innervation gives good elevation of the ptotic lid when the patient looks away from the palsied side this may be utilised by recessing the lateral rectus and resecting the medial rectus of the *un*affected eye. The patient exerts

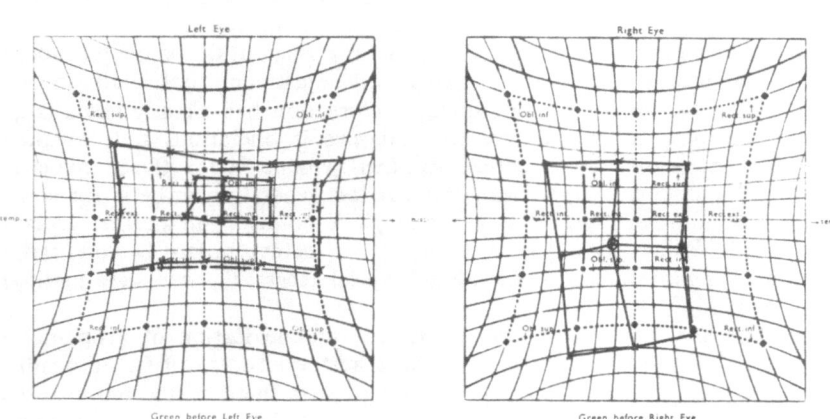

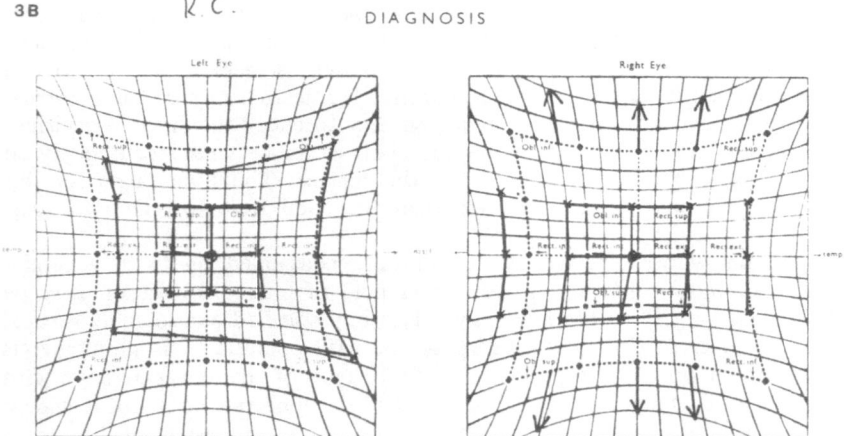

Fig. 3A and B.

gaze effort to centralise this eye which now elevates the ptotic lid in the primary position.

An even more interesting development in third nerve palsies is the use of very weak pilocarpine drops which directly stimulate the iris sphincter and the ciliary muscle (Flynn 1981). I find 0.1% G. pilocarpine used three times daily gives adequate miosis and improved accommodation, particularly if the patient is normally hypermetropic. Careful refraction before and at different times after the pilocarpine may allow a single focus convex lens to be used which gives good vision at all distances. This eight year old boy suffered a traumatic partial third nerve palsy eight

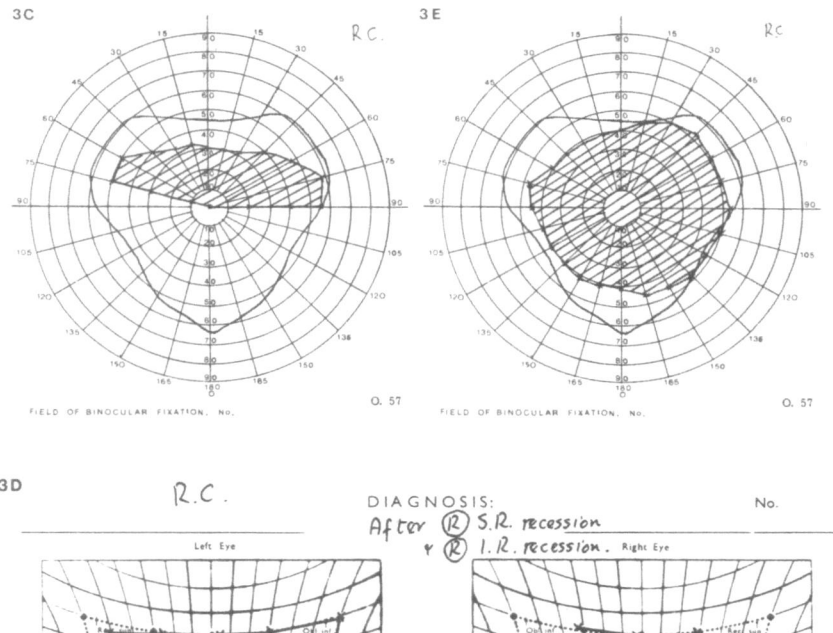

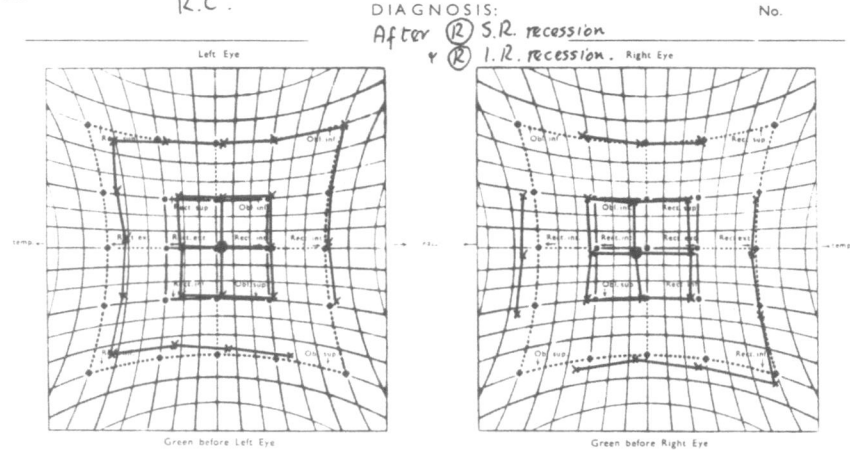

Fig. 3. A. Hess chart of boy who had reduced vertical movements of his left eye before any surgery was done. B. Hess chart after left orbital floor surgery gave improvement, but still much overaction of right vertical recti. C. Field of binocular single vision is still very restricted vertically. D. Hess chart after surgery to *right* eye where the superior and inferior recti were each recessed 5 mms. E. Enormously enlarged field of binocular single vision produced.

months ago. Wearing a +2.25 D.S./−0.50 D.C. axis 160° lens he sees 6/5 distance and N10 for near with the pilocarpine drop in use. The Hess chart also shows improved binocular control but whether this can also be attributed to the local cholinergic drug or not remains to be established (Fig. 4).

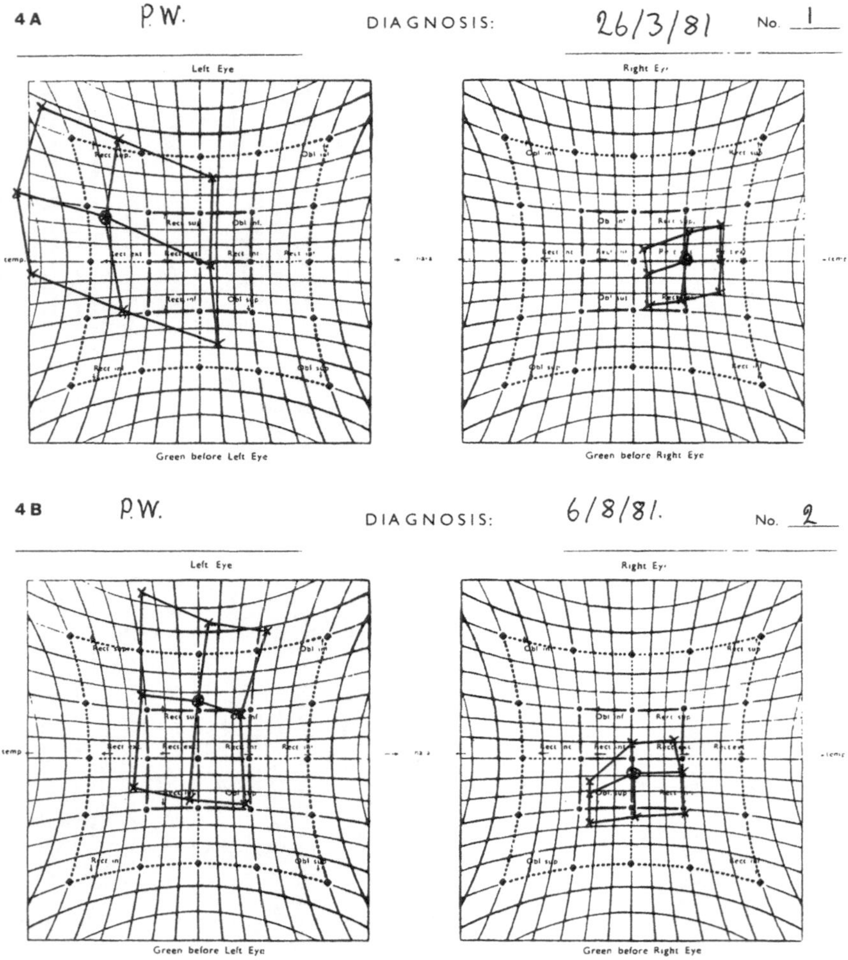

Fig. 4. A. Hess chart of 8 year old boy with traumatic partial left third nerve palsy four months after injury. B. Improved Hess chart eight months after injury and having used G. Pilocarpine 0.1% three times a day for preceeding three weeks.

CONCLUSION

I would like to remind you that better understanding of the changes in the orbital connective tissue and the ocular muscles is enabling appropriate surgery where indicated to be used at the time dictated by the natural history of the condition. Adjustable sutures are giving the surgeon a new confidence in gaining the best results for the patient. Central nervous system control and fusion may be hopelessly affected in some conditions but better understanding of the basic mechanisms of nerve regeneration and re-innervation points the way ahead. There is still a long way to go before we can begin to offer restoration of binocular control to everyone who needs it.

REFERENCES

Carlson, M.R. & A. Jampolsky. An adjustable transposition procedure for abduction deficiencies. Am. J. Ophthal. 87, 382 (1979).

Dichgans, J., G.M. von Reutern & U. Rommelt. Impaired suppression of vestibular nystagmus by fixation in cerebellar and non-cerebellar patients. Arch. Psychiat. Nerverkr. 226, 183 (1978).

Fells, P. Vertical rectus muscle transplantation to restore abduction in 'Orthoptics: Proc. second International Orthoptic Congress, Amsterdam 1971', ed. by J. Mein, J.J.M. Bierlaagh and T.E.A. Brummelkamp-Dons, p. 229 Excerpta Medica, Amsterdam.

Fells, P. The rôle of the oblique muscles. Trans. of Ophthal. Soc. U.K. 92, 705 (1972).

Fells, P. & E. Waddell. Ocular muscle involvement in dysthyroid disease in 'Secondary Strabismus: Proc. tenth meeting of the C.E.S.S.D., Athens' p. 83 (1979).

Fells, P. Anterior segment ischaemia: lens changes after strabismus surgery. Trans. of Ophthal. Soc. U.K. 100, 398 (1980).

Flynn, J.T. Personal communication (1981).

Hart, C.T. Disturbances of fusion following head injury. Proc. Roy. Soc. Med. 62, 704 (1969).

Heinze, J. Cranial nerve avulsion and other neural injuries in road accidents. Med. J. Australia 2, 1246 (1969).

Jensen, C.D.F. Rectus muscle union: a new operation for paralysis of the rectus muscles. Trans. Pacif. Coast Oto-ophthal. Soc. 45, 359 (1964).

Metz, H.S. The adjustable Harada-Ito procedure. Arch. Ophth. 99, 624 (1981).

Scott, A.B. Extra-ocular muscle forces in strabismus in 'The Control of Eye Movements' ed. by P. Bach-y-Rita, C.C. Collins and J.E. Hyde, p. 327. Academic Press (1971).

Scott, A.B. Transposition of the superior oblique. Amer. Orthoptic J. 27, 11 (1977).

Stanworth, A. Defects of ocular movements and fusion after head injury. Brit. J. Ophthal. 58, 288 (1974).

Waddell, E. Brown's syndrome revisited. Brit. Orthoptic J. (1982 in press).

Author's address:
Moorfields Eye Hospital
London, U.K.

USE OF ADJUSTABLE SUTURE TECHNIQUE IN SURGICAL MANAGEMENT OF NON-COMITANT SQUINT

J. SJÖSTRAND

(*Göteborg, Sweden*)

ABSTRACT

The adjustable suture technique as described by Jampolsky (1978) was used in order to manage surgically different types of ocular motility problems. The goal of surgery was to produce alignment in primary position and a binocular visual field as large as possible. The results of 22 cases with disturbed motility following thyroid myopathy, orbital processes, strabismus operations and neurological disorders will be presented. The technique was considered to be favourable in the majority of these cases with a low reoperation rate.

INTRODUCTION

In the management of non-comitant squint the use of adjustable sutures have been advocated by several authors (Rosenbaum et al. 1977; Scott et al. 1977; Jampolsky 1979; Scott & Thalacker 1981) during the last decade. By this adjustable suture technique the surgeon can either adjust the recession during operation under topical anesthesia (Thorsen & Jampolsky 1966; Boergen 1981) or early postoperatively following operation in general anesthesia (for review, see Jampolsky 1979). The second approach, which represents a two-stage technique and gives the surgeon a second chance to alter the effect of operation, was used in this study.

Cases of squint were selected, where I knew that the results with ordinary techniques were unpredictable. The goal of the surgery was to produce alignment in primary and reading positions and a binocular field as large as possible. The result of this study supports the results of others that the adjustable suture technique is the method of choice in certain cases of non-comitant squint.

MATERIAL AND METHODS

In my series of 22 cases the age varied between 18 and 80 years. With the adjustable suture technique as described by Jampolsky (1978) I have operated on both horizontal and vertical recti in four different groups of non-comitant squint: (1) Thyroid myopathy; (2) Acquired orbital restrictions; (3) Different types of paralytic strabismus, gaze palsies or skew deviation; (4) Reoperations with restrictions and incomitance (Table 1).

Thus almost all of my patients (except group 4) had an acquired type of adult strabismus and a good potential for fusion could be anticipated preoperatively. Preoperatively and one to several months postoperatively the deviation was recorded by use of Lee's screen and by prism cover testing and video recording in all cardinal directions. In some cases the binocular diplopia field was measured by using Goldmann perimetry.

During operation forced duction testing is carried out to identify restrictions. The muscle to be recessed with an adjustable suture is identified and a single, double-armed 6-0, dyed Vicryl is inserted into the muscle near its insertion. The muscle is cut and the needles are passed like two 'crossed

Table 1. Summary of patient data.

Group of non-comitant squint	Number of patients	Number of adjustable sutures in each patient	Postoperative adjustment of sutures in mm.	Improvement* postoperatively		
				0	partial	complete
Thyroid myopathy	7	1–4	0–4		4	3
Orbital restrictions	4	1	0–2		2	1
Neurological dys-functions:						
nerve palsies	6	1	0–2		2	4
supranuclear dis-orders	3	1–2	2–4	2	1	
Reoperations (secondary strabismus)	2	1	0		1	1

*Alignment in primary and reading position = *complete*; alignment with prisms (≤ 6△) = *partial* and no change = 0.

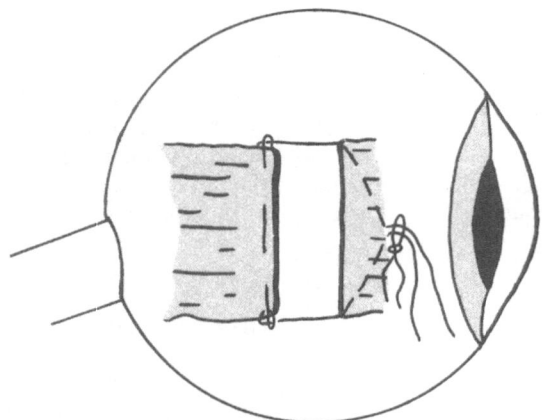

Fig. 1. Schematic drawing of the adjustable suture technique used.

210

swords' through the original insertion and the sclera anterior to it (Fig. 1). A sliding knot of the same suture material, secured with four knot ties, is used to adjust the suitable amount of recession determined by the surgeon on the basis of preoperative measurements and the passive forces during surgery. The general rule used by me has been to do more recession than ordinary estimated in conventional surgery. At the end of the operation the conjunctiva is recessed and sutured to the original muscle insertion and the episclera. This leaves the sclera bare in front of the muscle insertion. The sliding knot, securing the adjusted sutures, are therefore exposed and easy to grasp and adjust postoperatively. In 18 patients one muscle has been adjusted and in some patients two adjustable sutures have been placed, one in each eye or on two adjacent muscles in one or two eyes (4 patients).

It is important to dissect sharply through Lookwoods ligament, when supramaximal recessions of the inferior rectus are performed, otherwise lower lid retraction may be produced.

The morning following surgery adjustment of the suture(s) was made to eliminate persisting diplopia in primary position (Fig. 1). Postoperative adjustment was needed in 12 of the cases and in these cases the suture was loosened or tightened to correct an overcorrection or undercorrection before the suture finally was tied down and cut.

RESULTS AND COMMENTS

Thyroid myopathy

Following preoperative evaluation operation was delayed until the medical condition and motility status were considered stable for at least six months. In all the seven patients operated upon preoperative diplopia in primary position was present and restrictions especially in vertical gaze could be diagnosed. Supramaximal recessions of up to 10 mm was carried out on the vertical recti in most patients.

Fig. 2A shows a typical patient with thyroid myopathy with marked restriction of the right inferior rectus as visualized in this figure on attempted upgaze. In this case I performed a recession with an adjustable suture on the right inferior rectus. Following operation and adjustment of the suture on the first postoperative day a stable alignment in primary and reading position was obtained with some added prism. Fig. 2B demonstrates the improved elevation of the right eye following operation. In some other cases, however, the balancing of forces of the restricted superior recti and restricted inferior recti was considered so complicated that I decided to do an adjustable on two muscles in one or two eyes. In cases complicated with a marked horizontal misalignment in addition to the vertical one I combined an adjustable recession on one horizontal and one vertical rectus on the same eye.

In three of the cases with thyroid myopathy I achieved to adjust the binocular field to be positioned in an area surrounding primary position and reading position (Table 1). Fig. 3 shows the binocular field obtained by perimetry testing postoperative in a patient with a small preoperative field

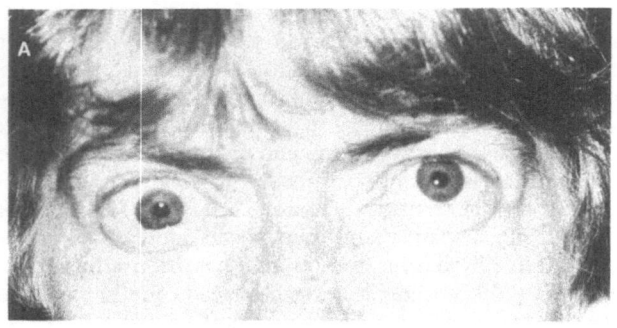

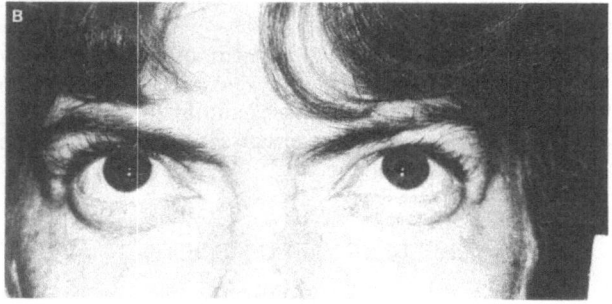

Fig. 2. Case with thyroid myopathy. The marked restriction of the right inferior rectus preoperatively is observed on attempted upgaze (A). Postoperatively marked improvement of elevation of the right eye is observed on upgaze (B).

centered around the extreme (50°–60°) downgaze position. In four cases a small amount of prism was needed to obtain single vision in both primary and reading positions.

Scott & Thallacker (1981) have similarly demonstrated the importance of adjustable sutures in the surgical management of thyroid myopathy.

Orbital restrictions

My goal to achieve binocular vision in primary and reading positions was also fulfilled in the four cases with orbital restrictions due to inflammation or fracture.

Neurological disorders

Good postoperative results were obtained in all five cases with acquired superior oblique palsy, where I included an adjustable vertical or horizontal rectus recession to eliminate a marked vertical and/or horizontal deviation in primary position. The surgical goal (see above) was also reached in one case with a partially recovered abducens paralysis, where an adjustable recession of the medial rectus was performed.

212

(a)

(b)

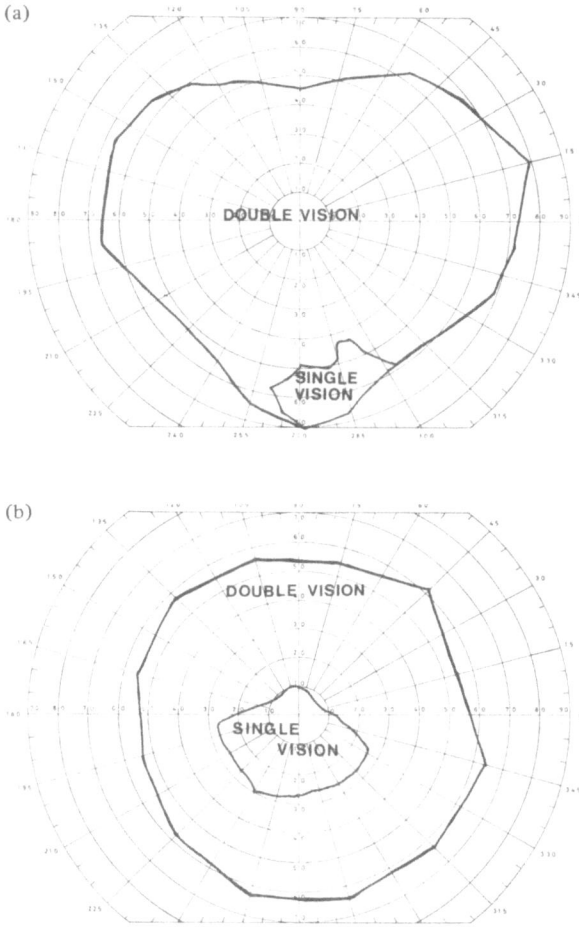

Fig. 3. Pre- and postoperative (3 months) visual fields with single or double vision in one representative case with thyroid myopathy. Postoperatively the field with single vision is well centered even though it is restricted due to the persisting stiffness of the muscles. Binocular diplopia fields were measured with stimulus II:4 using the Goldmann perimeter.

However, in the three cases with supranuclear disorders (gaze palsies, skew deviation) the results were discouraging. Besides minor improvement in one case no postoperative effects were seen.

Reoperations

Previous studies have shown that adjustable recession technique is a practical and effective means to use in complicated reoperation cases (Rosenbaum et al. 1977). In the present study adjustable sutures were used on two cases with

213

restrictions and non-comitant squint following previous strabismus operations. For example, in one case with secondary exotropia, restrictions and constant diplopia following previous surgery for primary oblique muscle dysfunction, reoperation could align the deviating eye in a diplopia-free position in the primary position. Therefore, when diplopia is feared postoperatively in adult cases, adjustable sutures could be indicated even in cases without restrictions.

In conclusion, my study demonstrates that adjustable sutures are indicated when alignment in primary and reading positions is difficult to obtain in one operative session with conventional techniques. Since the amounts of recession needed are difficult to estimate in patients with restrictions, these patients are the favourite group for the surgeon using adjustable sutures. It gives him a second chance to adjust early postoperatively and no lasting overcorrection has to be feared, when supramaximal recessions are performed at operation.

The surgical effect of adjustable sutures on three cases with supranuclear disorders, such as gaze palsies and skew deviations were negligible. However, since only three patients with supranuclear disorders have been operated on I plan to extend this group in order to test the relevance of the negative finding obtained in this study.

ACKNOWLEDGEMENTS

I am grateful to Dr. Lars Frisén for preoperative evaluation and referral of the major part of the patients and to Maths Abrahamsson for help with the schematic drawings.

REFERENCES

Boergen, K.-P. Operation in Oberflächenanästhesie bei endokriner Orbitopathie. Klin. Mbl. Augenheilk. 178, 453–456 (1981).
Jampolsky, A. Adjustable strabismus suture techniques. In: The New Orleans Academy of Ophthalmology Symposium on Strabismus, Mosby, St. Louis. (1978).
Jampolsky, A. Current techniques of adjustable strabismus surgery. Am. J. Ophthalmol. 88, 406–418 (1979).
Rosenbaum, A., H. Metz, M. Carlson & A. Jampolsky. Adjustable rectus muscle recession surgery. Arch. Ophthalmol. 95, 817–820 (1977).
Scott, W., A. Martin-Casals & O. Jackson. Adjustable sutures in strabismus surgery. J. Pediatr. Ophthalmol. 14, 71–75 (1977).
Scott, W.E. & J.A. Thalacker. Diagnosis and Treatment of thyroid myopathy. Ophthalmol. 88, 493–498 (1981).
Thorsen, J. & A. Jampolsky. Topical anesthesia for strabismus surgery. Trans. Am. Acad. Ophthal. Otolaryngol. 76, 968 (1966).

Author's address:
Department of Ophthalmology
Sahlgren's Hospital
S-41345 Göteborg, Sweden

DUANE'S RETRACTION SYNDROME: DIAGNOSIS AND THERAPEUTIC CONSIDERATIONS IN 150 CASES

K. KRZYSTKOWA, J. PAJAKOWA, C. BILSKA & J. PYZOWSKI

(Cracow, Poland)

ABSTRACT

In a period of 9 years (1972–1981) 150 patients with Duane's retraction syndrome (DRS) were treated in the Department of Pathophysiology of Vision and Neuroophthalmology Copernicus Academy of Medicine in Cracow.

The syndrome was more frequent in women and in the left eye. Patients were divided into 3 groups depending on the type of DRS. This congenital eye movement disorder was characterized by abduction deficiency (except Type II), adduction limitation, globe retraction, and palpebral fissure narrowing on attempted adduction. Compensatory head posture was observed in most patients.

Apart from complete ophthalmological examination in a group of these patients electromyography and oculomyodynamometry were performed.

Surgical treatment was applied in 47 cases with large squint and marked retraction of the eyeball, or compensatory head posture. Operations were performed on the horizontal rectus muscles of the affected and sound eyes. According to the indications in some cases Cüppers' posterior fixation suture was used for the hyperactive muscles of the sound eye, and in others Hummelsheim's transposition procedure on the affected eye.

The results obtained in 46 surgical patients are reported.

The congenital retraction syndrome was first described by Williams (1875), then by Stilling (1887) and Türk (1896). Duane (1905) presented the clinical symptoms in 54 cases (Burian & von Noorden 1974).

In the Polish literature the retraction syndrome was described by Orłowski et al. (1960) as well as by Michniowska-Leonowicz & Krych (1960), Maciejasz (1968) and Krzystkowa et al. (1980).

This syndrome in its classic form is characterized by the following features: 1) severe limitation or absence of abduction, most often of the left eye, or occasionally both eyes; 2) limitation of adduction differing in degree; 3) globe retraction and the narrowing of the palpebral fissure on adduction; 4) frequently associated elevation or depression in adduction.

The retraction syndrome is congenital and may be hereditary. According to Malbran (1953) three types may be distinguished. This division may be of importance in deciding the indications for surgery.

Docum. Ophthal. Proc. Series, Vol. 32, ed. by A.Th.M. van Balen & W.A. Houtman 215
© 1982, Dr W. Junk Publishers, The Hague. ISBN 90 6193 728 0

Type I (the classical) is the most frequent and exhibits all the symptoms listed above; esotropia or orthophoria occurs in the primary position. Type II exhibits limitation of adduction and slight exotropia, though usually abduction is intact. On attempted adduction retraction and palpebral fissure narrowing also occur. Frequently, the adducted eye moves upward, more seldom downward. Type III (Malbran 1953) is characterized by esotropia and narrowing of the palpebral fissure in the primary position, limitation or absence of elevation and depression, and globe retraction on adduction.

Huber (1964) has distinguished three types of DRS based on electromyographic recording. The Duane I type shows limited or absent abduction with relatively normal adduction; Duane II, limited or absent adduction with relatively normal abduction; and Duane III, limited or absent abduction and adduction. Huber considers that Duane III might be caused by an absent abducens nerve with oculomotor innervation to the lateral rectus muscle. Dual innervation of the lateral rectus muscle by both the abducens and the oculomotor nerves could account for Duane II. Duane I may be due to a partial double innervation of the lateral rectus muscle.

The retraction syndrome is often associated with other ocular lesions and systemic congenital malformations.

Various theories of its pathogenesis have been based on surgical, electromyographical and post mortem data (Malbran 1953; Lyle 1970). Possible aetiological factors include fibrosis of the lateral rectus muscle, with a resultant inelastic fibrous band, or paradoxical innervations because of anomalous peripheral or internuclear connections. In the latter cases it has been shown that there is co-contraction of the medial and lateral rectus muscles on attempted adduction, resulting in retraction of the globe. On attempted abduction the lateral rectus muscle is not innervated; this has been documented electromyographically (Papst & Esslen 1960; Wójtowicz 1968) or by oculomydynamometry (Mądroszkiewicz 1978).

Here we shall not discuss aetiological problems, but only mention that recently Hotchkiss et al. (1980) have described a well documented case of the bilateral retraction syndrome based on surgical and autopsy studies. Both abducens nuclei and nerves were absent from the brain stem and the lateral rectus muscles were partially innervated by branches from the oculomotor nerves.

MATERIAL

Our material from 1962 to 1981 includes 150 cases of retraction syndrome. The sex and age are given in Table 1.

The left eye was more often affected (100 cases) than the right, (32 cases), and bilateral forms (18 cases) are more often seen in males (12 cases) than in females. Our material was divided into three types, following Malbran (1953) (Table 2).

Visual acuity and refraction are shown in Tables 3 and 4. Normal visual acuity and slight amblyopia were very frequently observed, as were slight hyperopia and emmetropia. Anisometropia was found in 28 cases (18.6%). Eyeball position differed according to the type.

216

Table 1. Duane's Retraction Syndrome (D.R.S.). Material (1962–1981).

No. of patients	Sex		Age in years	
	♀	♂	4–15	16–30
150	105	45	125	25
100.0%	70.0	30.0	83.3	16.7

Table 2. Classification of patients with D.R.S.

Type of D.R.S. after Malbran	No. of patients	
	n	%
I	130	86.7
II	17	11.3
III	3	2.0
Total No. of patients	150	100.0

Table 3. Visual acuity in 150 cases of D.R.S.

No. of patients	Visual acuity		
	0.5–1.0	0.1–0.4	>0.1
150	131	14	5
100.0%	87.3	9.3	3.4

Table 4. Refraction in 150 cases of D.R.S.

No. of patients	Refraction in dptrs					
	0–+3.0	+3.5–+5.0	>+5.0	0––3.0	–3.5––5.0	>–5.0
150	109	23	8	7	–	3
100.0%	72.7	15.3	5.3	4.7	–	2.0

Table 5. Type and number of operation in 47 cases of D.R.S.*

Affected eye

Type of D.R.S. No. of patients	med. rect. m. recession	lat. rect. m. recession	inf. obl. m. recession or myectomy	inf. rect. m. recession	lat. rect. m. resection	transposition of vertical rect. m. m. (Hummelsheim)
I 40	40	–	13	–	12	19
II 4	–	4	4	–	–	–
III 3	–	–	–	2	–	–

*Several operations were often performed on one patient.

217

Table 6. Type and number of operations in 47 cases of D.R.S.*

Unaffected eye						
Type of D.R.S. No. of patients	med. rect. m. recession	med. rect. m. resection	lat. rect. m. recession	lat. rect. m. resection	inf. obl. m. recession or myectomy	Cüppers' posterior fixation suture
I 40	7	–	–	4	1	4
II 4	–	–	2	–	3	3
III 3	1	1	1	–	2	1

*Several operations were often performed on one patient.

In type I (130 cases) orthoposition without torticollis ocularis was present only in 22 cases (16.9%), esotropia with an angle from +5 to +10° in 57 cases (43.9%), and more marked esotropia with an angle over +10° in 51 cases (39.2%).

In Type II (17 cases) exotropia to –10° was present in 13 cases (76.5%), and over –10° in 4 cases (23.5%). In all cases the adducted eye moved upward; less frequently the eye moved downward.

In Type III (3 cases) there was marked esotropia, over +35°, and retraction with absence of horizontal and limitation of vertical motility. In all patients the main symptom was retraction.

Binocular vision was found by means of polaroid tests, as well as the Worth- and Bagolini tests in 95 patients (63.3%); in 73 of these cases torticollis ocularis was present. By means of the synoptophore (haploscopic examination) binocular vision was found in a greater number of patients (115–76.6%).

No patient exhibited spontaneous diplopia, and provoked diplopia was found in only 10 patients, while unilateral suppression, at gaze on the paretic side, was observed in all other patients.

METHODS AND RESULTS OF SURGICAL TREATMENT

Surgery was performed in 47 cases out of a total of 150.

Types and number of operations performed are presented in Tables 5 and 6. Type 1 was found in most surgical patients (40 cases – 85.1%).

Surgery was indicated only when there was a significant deviation in the primary position, marked retraction, or the anomalous head position was intolerably disfiguring. Operations were performed on the affected and unaffected eye.

When esotropia was present in the primary position, recession of the medial rectus muscle was usually performed (40 cases), accompanied only occasionally by resection of the lateral rectus muscle (12 cases). Resection was performed only in those cases in which paradoxical innervation was excluded by EMG examination or a negative forced duction test. If there was resistance on passive adduction, the lateral rectus muscle might be fibrotic, and a small resection (5—6 mm) of this muscle might enhance the effect of the recession.

If marked esotropia was present in the primary position, a large recession of the medial rectus (5 to 6 mm) was combined with vertical muscles transposition to the lateral rectus muscle (Hummelsheim). In 13 patients with marked elevation on adduction, recession or myectomy of the inferior oblique muscle was performed. On the unaffected eye the recession of the medial rectus muscle was performed in 7 cases, combined with resection of the lateral rectus muscle in 4 cases, of significant esotropia. Cüppers' posterior fixation suture was performed in 4 cases, on the principle of paresis versus paresis. In 7 cases operations were carried out on both eyes.

All surgical patients with Type II were subjected to recession of the lateral rectus muscle and the inferior oblique muscle in the affected eye. In the unaffected eye, Cüppers' posterior fixation suture on the lateral rectus muscle was applied in 3 cases, in 2 with simultaneous recession of this muscle. To compensate vertical deviation, recession of the inferior oblique muscle was performed in 3 cases.

Patients with Type III (3 cases) were the most difficult to treat. Most frequently the sound eye was operated on: in one case recession of the medial rectus, in two cases recession of the inferior oblique muscle, and in one Cüppers' posterior fixation suture on the superior rectus muscle. In the affected eye, recession of the inferior rectus muscle was performed in 2 cases.

The best surgical results were obtained in Types I and II. Orthophoria in the primary position was obtained in 39 cases (83.0%), reduction of the angle in 8 cases (17.0%), but only slight improvement in abduction could be achieved in 14 cases of Type I (29.8%).

DISCUSSION AND CONCLUSIONS

Our studies confirm the opinion of most authors that DRS occurs more often in the left eye and in females. Bilateral forms are infrequent and most often found in men. Visual acuity was normal in most cases, and hyperphoria of slight degree was very frequent (Burian & van Noorden 1974), as well as anisometropia (28 cases — 18.6%).

There are various opinions on surgical indications and methods. The results of surgical treatment of the retraction syndrome have often been disappointing. For this reason, we prefer not to operate when binocular vision is present in the primary position of the eyes, or if it can be maintained with a slight head turn. Surgery is indicated only when there is a significant deviation in the primary position or if the torticollis ocularis is intolerable from an aesthetic point of view, or if significant retraction is present.

There are different methods of operation (Orłowski 1961; Lyle 1970; Krzystkowa et al. 1972; Burian 1974; Krzystkowa et al. 1980). Limited passive adduction indicates fibrosis and loss of elasticity in the lateral rectus muscle. If esotropia is present in the primary position, a large recession of the medial rectus muscle is indicated. This may be combined with a small resection of the lateral rectus muscle or transposition procedure according to Hummelsheim or Jensen. Unrestricted passive adduction indicates a central or peripheral neural basis of retraction, such as co-contraction of the medial and lateral rectus muscles on attempted adduction. In this instance resection of the lateral rectus muscle is contraindicated, for it may increase retraction on adduction. If there is esotropia in the primary position, recession of the medial rectus is recommended (von Noorden 1973).

In some cases operations on the unaffected eye are advisable in order to enable orthophoria in the primary position or more symmetrical eye movements to be obtained on the principle of paresis versus paresis.

REFERENCES

Burian, H.M. & G.K. von Noorden, Binocular vision and ocular motility p. 368. Mosby, St. Louis (1974).

Cüppers, C. Die sog. Fadenoperation. In: BVA, Arbeitskreis Schielbehandlung, Wiesbaden (1974), p. 206, 7. Nürnberg (1975).

Hotchkiss, M.G., N.R. Miller, A.W. Clark & W.R. Green, Bilateral Duane's Retraction Syndrome. Arch. Ophthal. 98, 870 (1980).

Huber, A. et al. Zum Problem des Duane-Syndroms. Graefe Arch. Ophthal. 167, 169 (1964).

Krzystkowa, K. Operacyjne leczenie oczopląsu i zeza sposobem Cüppersa. Klin. Oczna. 48, 501 (1978).

Krzystkowa, K. & B. Huczyńska. Operacyjne leczenie niektórych postaci zezów porażennych. Klin. Oczna., 42, 461 (1972).

Krzystkowa, K., J. Pająkowa, Cz. Bilska & A. Mądroszkiewicz, Zespół Stilling-Türka-Duane'a: Diagnostyka kliniczna i wyniki leczenia operacyjnego. Klin. Oczna. 82, 45 (1980).

Lyle, T.K. Surgical management of congenital musculofacial anomalies. In: Strabismus, 69. Proceedings Europ. Strab. Studio. Ded. Congress. p. 119. Kimpton, London. (1970).

Maciejasz, A. Postać pionowa zespołu Stillinga-Türka-Duane'a. Klin. Oczna. 38, 223 (1968).

Malbran, J. Strabismes et paralysies. (Heraly, Charleroi). 596 (1953).

Mądroszkiewicz, M. Okulomiodynamometr tarczowy. Klin. Oczna. 48, 523 (1978).

Michniowska-Leonowicz, J. & J. Krych, Zespół Stillinga-Türka-Duane'a. Klin. Oczna., 30, 59 (1960).

Noorden, G.K. von. Atlas of strabismus surgery. Mosby, St. Louis. (1973).

Orłowski, W.J. Leczenie chirurgiczne zespołu Stillinga-Türka-Duane'a. Klin. Oczna., 31, 41 (1961).

Papst, W. von. & E. Esslen. Zur Ätiologie der angeborenen Abduzenslähmung. Klin. Mbl. Augenhk. 137, 306 (1960).

Wójtowicz, S. Elekromiografia w neuropochodnych i rzekomo neuropochodynch zaburzeniach ruchomości oczu. A.M. Poznań (1968).

Authors' address:
Department of Pathophysiology of Vision and Neuroophthalmology
Copernicus Academy of Medicine
Kopernika str. 38
Cracow, Poland

220

LA CHIRURGIE DU GRAND OBLIQUE
Etude des voies d'abordage nasal et temporal

J.C. CASTIELLA, J. ORBEGOZO, M.A. ZATO & G. CASTIELLA

(*Bilbao, Spain*)

D'après le procédé chirurgical chaque jour plus fréquent sur l'oblique supérieur, il n'est pas rare de trouver dans la phase pos-opératoire, des tableaux qui ressemblent à la paralysie de l'oblique inférieur (Pseudo-Brown), étant d'apparition précoce ou tardive, c'est pourquoi certains auteurs parlent de 'l'alerte' à l'oblique supérieur (Lavat).

La plupart (Arruga 1961; Burian & von Noorden 1974; Costenbader 1970; Hervouet 1970; Hugonnier 1970; Parks 1975) préfère la voie d'abordage temporale (Technique de Mac Lean) et d'autres (Castanera 1968; Fink 1962; Mocorrea & Locascio 1978) la nasale (Technique de White et Berke), sans spécifier ni les uns ni les autres le pourquoi de cette préfèrence.

Seul Arruga explique le choix de la voie temporale, le procédé opératoire pouvant se dédoubler sur le composant torsionnel (Technique de Harada et Ito) ou sur le vertical alors que du côté nasal le procédé est obligatoirement global.

Nous, nous avons employé au début la voie nasale de realisation plus facile, l'ayant laissée actuellement à cause des tableaux de Pseudo-Brown qui sont apparus plus tard.

Peu d'auteurs ont expliqué la pathogénie de ces tableaux. Ainsi pour Crone (1973) c'est dû à la réalisation d'un plissement excessif, alors que Parks (1975) y implique un phénomène d'adhérence dans le quadrant nasal supérieur. Pour Mocorrea et Col (1978) c'est dû à l'introduction d'éléments qui ne sont pas le tendon dans la zone plissée, ou à la lésion des gaines.

Spielman se référant à Cüppers, l'attribue à une contracture de l'oblique inférieur aggravée par le renforcement d l'antagoniste oblique supérieur.

Nous, nous avons établi la pathogénie mécanique à partir de l'observation d'un Pseudo-Brown dans la phase post-opératoire immédiate à une intervention du plissement de l'oblique supérieur par la voie nasale, tableau qui a cédé avec le temps, et dans lequel, ayant été nécessaire d'intervenir à nouveau, nous avons trouvé que la zone plissée était au-dessous du droit supérieur.

TECHNIQUES

En essayant d'éclaircir la pathogenie de ces syndromes yatrogéniques nous avons réalisé, sur des cadavres, des plissements nasaux comme temporaux, par une voie d'abordage intra-craniènne, pour constater ce qui se passait au moment de faire les différents mouvements de duction.

Technique de White et Berke

Avec cette technique nous avons un plus grand champ chirurgical, bien qu'elle ait l'inconvénient de devoir isoler le tendon de sa gaine qui, à ce niveau est composée de ses trois couches.

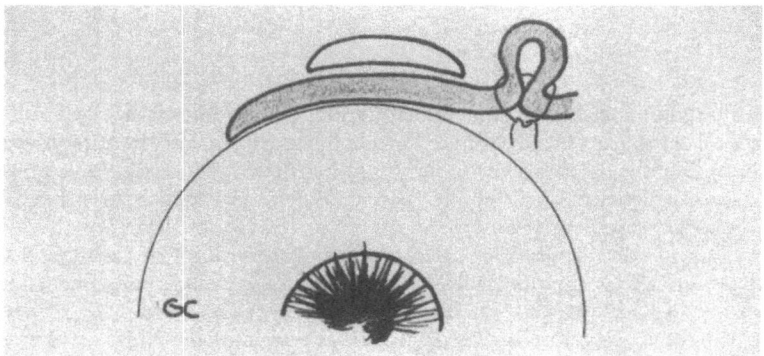

Fig. 1.

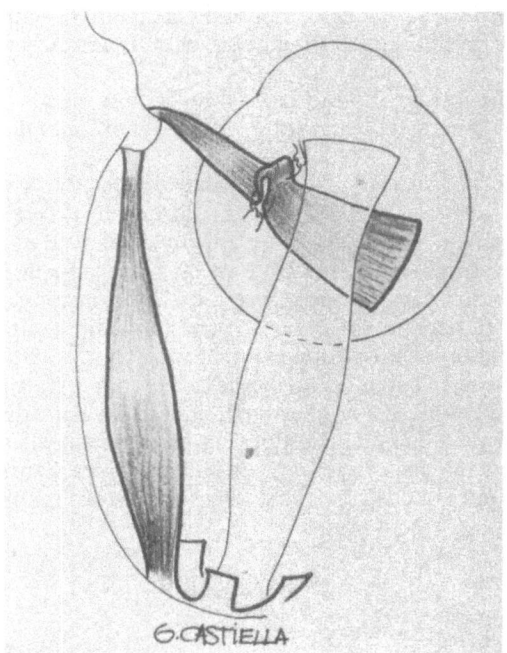

Fig. 2.

Après avoir réalisé le plissement (Figs. 1, 2), nous avons fait le test de duction en essayant d'amener le pôle postérieur vers le dehors et en bas, ce qui exige un relâchement maximum du tendon réflexe de l'oblique supérieur, constatant comment la base du plissement, en effectuant cette manoeuvre choque (Figs. 3, 4) contre le bord nasal du droit supérieur, barrant le passage de la zone plissée, ce qui rend impossible l'alongement de l'oblique supérieur, et par conséquent l'élévation du globe en adduction. Si nous forçons cette situation nous voyons que la difficulté disparaît quand la zone plissée passe sous le droit supérieur.

Technique de Mac Lean

Nous avons beaucoup moins de champ chirurgical puisque pour la réaliser il faut refouler le droit supérieur vers la zone nasale, ayant pour avantage le peu de gaine que présente l'oblique supérieur après être passé au dessous du droit supérieur.

Nous avons essayé de pourvoir à ce que la base du plissement soit le plus près possible de l'insertion de l'oblique supérieur, rabattant son sommet qui s'accroche à un point dans la sclère.

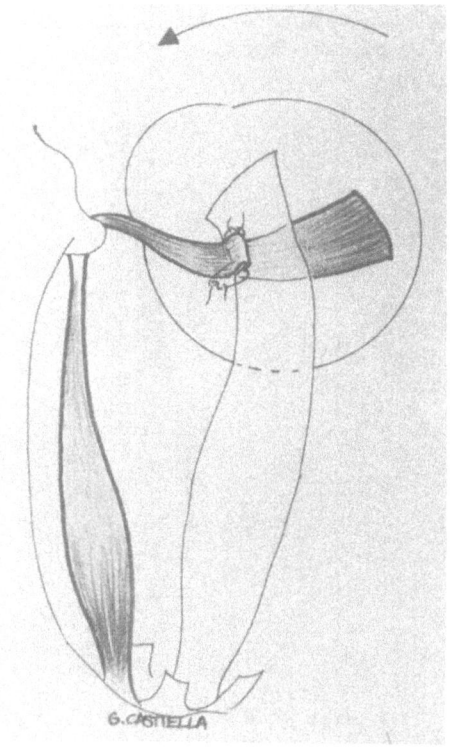

Fig. 3.

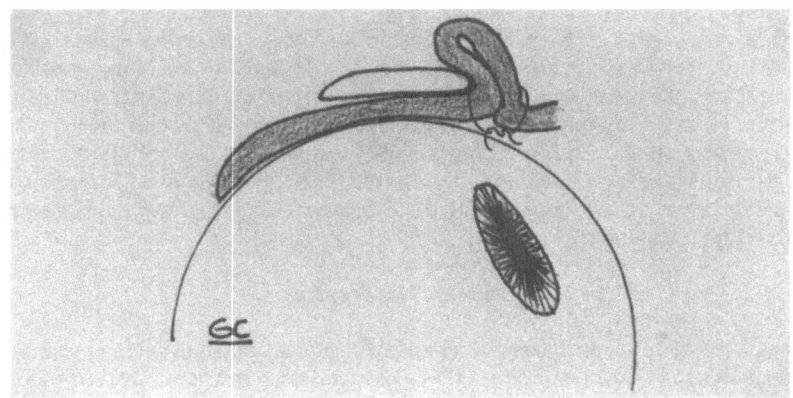

Fig. 4.

Ici nous voyons comment la zone plissée se place sous ou juste au bord temporal du droit supérieur (Figs. 5, 6). C'est pour cela, lorsqu'on réalisé le test de duction, comme nous l'avons fait avant nous ne nous heurtons à aucune difficulté en voyant comment la zone plissée apparaît par le bord temporal du droit supérieur. (Fig. 7).

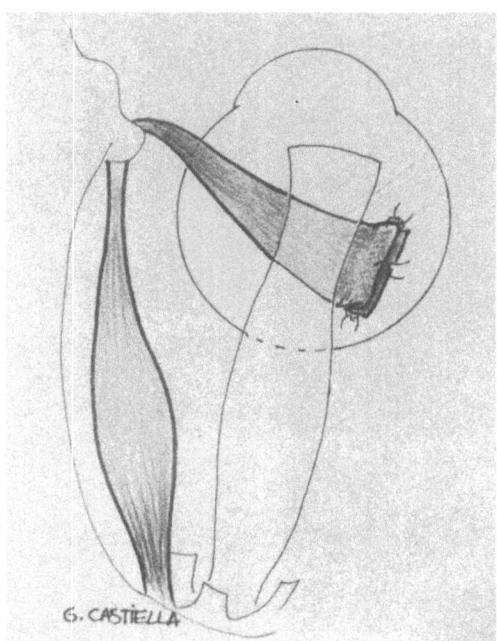

Fig. 5.

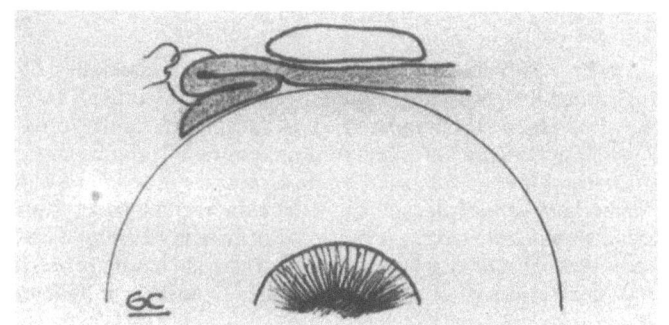

Fig. 6.

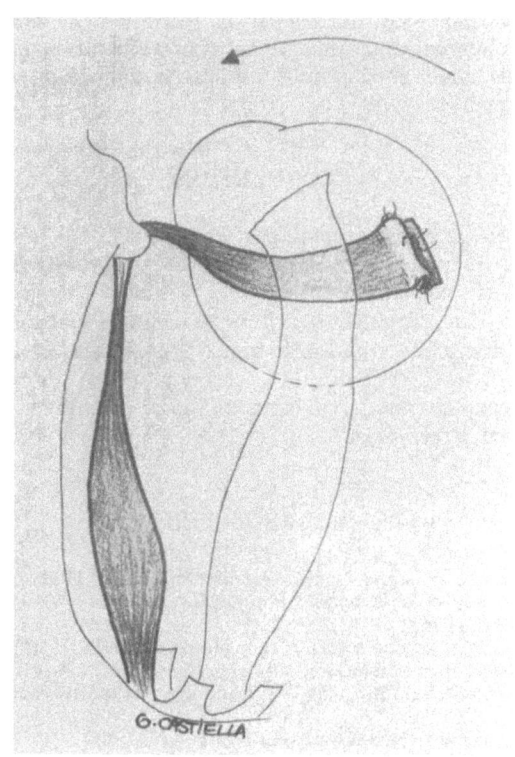

Fig. 7.

225

DISCUSION

Malgré l'existence de deux techniques chirurgicales classiques de renforcement par plissement de l'oblique supérieur (Berke & Mac Lean 1946), la seule différence entre les deux n'apparaît que dans la difficulté plus ou moins grande de procédé chirurgical, n'ayant donc pas de difference dans ses indications, sauf lorsqu'on veut dissocier les deux actions (torsion et dépression de l'oblique supérieur) en déplaçant son insertion vers la partie antérieure ou postérieure, où nous nous verrions obligés d'utiliser la technique de Mac Lean, étant la seule se réalisant dans l'insertion, car dans le cas de procéder pareillement sur la dépression et la torsion on pourrait utiliser indifféremment les deux techniques.

Nous pensons que nous n'avons pas seulement à choisir une technique chirurgicale pour sa difficulté plus ou moins grande mais aussi pour les moindres complications qu'elle pourrait avoir, donc d'après ce que nous avons vu sur les cadavres nous devons rejeter l'abordage nasal comme technique de renforcement de l'oblique supérieur.

Actuellement la tendance des auteurs c'est d'utiliser la technique de Mac Lean (Arruga 1961; Burian & von Noorden 1974; Helveston 1973; Hervouet 1970; Hugonnier 1970; Parks 1975) non seulement pour la possibilité de différencier son action sur la torsion et la dépression ou pour pouvoir réaliser une chirurgie plus ou moins réglable les jours suivants l'opération (Spielman), mais aussi pour éviter des complications post-opératoires du gendre de Pseudo-Brown.

CONCLUSION

Le Pseudo-Brown aprés plissement par voie nasale peut être dû à l'obstacle mécanique entre la zone plissée et le bord nasal du droit supérieur qui empêche l'allongement du tendon.

Le Pseudo-Brown disparaît quand la zone plissée se place sous le droit supérieur produisant une grande adhérence à ce niveau, ce qui rend difficile les réopérations.

C'est pour cela que nous croyons qu'il faut employer la technique de Mac Lean d'abordage temporal.

BIBLIOGRAPHIE

Arruga, A. Estrabismos. Arch. Soc. Oftal. Hispano Americana. 1961.
Berke, R.N. Tenotomy of the superior oblique for hipertropia. Trans. Amer. Ophthal. Soc. 44, 304–342 (1946).
Brown, Anomalias musculares estructurales congénitas. Mosby Co. St. Louis, 219 (1950).
Brown, Syndrome del oblicuo Superior. J. Michigan. Med. Soc. 50, 509–549 (1961).
Burian, & G.K. von Noorden. Binocular Vision and Ocular Motility. Mosby Co. St. Louis (1974).
Castanera, A. Estrabismos y Heteroforias. Paz Montalvo (1968).
Castiella, J.C. Indicación quirúrgica a partir de la gráfica de Hess-Lancaster y Sinoptómetro. Acta Estrab. (1977).

Castiella, J.C. Evolución de las parálisis del oblicuo superior por medio de la pantalla de Lancaster y del Sinoptómetro. Archi. Soc. Esp. de Oftal. Tomo XXXVII, no. 12 (1977).

Catford, & Hart. Superior oblique tendom Syndrome. An electromyographical study. Brit. J. Ophtal. 55, 155 (1971).

Crone, R.A. Diplopia. Excerpta Medica, Amsterdam (1973).

Costenbader, A. Spontaneous regression of pseudoparalysis of the inferior oblique muscle. Arch. Ophtal. 59, 607 (1958).

Dyer, Superior Oblique Tendom Sheat Syndrome. Ann. of Opht. 2, 8, 791–792 (1970).

Espesson, & Coll. Syndrome et pseudo syndrome de Brown. Bull. Soc. Ophtal. Fr. 69, 812–815 (1969).

Fink, W. Surgery of the vertical muscles of the eye. Charles C. Thomas. 20 ed. (1962).

Folk, E. Superior oblique tendom sheat syndrome. Arch. Ophtal. 57, 39 (1957).

Girard, Pseudo paralysis of the inferior oblique muscle. South M.S. 49, 342 (1956).

Hardesty, Surgery of the vertical muscles of the eye. Charles C. Thomas 20 ed. (1962).

Helveston, Atlas of Strabismus Surgery. Mosby C.V. St. Louis. (1973).

Hervouet, & Chevannes. Le Syndrome de la gaine du grand oblique. Ann. Ocilist. 199, 9, 857–865 (1966).

Hervouet, Atlas practique de la chirurgie du strabisme. Mason, New York (1970).

Hugonnier, Strabismes, Mason, New York (1970).

Mocorrea, & Locascio. Clinica y cirugía del estrabismo. Ateneo (1978).

Parks, Ocular motility and strabismus (1975).

Sandford, & Smith. Intermittent superior oblique tendom sheath syndrome 53, 6, 412–418 (1969).

Spielmann, Plicature regalble du grand oblique. Jour. Fr. D'Ort. (1981).

Yamazaki & Ishikawa, Superior oblique tendom sheath syndrome with hito-pathological observation. Jour. Ped. Ophtal. 4, 1, 12–21 (1966).

Authors' address:
Gardoqui no. 1
Bilbao 8-Vijcaya, Spain

227

CONSIDERATIONS ON THE SURGICAL MANAGEMENT OF ISOLATED OCULO-MOTOR PALSIES

M. DELLER

(*Lausanne, Switzerland*)

Under normal conditions, the two eyes as a pair enjoy an innervational balance characterized by parallel ocular axes and harmonious conjugated movements. Static and dynamic elements are attuned to the benefit of binocular single vision.

Paresis of one of the muscle pair causes an innervational imbalance and hence an incomitant deviation. The static disorder is uniquely due to disturbance of the dynamic motor function. A break in this team is troublesome from the cosmetic point of view, and even more so functionally due to the resulting diplopia.

The counter parade of traditional surgery far from satisfies the requirements of an ideal surgical correction, these being in order as follows: A. Suppression of diplopia and recovery of binocular single vision with satisfactory or complete restoration of binocular field. B. Disappearance of torticollis. C. Cosmetic improvement.

It would be only a slight exaggeration to say that even now the order of priorities is reversed, that there are still many authors for whom 'the surgical goal is stable alignment in the primary position (Jampolsky 1975)'. These are satisfied with an essentially cosmetic result, as the diplopia is only eliminated in the primary position. The insufficiences of this surgery are perfectly understandable when the historical development is reviewed.

The original error comes from an unfortunate amalgamation of so-called concomitant and paralytic squints, whereby the rules governing the former are applied to the latter. The desire to correct the deviation by essentially static surgery remains, in spite of the principles for more logical management of oculo-motor palsies having been laid down at the beginning of this surgery by Albrecht von Graefe in 1864.

Over a century passed before exploitation of these principles be made possible in clinical practice, thanks to the efficacy of contact arc surgery introduced in 1974 by Cuppers' retro-equatorial myopexy.

Without doubt also a cosmetic problem, the paretic deviation is particularly troublesome because of the resulting diplopia. This latter remains the same type, but is of varying separation according to the direction of gaze.

As initial operation, the so-called surgical balancing procedure (Albert Graefe) is commonly recommended. This consists of weakening the ipsilateral antagonist to the paretic muscle, according to 'the principle of balancing equally dead forces (Jampolsky 1975)'. The paretic eye may be recentered by these means, but the initial incomitance remains, in addition to the surgically induced incomitance. This has unpleasant consequences, as is seen on the resulting diplopia. Association with a strengthening procedure of the paretic muscle only modifies the position of reversal of diplopia. In both the above cases, the field of binocular single vision initially restricted in the gaze dependant on the paretic muscle becomes also restricted on the opposite gaze.

Albrecht von Graefe was aware of these various inconveniences, and to alleviate them proposed weakening of the associated muscle in the sound eye. In passing, may we pay respects to this emminent master's shrewdness, he being the first to consider an associated gaze function of muscle pairs at a time when neither Hering's law of 1864, nor Sherrington's of 1894 were known. Unfortunately for von Graefe's logical compensatory operation, the best weakening procedure known at the time was unable to produce perfect results. Muscle recession certainly provides a reduction in the motor function of the operated muscle, but is accompanied by a regrettable modification in the static and innervational balance of the sound eye. This produces the same inconveniences as in the first surgical proposals, although to a lesser degree.

Cüppers' retro-equatorial myopexy presents none of these faults, and allows henceforward the application of the only logical surgical procedure. Any muscle having undergone a retro-equatorial myopexy no longer has the same effective rotating force, or torque. The response therefore, to normal motor stimulation, is no longer a normal rotation. Thus the more posterior the anchoring, the more important will be the paretic effect. Cüppers has shown that this latter may be calculated.

One would expect a surgeon to exploit the multiple possibilities of this paretic effect. Progressive restriction of the motor response may be calculated and dosed, without modification of the position of the operated eye. Motor incomitance is eliminated by opposition of the paretic muscle with an artificial palsy of the conjugated muscle. Further, there is gaze stimulation by proprioceptive increase of nervous influx in the conjugated muscle pair.

In clinical terms, this means a reduction or suppression of the paralytic deviation, disappearance of the diplopia, and an improvement if not normalization of the field of binocular single vision. In other words, a restitutio ad integrum.

The originality of Cüppers' surgical procedure is that it introduces a dynamic concept to the management of a kinetic disorder. The ideal surgical protocol for any isolated oculo-motor palsy must provide a simultaneous effect on the binocular muscle pair involving the paretic muscle. This means a strengthening of the latter, combined with a retro-equatorial myopexy of the contra-lateral synergist, the accent being on the myopexy. This latter plays the principal, the motor role. The strengthening of the paretic muscle has a purely mechanical effect. It straightens the eye, and the muscle being put under a passive tension prevents over-action of the ipsilateral antagonist. The retro-equatorial myopexy has on the other hand a dynamic effect, which allows harmonization of the conjugate binocular innervation. This dynamic effect is clearly shown by the fact that the immediate post-operative result is usually incomplete. With time, an adjustment takes place, producing nearly always an ideal final result. This would be inexplicable except by innervational mechanisms.

Further advantages of this protocol are firstly that the choice of muscles operated is not influenced by the fixing eye. Secondly, a single operation is generally sufficient, contrary to the multiple operations usually necessary with traditional surgery.

Thus angle-of-deviation surgery may finally be replaced by the only logical surgery, that is, surgery of direction of gaze.

REFERENCES

Cüppers, C. Die sogenante Fadenoperation. BVA Arbeitskreis Schielbehandlung, Wiesbaden 1974. Freigang, Nürnberg, (1975).

Graefe, A. Die Lähmungen der Augenmuskeln. In Handbuch der Gesamten Augenheilkunde, 2ème édition, Vol. 8, chapitre XI, Berlin Verlag von Julius Springer, p. 81, (1939).

Von Graefe, A. Aphorismen über Tenotomie in Sonderheit gegen paralytische Diplopie. Klinische Monatsblätter für Augenheilkunde, p. 1–22, (1864).

Jampolsky, A. Management of acquired (adult) muscle palsies. In Transactions of the New Orleans Academy of Ophthalmology. Symposium on neuroophthalmology. The C.V. Mosby Company, St. Louis, p. 148–167 (1976).

Author's address:
Monbenon 2
CH-1003 Lausanne, Switzerland

SURGICAL SYMMETRIZATION OF KINETICAL INCOMITANCES

G. SALVI, R. FROSINI & M.C. BOSCHI

(*Firenze, Italy*)

INTRODUCTION

Two years ago at the meeting held in Athens we talked about the first results obtained from our experience in a new surgical procedure on the eye muscles. This procedure is intended to weaken the muscular action and it consists of the lengthening of the tendon by means of fascia lata graft.

At that time we reported the favourable results obtained in cases of gross strabismus or in excess of resection associated with movement reduction. We also reported the first results obtained by the surgical correction of pendular nystagmus, of jerky nystagmus with torticollis and in concomitant strabismus.

Since then our case history has greatly increased. We have also been able to check the effects of this surgical procedure on the so-called kinetical incomitances.

This term refers to the alterations of eye movements which are brought out by motor electrooculography. One of the main syndromes that can be observed by this technique is the so-called dissynergy, which can be either alternating or monolateral.

It consists of a sharp reduction in the movement of the occluded eye and it appears as a decrease in the amplitude of the electrooculogram.

This reduction in amplitude occurs in each eye when occluded in the alternating form. In the monolateral dissynergy the same happens in only one eye, when occluded.

This phenomenon occurs quite frequently in concomitant strabismus and is one of the chief characteristics of the so-called blockage syndrome. The normalisation of the tracing, together with the elimination of the static angle are regarded as signs of motor normalisation.

The aim of our study has been to evaluate the effects of the lengthening of the tendon also in this particular case of strabismus.

SURGICAL TREATMENT

Let us briefly recall the main technical points of the operation.

First a strip of fascia lata 4 mm in width is prepared and somewhat thinned. Two 5/0 vicryl stitches are applied at one end. After opening the conjonctiva with a paralimbar cut, the muscle is exposed up to the foramen and it is blocked with a myostat. Two 5/0 vicryl stitches are applied near the scleral insertion and the insertion is cut. The fascia lata strip previously prepared is then fixed with the two stitches at the ventral face of the muscle at 4 mm from the muscular end which is kept stretched by the two threads applied to it. The muscle end is then sutured to the fascia lata by means of these threads in a way that the two overlap by 4 mm. The strip is then cut to the required length and sutured to the normal scleral insertion of the muscle. Then the conjunctival wound is closed with one or two stitches.

We planned the operation taking into account only the amplitude of the static angle and subdividing the extent of the surgical correction between the two eyes in case of alternating dissynergy.

Our previous experience had shown that esodeviations up to 20 diopters required grafts up to 7 or 8 mm in length. Above this size it was necessary to associate a resection of the lateral rectus of 3 to 4 mm for angles up to 35 diopters and of 7 to 8 mm up to 60 or 70 diopters. The result of this procedure could be enhanced by lysis of the check ligaments.

Patients

One hundred and fifty four out of 512 patients operated on with the above technique, showed electrooculographic signs of dissynergy before surgery.

Fourty-eight of these patients presented alternating and 106 monolateral dissynergy. However, they were all esotropias and their angle varied from 20 to 70 diopters.

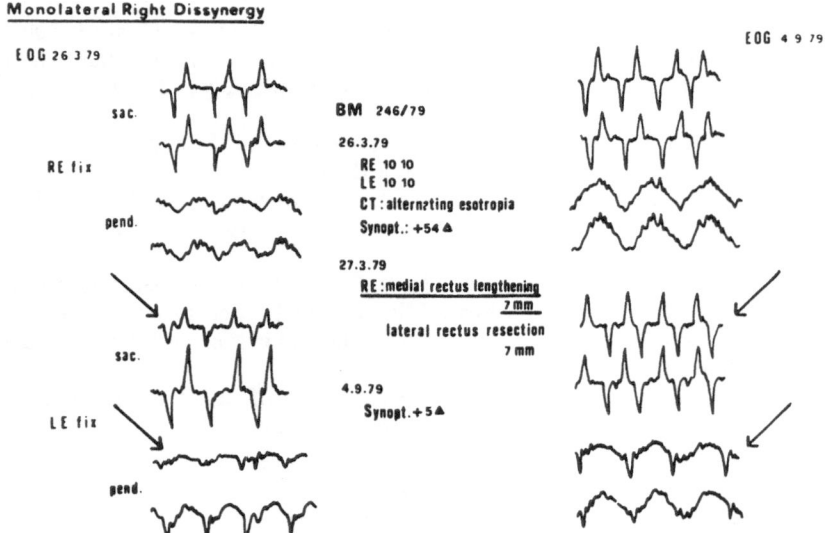

Fig. 1. Effect of fascia lata graft lengthening procedure in a case of left monolateral dissynergy (left) before and (right) after surgery.

234

RESULTS

These were the criteria followed for the evaluation of the effects of the surgical procedure: a) the presence of a residual static angle of deviation; b) the behaviour of the dissynergy.

We noticed that the lengthening alone produces an average angle reduction up to about 20 diopters. Each millimeter of medial rectus lengthening produces an average angular effect of about 3 diopters.

Above 20 diopters a resection of the antagonist lateral rectus must be added: each millimeter of lateral rectus resection produces an addictional effect of about 5 diopters on the statical angle.

Fig. 1 shows the effect of the operation on one case of left monolateral dissynergy before and after surgery.

Table 1 shows the total results from our 154 cases. If we take into account both the elimination and the marked postoperative reduction of dissynergy, we can see that 121 cases out of 154 (78,5%) showed positive results.

Only in 7 cases surgery had no effect whatsoever.

Table 1. Results of 154 fascia lata graft lengthening procedures.

DYSSYNERGIA					
Preoperative		Postoperative			
N°		unchanged	reduced+	reduced++	eliminated
48	Alternating	2	8	28	10
106	Monocular	5	18	56	27

CONCLUSION

The results obtained in 154 patients operated on for lengthening of the tendon according to Focosi's technique, lead to the consideration that this type of strabismus shows the same angular effect that in 'normal' strabismus, but that this operation has nearly always proved valid in reducing kinetical incomitances.

There is a symmetrization of the eye movements as obtained in the more widely known Faden-operation.

However, when compared to the latter technique, the lengthening of the distal tendon has remarkable advantages: a) it is easier to perform, b) there is absence of postoperative complications, c) the feasibility of re-operation is ample, d) the normal anatomical scleral insertion and the normal arc of contact are fully preserved and consequently is fully preserved the normal anatomo-functional situation between the muscle-tendon apparatus and the eye, e) gross muscular alterations are absent.

REFERENCES

Focosi, M., G. Salvi & R. Frosini. Tendon lengthening by fascia lata graft to weaken action of extraocular muscles. Xth meeting of C.E.S.S.D. Athens (1979).

Focosi, M. & P. Ruzzi. Su di una nuova tecnica di indebolimento muscolare mediante l'innesto tendineo. Boll. Ocul. 57, 3–12 (1978).

Salvi, G., R. Frosini & M.C. Boschi. L'allongement du tendon selon Focosi dans les syndromes de blocage. Mecanisme d'action et tecnique chirurgicale. J. Fr. Ophtal. 4/2, 127–132 (1981).

Salvi, G., R. Frosini & M.C. Boschi. Congenital cataract induced nistagmus: surgical management by means of tendon lengthening. IInd International Congress On Cataract. Florence 17–20 June 1981.

Quéré, M.A., A.M. Larmande & M.P. Delplace. Incomitances des mouvements pendulaires de poursuite dans les paralysies oculo-motrices et les strabismes fonctionnelles. Bull. Soc. F. 124, 536–576 (1971).

Quéré, M.A. & M.P. Delplace. Les incomitances des esotropies fonctionelles. Ann. Ocul. Paris. 205, 533–548 (1972).

Cüppers, C. Die Fadenoperation, theorische Grundlagen, Indikationen und Technik. Bologna 1975, Sec. Inter. Symp. of Eye Surgery.

Cüppers, C. The so-called 'Faden-operation' (surgical correction by well-defined changes in the arc of contact). Sec. Congress of the International Strab. ass., Ed: P. Fells, Marseille Diffusion Generale de Librairie p. 394, (1976).

Cüppers, C. Erganzugen zur Indikation der Fadenoperation. Arbeitskreis Schielbenhandlung, 9(2), 98 (1977).

Authors' address:
Istituto di Clinica Oculistica
Cattedra di Ottica Fisiopatologica
Università degli Studi di Firenze
Firenze, Italy

236

RETRO-EQUATORIAL MYOPEXY OF THE VERTICAL RECTI IN TRAUMATIC DIPLOPIA

L. KOORNNEEF, R.A. CRONE & A.M. NOORDENBOS

(Amsterdam, The Netherlands)

ABSTRACT

Limited deorsumduction was treated in 12 patients by myopexy of the contralateral inferior rectus, if necessary combined with a recession. Ten cases improved clinically. The average secondary overaction of the contralateral eye, when the affected eye moved 25° downwards, was 11°. The average effect of the myopexy, 10 to 15 mm behind the insertion, was 7°. There was little correlation between the place of the fixation sutures and the effect of myopexy. Five other patients were treated by myopexy of the superior rectus (11–15 mm). The effect was negligible in three, but there was a serious overcorrection in two patients.

INTRODUCTION

Disorders of ocular motility caused by orbital trauma are always highly incomitant. The results of muscle surgery on the affected eye are generally disappointing because of fibrous adhesions. These adhesions make surgery on the affected eye complicated and unattractive; therefore an operation on the normal eye is the best strategy.

Often a recession is needed to align the eyes in the primary position, but this does not result in an important decrease of the incomitance. To annul the hyperfunction of the contra-lateral vertical rectus a retro-equatorial myopexy, using the method of Cüppers, seems to be the operation of choice. We have performed this operation in 17 cases, twelve times on the inferior rectus and five times on the superior rectus. Table 1 illustrates the causes of

Table 1.

Myopexy superior rectus		Myopexy inferior rectus	
Orbital fractures	2 cases	Orbital fractures	5 cases
Operation orbital tumour	1	Stab wounds	3
Strabismus operation	1	Operations orbital tumour	2
Detachment operation	1	Strabismus operations	2
	5		12

Docum. Ophthal. Proc. Series, Vol. 32, ed. by A.Th.M. van Balen & W.A. Houtman 237
© *1982, Dr W. Junk Publishers, The Hague. ISBN 90 6193 728 0*

muscle imbalance in the different patients. The number of patients is small of course, but in the literature there are comparatively few quantitative data on this subject.

MYOPEXY OF THE INFERIOR RECTUS

The muscle was attached to the sclera at 10 to 15 mm from the insertion. In four cases a moderate recession was performed simultaneously.

The effect of the myopexy was evaluated in the following way: The excursion of the good eye was measured on the Maddox cross with a Maddox rod while the affected eye moved from the primary position to 25° downwards. The postoperative decrease of the overaction was the degree for the effect of the myopexy.

Fig. 1 shows the relationship between the fixation spot of the posterior suture, in mm from the insertion, and the effect on the incomitance. As you see there is some correlation, still there is no question of a predictable effect.

Most cases improved clinically. In four the result was excellent, in six reasonable to moderate, and in two cases almost nil. Because we cannot report on all individual cases we will discuss one highly and one moderately successful one.

The first patient (Fig. 2a, 2b) was operated on in 1977 because of a tumour located in the upper-nasal part of the orbit. Fig. 2a shows the preoperative condition, Fig, 2b the situation a few months after myopexy of the inferior rectus. The procedure also had a favourable effect on the hypertropia during head tilt. We saw the same effect on the Bielschowsky test in three other patients. The postoperative field of binocular single vision became almost unlimited in this patient.

In the second patient we achieved a moderate, but not satisfactory result. In 1949 the patient sustained a stab injury in the trochlear area, which

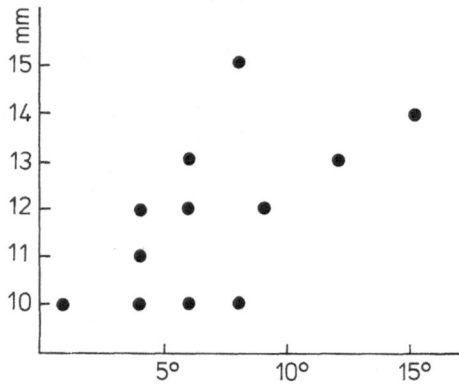

Fig. 1. The effect of myopexy in different patients. The ordinate indicates the distance between insertion and myopexy in mm. The abscissa shows the decrease of incomitance in 25° deorsumduction.

238

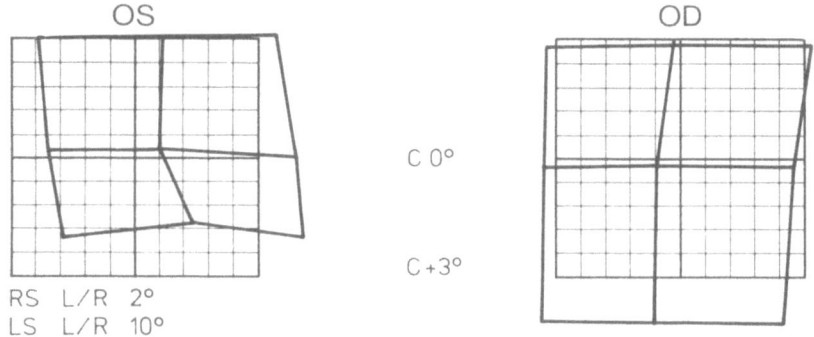

Fig. 2a. First patient. Motility diagram after extirpation of orbital tumour. Each small square = 5°. C: cyclotropia, in primary direction of gaze and 25° deorsumduction. RS, LS: hypertropia in primary direction of gaze during head tilt to right, left, shoulder.

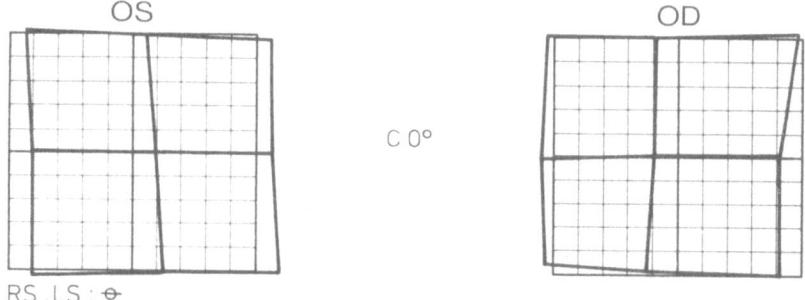

Fig. 2b. First patient, after 15 mm myopexy of R inferior rectus.

led to an atypical paralysis of the superior oblique (Fig. 3a, 3b). The effect of myopexy was 9° in this case. There was a limited but useful field of binocular single vision (Fig. 4a, 4b).

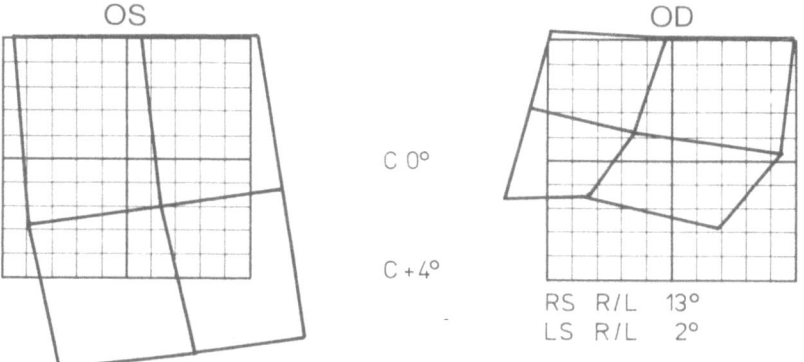

Fig. 3a. Patient after sustaining a stab injury on the right in the trochlear area.

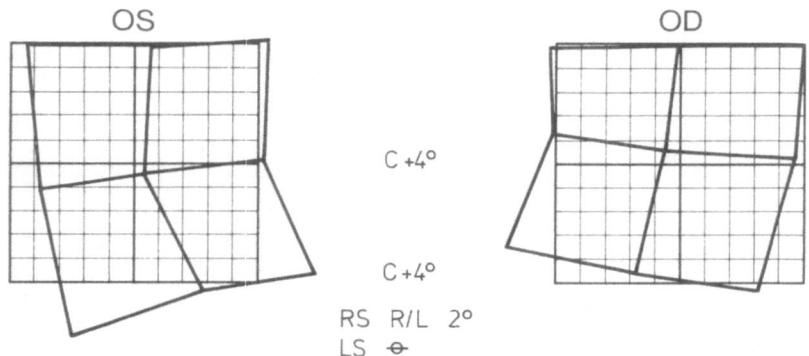

OS
OD
C +4°
C +4°
RS R/L 2°
LS ⊖

Fig. 3b. Same patient one year after a 4 mm recession of the left inferior rectus and myopexy at 12 mm from the original insertion.

30
20
10
(a)
30
20
10
(b)

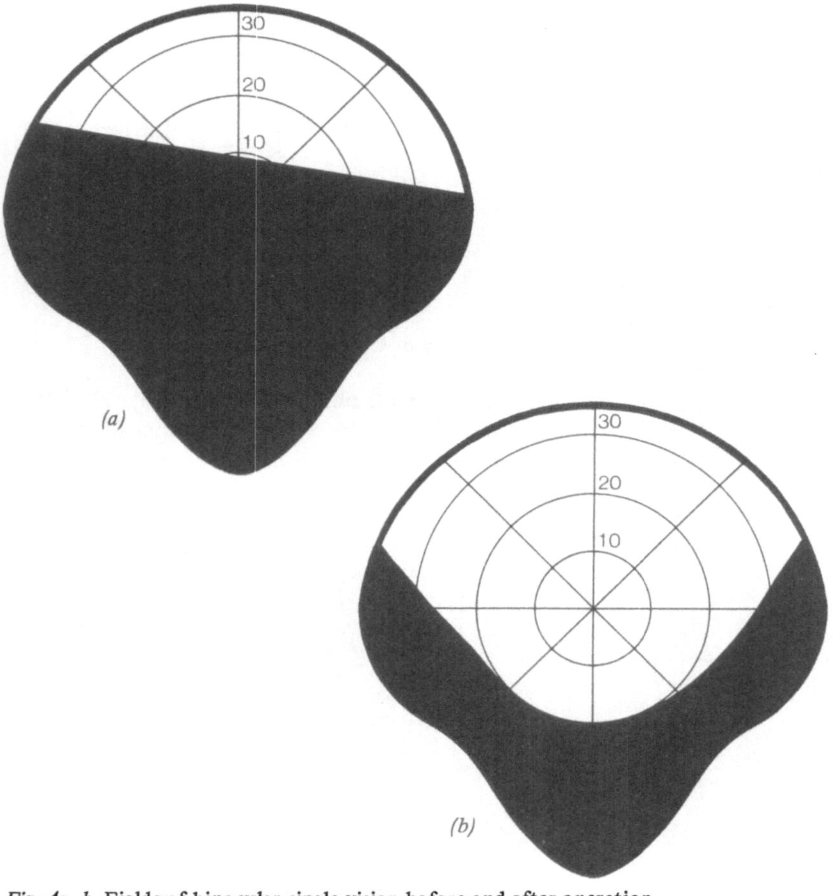

Fig. 4a, b. Fields of binocular single vision before and after operation.

The procedure was combined with a recession in four of the five cases. The site of the posterior fixation suture was 12–14 mm behind the insertion. The effect was negligible in three cases, in the two other cases the

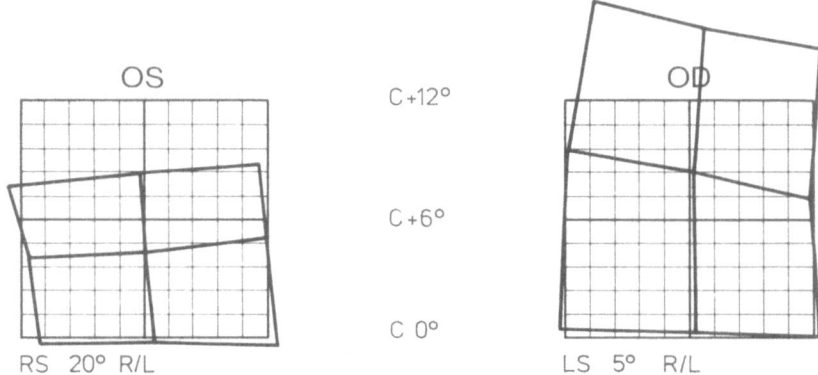

Fig. 5a. Motility scheme of a patient with diplopia after two retinal detachment operations.

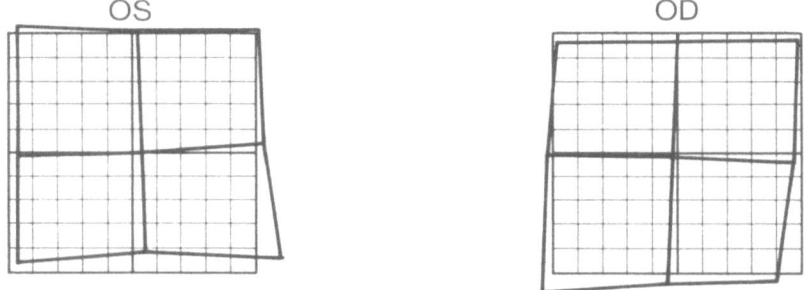

Fig. 5b. Motility scheme three weeks postoperatively after 4 mm recession left superior rectus and myopexy 14 mm behind original insertion.

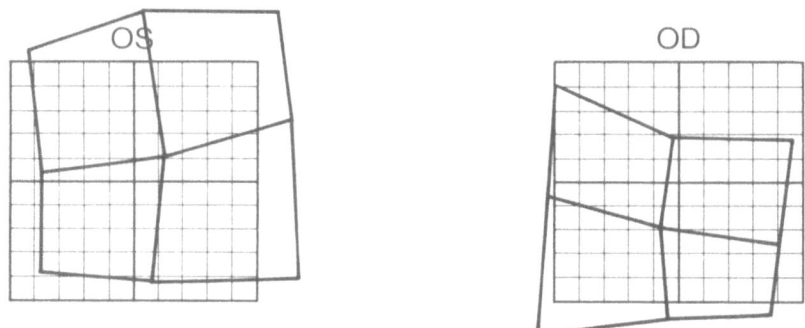

Fig. 5c. Serious overcorrection two months postoperatively.

241

initial result was excellent, but after a few weeks a serious overcorrection developed (Fig. 5a, 5b, 5c).

DISCUSSION

It is not clear why all of our five cases of superior rectus myopexy failed. Perhaps interference with the superior oblique muscle tendon running between the superior rectus and the globe explains the disappointing results. Undoubtedly Faden-operations are not easy, but all operations have been performed by one surgeon, experienced in muscle and detachment surgery. A head lamp was used for good visualization of the field of operation. Still the bad results are suprising because other authors report excellent results of superior rectus myopexy, for instance in cases of alternating hyperphoria.

The results of inferior rectus myopexy, on the other hand, were quite gratifying. The average effect of Cüppers' operation was a decrease of overaction up to seven or eight degrees.

In view of the unpredictability of the effect, there is little justification for subtle mathematical or pathophysiological reflections. From our data it is impossible to decide whether myopexy is actually 'contact arc' surgery or just another way of weakening a muscle. The Faden-operation was the first systematically developed method of muscle weakening and as such a great asset in squint surgery. That should not, however, keep us from looking for better and easier methods.

Authors' address:
Oogheelkundige Kliniek
Academisch Ziekenhuis
Universiteit van Amsterdam
le Helmersstraat 104
1054 EG Amsterdam, The Netherlands

L'ARRACHEMENT ET LA MIGRATION ANTERIEURE DU FIL DANS LA FADENOPERATION DE CÜPPERS

A. PECHEREAU & M.A. QUÉRÉ

(*Nantes, France*)

RESUME

Sur une série de 1106 Fadenoperations les auteurs ont relevé un groupe particulier de 52 cas d'ésotrophies fonctionnelles dont la cure chirurgicale a été suivie d'un échec manifeste qui a nécessité une réintervention sur le muscle soumis précédemment à la myopexie rétro-équatoriale.

Ils ont pu constater que la Fadenoperation donne des réactions capsulo-musculaires focales nettement plus marquées que les techniques classiques gênant les réinterventions. En revanche, elle a des conséquences iatrogènes beaucoup moins importantes sur l'ensemble du muscle que les récessions isolées.

Les échecs différés de la Fadenoperation sont expliqués par un défaut de neutralisation des facteurs visco-élastiques constitutionnels conjugué aux effets de la force perpendiculaire créée par la myopexie rétro-équatoriale. Il en résulte souvent un arrachement du Fil ou sa migration antérieure.

Les règles pratiques pour éviter ces échecs sont indiquées.

SUMMARY

In a series of 1106 Fadenoperations the authors observed 52 cases of functional esotropia with a particular course. The surgery was followed by an obvious failure which required a new operative step on the muscle previously submitted to retro-equatorial myopexy.

It was noticed that the Fadenoperation causes more scarring of the muscle and the fascia than classical procedures, making reoperations more difficult. On the contrary, its iatrogeneous effects on the muscle are as a whole less heavy than by sole recession procedures.

The delayed failures are explained by a lack of surgical neutralization of abnormal muscle elongation associated with the effects of perpendicular muscle force, caused by the equatorial myopexy. It frequently results in a pulling up or a slipping foward of the thread.

Various practical rules are given to avoid such failures.

INTRODUCTION

L'opération du Fil ou myopexie rétro-équatoriale a été proposée par Cüppers en 1972 et en 1974. Ses mécanismes d'action sont radicalement différents de tous les autres procédés opératoires. Elles provoquent la décomposition de la force musculaire en deux composantes: une force perpendiculaire sans aucun effet rotatoire – une force tangentielle qui seule assure la rotation du globe.

La valeur de la force tangentielle dépend de deux paramètres: 1) tout d'abord de la distance du point d'amarrage. Plus il est postérieur, plus elle est diminuée; 2) par ailleurs, de la position du globe. Plus le muscle est sollicité dans son champ d'action – c'est-à-dire plus la force développée est élevée – plus la valeur relative de cette composante tangentielle est faible. La composante perpendiculaire subit une évolution inversement proportionnelle à ces deux paramètres.

MATERIEL ET METHODES

Nous ne reviendrons pas sur les détails de la technique qui ont été exposés par Cüppers. Nous voulons seulement rappeler que l'utilisation du microscope est essentielle pour le contrôle minutieux de la distance d'amarrage, la profondeur des passages scléraux, enfin pour l'épargne maximum des gaines et des fascias.

Pour des raisons que nous avons déjà exposées, la très grand majorité des myopexies ont été faites sur le droit interne délibérément à 13 mm de l'insertion. Cette distance n'a été inférieure que dans les globes de petits diamètres chez quelques très jeunes enfants et les forts hypermétropes.

En 6 ans nous avons fait 1106 Fadenoperations dans divers syndromes oculomoteurs présentant des dérèglements innervationnels. Notre propos est de vous parler d'un group très particulier de 52 ésotropies dont la cure chirurgicale par la Fadenoperation a été suivie d'un échec manifeste qui nous a contraint à réintervenir sur le muscle primitivement soumis à la seule myopexie.

Cette série comporte deux types d'évolution postopératoire: les échecs immédiats et les échecs différés.

Les échecs immédiats

Ils sont au nombre de 8. Dès la première semaine l'échec a été évident. La réintervention a été effectuée dans un délai inférieur à 2 mois et nous avons toujours constaté la même faute technique: c'est-à-dire un amarrage insuffisant qui a lâché.

Les échecs différés

Nous avons eu 44 réinterventions différées dans un délai de 3 mois à 5 ans avec un délai moyen de 23 mois. Chez tous ces patients l'évolution postopératoire a été identique. Après un résultat immédiat satisfaisant, nous avons assisté dans les semaines et les mois suivants à une récidive inexorable, d'abord lente, puis progressivement accélérée de la plus grande part de la déviation initiale. Contrairement aux échecs immédiats, leurs causes sont loin d'être évidentes.

Les constatations opératoires dans les échecs différés

Nous avons retenu trois causes possibles, d'ailleurs le plus souvent associés: 1) les cicatrices capsulo-musculaires; 2) l'élongation musculaire anormale; 3) l'arrachement ou la migration du Fil.

Les cicatrices capsulo-musculaires. Toutes les techniques sans exception provoquent des cicatrices capsulo-musculaires au niveau de foyer opératoire, mais elles sont particulièrement évidentes avec la Fadenoperation dans plus de la moitié des cas.

En ce qui concerne le muscle lui-même, nous avons observé: a) dans 24 cas (55%) un aspect normal; b) dans 16 cas (36%) un certain degré de fibrose de la portion en amont du Fil; c) dans 4 cas (9%) un sclérose complète de toute la portion du muscle chirurgicalement accessible.

L'élongation musculaire anormale. Rapidement de facteur nous est apparu comme essentiel.

Au début nous l'avons totalement méconnu et nous nous contentions de la notion d'angle minimum. Nous n'avons mis au point et utilisé de façon systematique notre test d'élongation musculaire qu'au cours de deuxième semestre de 1977. Or, plus des 3/4 des échecs différés ont été opérés avant cette date. 9 réinterventions lui-sont antérieures. Dans tout les cas il s'agit de Fadenoperation sans recul du droit interne.

Dans 35 réinterventions postérieures à cette date nous avons trouvé: a) 13 cas (37%) d'élongation normale ou légèrement diminuée; b) 22 cas (63%) d'élongation nettement diminuée (Tableau 1). Nous n'avons constaté aucune élongation très diminuée, nulle ou negative.

La position du Fil. C'est la constatation la plus surprenante: a) dans 12 cas nous avons retrouvé le Fil à 13 mm de l'insertion; b) dans 12 cas il était arraché de la sclère et laissait toujours un sillon d'atrophie bleutée au niveau des passages scléraux primitifs; c) dans 20 cas, nous avons eu la surprise de constater sa migration vers l'avant à une distance variant entre 4 et 11 mm de l'insertion, la distance moyenne étant de 8 mm.

Tableau 1. Esotropies recidivantes – reinterventions etat de l'élongation musculaire du droit interne opere lors du 1er temps.

Groupes T.E.M.	8–12 mm	4–7 mm	0–4 mm	Negative	Total
Fadenoperations	13	22	0	0	35
Recessions isolées	3	12	10	7	32

DISCUSSION

La question essentielle est de savoir quelle est la part respective de ces 3 facteurs dans la récidive de la déviation.

L'arrachement du Fil ou sa migration. Ils sont dus à la force perpendiculaire. Leur rôle est apparemment évident. En somme ils ont provoqué la neutralisation de la Fadenoperation. Cependant, dans 12 échecs cette cause ne peut être invoquée.

Les réactions capsulo-musculaires. Les réactions focales sont nettement plus marquées dans la Fadenoperation que dans les techniques classiques, elles compliquent d'ailleurs les réinterventions. Au début nous leur avons attribué un rôle majeur dans les récidives.
Trois faits nous ont amené à changer d'avis:
Les récessions et les résections sont également génératrices de réactions capsulo-musculaires focales parfois considérables.
Les syndromes d'adhésion après les récessions sont observés aussi bien dans les ésotropies résiduelles que dans les fortes exotropies secondaires.
Dans les réinterventions pour décollement de la rétine, on constate souvent des réactions capsulo-musculaires exubérantes sans qu'il en résulté des conséquences motrices majeures.

Une élongation anormale méconnu. Elle a eu un rôle certain dans les deux tiers des cas. On peut toujours objecter que ces facteurs visco-élastiques anormaux sont secondaires à la Fadenoperation elle-même.
Un argument statistique prouve le contraire. Depuis que nous pratiquons le test d'élongation musculaire, et adaptons en conséquence le plan opératoire, la nécessité d'une réintervention in situ est devenue six fois moins fréquente.
En revanche, on ne peut en dire autant des récessions isolées qui sont terriblement iatrogènes. Comme le prouve le tableau no 1 elles sont génératrices dans plus de la moitié des cas d'élongations très diminuées, nulles ou négatives, choses que l'on ne constate jamais lors du premier temps opératoire ou après une Fadenoperation. Elles entraînent un relâchement intempestif et non équilibré qui a pour conséquence une mutilation et une rétraction de l'ensemble du muscle, et non pas seulement au niveau du foyer opératoire.

CONCLUSIONS

En pratique, 4 règles sont essentielles pour éviter les échecs:
1) Il faut systématiquement mesurer l'élongation du muscle soumis à la Fadenoperation et de son antagoniste direct afin de neutraliser les facteurs visco-élastiques anormaux en conséquence. 2) Tout recul musculaire doit être équilibré par un renforcement de l'antagoniste. 3) Quand après le 1er temps sur un oeil il persiste une déviation résiduelle importante, le deuxième temps sur l'autre oeil doit être effectué dans un délai très court, durant lequel il faut maintenir l'oeil qui vient d'être opéré fixateur afin de ne pas

solliciter de façon exagérée la force perpendiculaire. 4) Enfin, il est impératif de maintenir de façon draconienne le traitement médical, en particulier la correction optique.

BIBLIOGRAPHIE

Cüppers, C. & F.E. Adelstein. Possibilidades de tratamiento quirurgico del nistagmus. Arch. soc. esp. Oftalmol. 32, 207–222 (1972).

Cüppers, C. The so called 'Fadenoperation' (Surgical corrections by well defined changes of the arc of contact). p. 168–170. International Strabismological Association 11 Meeting, mai 1974, Marseille. Fuery-Lamy, Marseille, p. 422 (1976).

Authors' address:
Clinique ophtalmologique universitaire de Nantes
Hôtel Dieu
44035 Nantes, France

OCULOMOTOR IMBALANCE IN CONGENITAL PTOSIS

A. CASTANERA MOLINA, A. CASTANERA PUEYO,
J. CASTANERA MOLINA & F. CASTANERA MOLINA
(Barcelona, Spain)

SUMMARY

We report the presence of against the rule vertical imbalances in several cases of unilateral or bilateral congenital ptosis possibly having a postural pathogenetic mechanism, causing a binocular dissociation that could be the origin of numerous so-called non-related Strabismus (eso or exotropias).

Burke (1949) and Anderson (1980) report the high incidence of Strabismus in patients with congenital ptosis, stressing the need for a careful examination of all ptotic patients to detect any form of oculomotor imbalance.

We report some forms of oculomotor imbalance not previously mentioned by either author.

In Anderson's series of 113 congenital ptosis, the overall incidence of strabismus is 32%, slightly higher than that of Burke (26.5%).

It is interesting to note that only 44% of these strabismus could be described as in association with ptosis: 6 cases of double elevator palsy, 4 cases of jaw-wink ptosis, 3 cases of IIIrd nerve palsy, 3 cases of cyclic IIIrd nerve palsy.

The remaining 56% of ptotic patients had a form of strabismus that could not be considered as an association to the lids condition.

From them 3.5% (3 cases) were considered as consecutive to Ptosis (exotropia developing from visual deprivation by the falling lid).

The rest of the patients had several different forms of strabismus, none of them in apparent relation to the ptosis (3 cases of Hypotropia, 3 cases of Hypertropia, 1 Brown syndrome, 3 Duane syndrome, 1 DVD Syndrome and 3 congenital esotropias).

REPORT OF CASES

We have been revising our population of ptotic patients and have found the same frequency distribution of different forms of strabismus as in strabismus without ptosis.

Docum. Ophthal. Proc. Series, Vol. 32, ed. by A. Th.M. van Balen & W.A. Houtman 249
© *1982, Dr W. Junk Publishers, The Hague. ISBN 90 6193 728 0*

Nevertheless we have found with some consistency the presence of a kind of oculomotor imbalance not mentioned by the previously cited authors that might be considered as secondary or consecutive to the lids anomaly:

Patient 1: D.A.O. A 2-year-old boy presenting left ptosis since birth and esophoria. In the clinical examination we found bilateral ptosis with poor levator function in both eyes (5 and 3 mm) presenting bilateral double elevator paresis, more prominent in the right eye, and marked bilateral superior oblique overaction. A bilateral superior oblique tenotomy was performed together with an upwards transposition of all horizontal recti, after which the condition improved leaving a slight overaction of both superior obliques.

Patient 2: D.A.L. A 6-year-old boy with bilateral congenital ptosis with levator function of 3/1 mm. He presented intermittent exotropia, DVD syndrome, bilateral superior oblique overaction and A syndrome with esotropia in upgaze and exotropia in downgaze.

Patient 3: D.E.R. A 2-year-old boy with left congenital ptosis without levator function. Presents right Brown syndrome with positive forced duction test under general anesthesia, causing marked upshoot of the left ptotic eye in attempted elevation of the dominant right eye.

A tenotomy and fasciectomy was performed in the right superior oblique with some improvement of the condition.

Patient 4: R.B.E. A 1-year-old boy presenting with left ptosis since birth without levator function. The parents appreciate the left eye moving up in a disproportionate manner on attempted upgaze without moving the left ptotic lid. The boy's mother presents the same condition in lesser extent.

After frontalis suspension procedure for the left lid a slight improvement of ocular elevation was noted in the right eye.

COMMENT

It is generally agreed that the oculomotor imbalance present in congenital ptosis is two-fold: a) Related or associated to ptosis: elevation deficiency in the ptotic eye either due to underaction or paresis of the elevators of the eye — superior rectus, inferior oblique — or overaction or contractures of the depressors of the eye — inferior rectus, superior oblique — b) Non-related strabismus: types of oculomotor imbalance apparently not related to the lid's anomaly.

It is noteworthy that the incidence of strabismus in the general population ranges from 1 to 5% according to different authors, whereas those 'non-related to ptosis' strabismus represent an incidence close to 18%.

This figure appears to be too high if we compare it with the figure of general incidence of strabismus in the normal population.

A relationship between both conditions must be present to lead to such high figures.

However, the kinds of oculomotor imbalances described by Anderson do not permit the establishment of any clear relationship between both conditions.

We have been looking for an explanation for the high incidence of strabismus among ptotic patients and have found a rather higher percentage of cases in which it was possible to demonstrate an 'against the rule' vertical imbalance: elevators deficiency or depressors overactions in the non-ptotic eye, or more prominent in the less ptotic eye, when bilateral.

A careful examination reveals a frequent pattern of superior oblique overaction in the non-ptotic eye or less ptotic eye and/or an elevation deficiency — double elevator paresis — in the same eye.

The pathogenetic mechanism for such vertical imbalance is not clear.

The presence since birth of a ptosis in one or both eyes leads to the need for a forced chin-up fixation position i.e. in constant contraction of the depressors of one or both eyes — the ptotic eye suppressed by the falling lid could well be in elevation due to Bell's phenomenon.

This situation maintained during the whole period of oculomotor immaturity could lead to a progressive dysfunction — overaction — of the depressors of the eye, which might in time become irreversible, being responsible for a binocular dissociation that favours the decompensation of any possible phoria.

The same forced position for fixation and the absence of any upgaze demand during this important period could also lead to a deficient integration or maturation of the mechanisms of elevation of the eye, being responsible for the deficit of elevation (pseudo double elevator paresis) present in the non-ptotic eye.

The surgical correction of ptosis in an early period permits a slight to marked improvement of elevation in one or both eyes eliminating the pseudo double elevator paresis, although the depressors overaction usually persists.

Nevertheless the dissociation present during the first years of life could have been important enough as to provoke the appearance of other oculomotor anomalies; decompensated phorias.

Authors' address:
Via Augusta 20
Barcelona 6, Spain

DIE BEDEUTUNG DER VERTIKALABLENKUNG BEI DER HORIZONTALEN BLICKLÄHMUNG

H.F. PIPER

(Lübeck, F.R.G.)

ZUSAMMENFASSUNG

Horizontale Déviationen und/oder Blicklähmungen können sich in unterschiedlicher Weise mit vertikalen Blickstörungen, insbesondere Rucknystagmus, kombinieren. In den vorgestellten 6 Fällen war diese Kombination in Rahmen völlig verschiedener Höhenlokalisationen und Ausbreitungsgrade im Zentralnervensystem aufgetreten. Diffus-doppelseitige Läsionen betonen die vertikale, einseitige die horizontale Blickstörung, wobei je nach Charakter des zugrundeliegenden Leidens die eine oder andere Komponente vorherrscht. Aus Reihung und Kombination lassen sich prognostische Schlüsse ziehen.

Die tierexperimentellen Arbeiten von Bender (1980), Pasik & Pasik (1964) sowie Kömpf (1978) haben bestätigt, daß es besonders empfindliche Zonen für die Auslösung horizontaler und vertikaler Augenbewegungen im Hirnstamm gibt: diese liegen für die horizontalen Blickbewegungen mehr kaudal, für die vertikalen mehr rostral. Die beiden Hauptbewegungsrichtungen unterscheiden sich aber nicht nur topographisch, sondern auch prinzipiell: Die horizontalen sind im Hirnstamm rechts/links antagonistisch und damit paramedian — einseitig, die vertikalen um die Mediane und damit im Prinzip doppelseitig organisiert.

Wenn vertikale Nystagmen horizontale Blicklähmungen begleiten, so ist anzunehmen, daß im Bereiche der parapontinen reticulären Formation (Bernsmeier & Friedburg 1980) oder in einer anderen Höhe des Hirnstamms beide Seiten betroffen sind. Klinische Beobachtungen sprechen aber auch dafür, daß horizontale Störungen primär vertikale begleiten können: Diffuse Hirnstammaffektionen äußern sich vielfach in einem Vertikalnystagmus; eine sekundäre Schwerpunktsbildung auf einer Seite führt erst zur horizontalen Blickstörung.

DÉVIATION CONJUGUÉE BEIDER AUGEN MIT VERTIKALNYSTAGMUS

Im akuten Stadium eines Insultes wird eine horizontale Déviation oft von einem heftigen Vertikalnystagmus begleitet, der — wenn sich das Bild wieder bessert – rasch verschwindet. Eine Sakkadierung der Führungsbewegungen kann erhalten bleiben (Mehdorn et al. 1977).

Fall 1. Herbert W., geb. 18.5.14; Untersuchung am 11.4.78 (Abb. 1).

Beide Augen sind nach rechts abgelenkt und können nur ruckweise zur Medianen und nach links bewegt werden. Das linke Auge steht höher (Hertwig-Magendiesche Schielstellung). Die Augen déviieren außerdem nach unten und federn ruckweise nach oben zurück. Aktiver Aufblick erzeugt einen kräftigen vertikalen Rucknystagmus nach oben, einen horizontalen die versuchte Linkswendung. Außerdem zeigt sich ein Horner-Syndrom rechts (und ein Fundus hypertonicusIII). Neurologisch besteht ein Trigeminusausfall rechts sowie eine Ataxie in Bereich der rechten und eine Hemianästhesie im Bereich der linken Extremitäten. Stimmbandlähmung. Sehschärfe gering durch Cataracta incipiens beeinträchtigt. Gesichtsfeld intakt.

Bei Lagerung des Kopfes zur linken Schulter nahm der Linksnystagmus zu, auf die rechte ab. Im Elektronystagmogramm erwiesen sich die Führungsbewegungen von rechts nach links sowie von unten nach oben sakkadiert. Ein besonders heftiger Nystagmus in der Vertikalen ergab sich im Dunkeln.

Die neurologische Diagnostik bestätigte das Wallenberg-Syndrom und die Durchblutungsstörung im Bereich der A. cerebelli posterior inferior. Nach zwei Tagen war der vertikale Spontannystagmus verschwunden, die horizontalen Blickstörungen und das Horner-Syndrom blieben jedoch weiterhin erkennbar. Weitgehende Restitution im Laufe der halbjährigen Nachbeobachtung; die Führungsbewegungen von unten nach oben behielten aber sakkadierten Charakter.

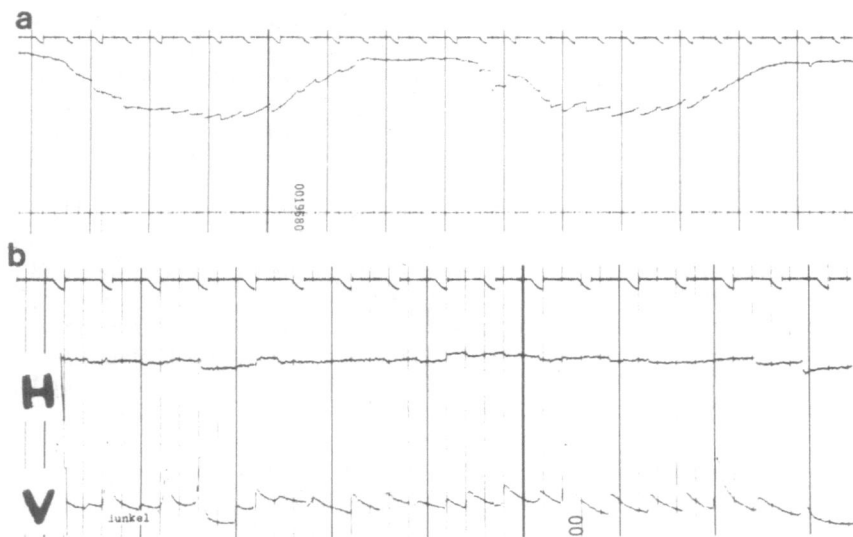

Abb. 1. a. Horizontale Führungsbewegungen: Blickparetischer Nystagmus begleitet die Linkswendung. b. Vertikaler (up-beat) Nystagmus im Dunkeln.

Im nachfolgenden Fall begleitet eher die horizontale eine vertikale schwere Blickstörung. Das Bild entspricht dem von Fisher (1967) bei Bewußtlosen beschriebenen Déviationssyndrom nach unten und führte unter rascher Verschlechterung zum Exitus. Der Hirnstammreflex ist — bei Schädigung übergeordneter Zentren — enthemmt.

Fall 2. Romedius, Pr., geb. 14.12.29; Untersuchung am 10.6.81 (Abb. 2).

Der durch ein Pankreasleiden sehr reduzierte Patient erlitt einen Apoplex und war benommen, jedoch ansprechbar. Beide Augen déviierten nach unten,

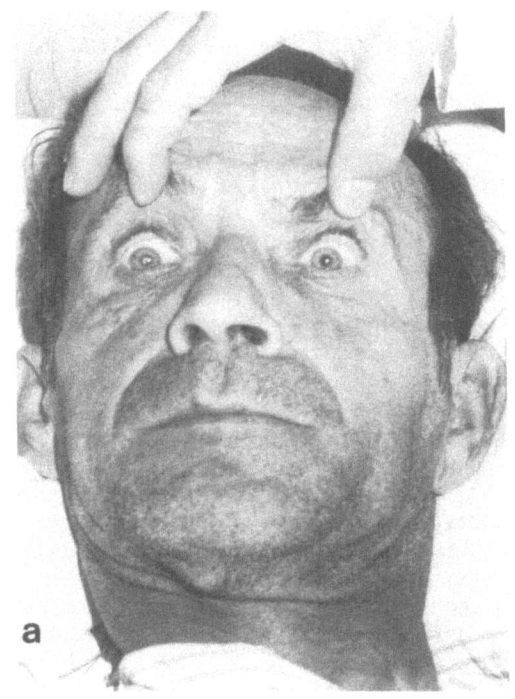

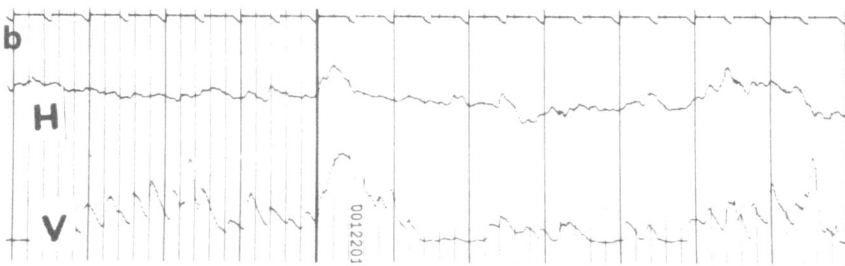

Abb. 2. a. Déviation der Augen nach unten. b. Up-beat-Nystagmus bei Déviation nach unten.

255

unterbrochen durch kurzzeitige Rückführungsintervalle zur Horizontalen, die sich durch grobe aufwärts gerichtete Rucke auszeichneten. Der Patient vermochte nur begrenzt nach rechts und links zu blicken. Die Blickhebung war unter Nystagmusverstärkung möglich, die aktive Senkung jedoch völlig aufgehoben. Neurologisch bestand eine Hemiparese links. Am 15.6.81 verstarb der Patient unter linksbetonten Krämpfen. Die Sektion ergab Hirnerweichung an der Unterseite beider Schläfenlappen polnah, alte Rindenprellherde und walnußgroße Zyste an der Unterseite des rechten Stirnlappens. Hirnstamm und zentrales Höhlengrau unauffällig. Mäßig ausgeprägtes allgemeines Ödem.

BLICKLÄHMUNGEN MIT NYSTAGMUS

Eines der bekanntesten Syndrome ist das des hinteren Längsbündels: Dissoziierter Nystagmus nur des jeweils abduzierten Auges und internukleäre Medialisparese. Im akuten Stadium gehört auch ein oft nur sehr kurz zu beobachtender Vertikalnystagmus zum Bild (Kornhuber, H.H. 1966).

Fall 3. Alfons W., geb. 4.5.08; Untersuchung am 24.3.81 (Abb. 3).

Der Patient, der unter Diabetes, Herzinsuffizienz, Bluthochdruck leidet, bemerkt seit dem Vortag Doppelbilder. Neben einer −VD von 5−8° (Senkerparese links) besteht eine linksseitige Parese des M. rectus internus für Seitwendung, nicht aber für Convergenz. An beiden Augen beobachtet man einen Abduktionsnystagmus in Sinne des dissoziierten Nystagmus. Die Augen tendieren ferner nach unten und werden ruckartig nach oben eingestellt; bei Blickhebung nimmt dieser Vertikalnystagmus zu. In der Wendung nach links kombinieren sich die Nystagmen zu rechtsrotatorischen Rucken, ausgeprägt besonders am linken Auge. Der optokinetische Nystagmus ist gut auslösbar, nach rechts gemindert. Pupillen gleichweit, reagierend.

Neurologisch: Abschwächung der Reflexe, insbesondere im Bereich der rechten Extremitäten, ferner eine periorale Sensibilitätsstörung. Diagnose: Weber-Syndrom (inkomplett). HNO-ärztlich normaler kalorischer Nystagmus auslösbar. Im Verlaufe einer zweiwöchigen Beobachtung bildete sich das Lähmungsbild zurück, zunächst die vertikale Blickstörung, dann die horizontale. Die Führungsbewegungen blieben sakkadiert.

Diffuse Encephalomyopathien zeigen nicht selten einen paretischen Nystagmus in allen Richtungen mit Überwiegen der vertikalen Oszillationen. Die nystagmusfreie zentrale Zone kann nach unten verlagert sein, so daß bei Geradeausblick ein ständiger aufwärts schlagender Rucknystagmus beobachtet wird.

Fall 4. Horst P., geb. 8.3.35; Untersuchung am 29.11.1975 (Abb. 4).

Die neurologische Diagnose lautete: Wernicke-Encephalitis; dementsprechend war der Patient stark reduziert und teilweise somnolent. Aufgrund einer ataktischen Gangstörung wurde eine toxische Polyneuropathie diagnostiziert. Ophthalmologisch zeigte der Pat. überweite, schlecht reagierende Pupillen bei Sehschärfe von 0,8 und intaktem Gesichtsfeld, aber Opticusab-

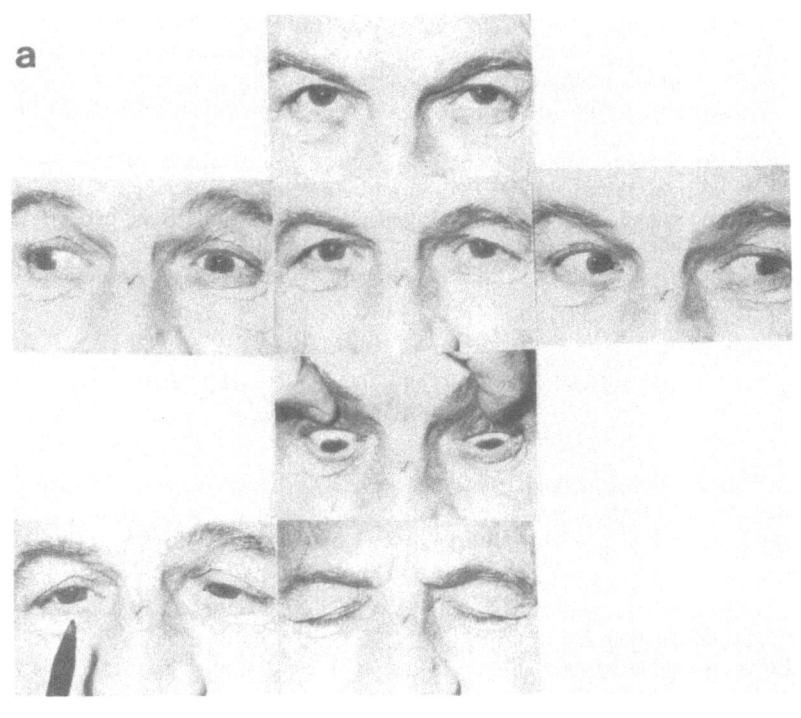

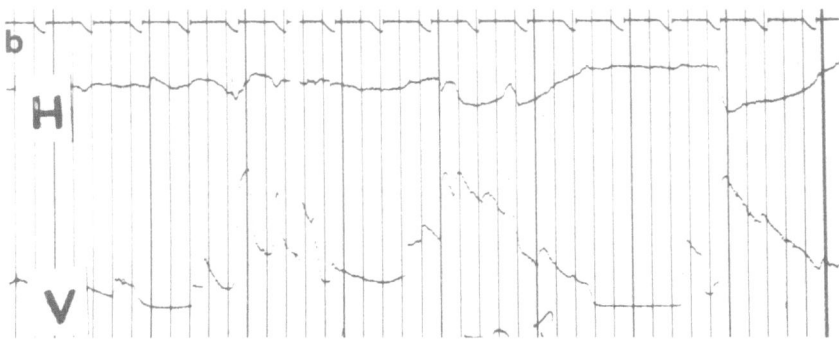

Abb. 3. a. Internucleäre Medialisparese: Das linke Auge wird bei Rechtswendung nicht, bei Convergenz jedoch adduziert. b. Grober Vertikalnystagmus beim Blick nach oben.

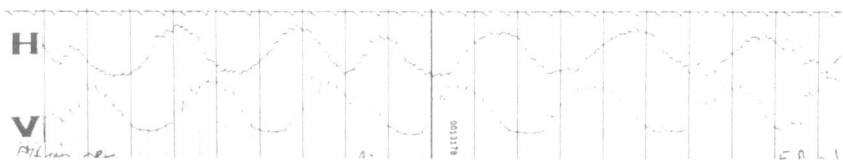

Abb. 4. Der Blick folgt einer Kreisbewegung: horizontale und vertikale Dyskinesen.

blassung, ferner einen vorwiegend vertikalen frequenten Rucknystagmus, der sich beim Blick nach oben verstärkte, beim Blick nach unten abnahm und bei extremem Abblick in Rucknystagmus nach unten überging. Ferner fand sich ein horizontaler Endstellnystagmus, der nach links stärker schlug als nach rechts.

Der neurologische Reflexstatus ergab schwach auslösbare Reflexe an den unteren Extremitäten, keine Pyramidenbahnzeichen aber eine ataktische Gangstörung. Die Pneumencephalographie zeigte einen Hydrocephalus internus mit vorwiegender Beteiligung des 3. Ventrikels (16 mm). Die Seitenventrikel wirkten verplumpt, die Stammganglienkante verstrichen, die Umschlagkante plump.

KOMBINATION VON DÉVIATION UND LÄHMUNGEN MIT NYSTAGMUS

Schwerste Encephalomalazien lassen sowohl Blicklähmungen wie Déviationen erkennen und vereinen Ausfälle in horizontaler und vertikaler Richtung. Als Beispiel sei ein Fall von Thrombose der A. basilaris vorgestellt.

Fall 5. Helmut Gr., geb. 20.12.14; Untersuchung am 6.8.81, drei Wochen nach apoplektischem Insult (Abb. 5).

Beide Augen sind nach links déviiert und werden aktiv nur etwa bis zur Mittellinie gewendet, begleitet von groben Rechtsrucken. Außerdem besteht eine vertikale Blicklähmung: Den Auftrag zur Senkung entsprechen grobe Rucke, die kaum unter die Horizontale führen. Ständiger Rucknystagmus nach oben, langsame Rückkehrkomponente zur Horizontalen. Die Augen können aber aktiv nach oben bewegt werden, wobei der Vertikalnystagmus zunimmt. Sehschärfe wahrscheinlich 0,2 und besser.

Die im Liegen vorgenommene Gesichtsfeldprüfung ergibt eine homonyme Hemianopsie nach rechts.

Computertomogramm: Corticale Hirnsubstanzminderung, kein Hinweis auf Parenchymläsionen.

Neurologisch bestand und entwickelte sich in den nächsten Tagen eine Tetraplegie, ophthalmologisch eine vertikale totale Blicklähmung bei Déviation der Augen nach links. Die neuroradiologischen Zusatzuntersuchungen ergaben einen Insult im Basilarisversorgungsgebiet, betreffend den Hirnstamm und das linke Occipitalhirn. Der Verschluß wurde damit relativ rostral lokalisiert und eine Beteiligung der A. cerebri posterior inferior angenommen. Zwei Tage später war der ophthalmologische Befund teils gebessert, teils verändert: Die Augen konnter jetzt auch nach rechts mit groben Rucken bewegt werden, die Blickhebung war erschwert und die Blicksenkung relativ frei mit blickparetischem Nystagmus jetzt nach unten, wobei das rechte Auge weiter zurückblieb und eine +VD entstand. Optokinetisch ließen sich nach rechts Rucke erzielen, nach links fehlte die Reaktion. Wieder zwei Tage später, am 10.8., entwickelte sich im Rahmen einer weiteren Verschlechterung

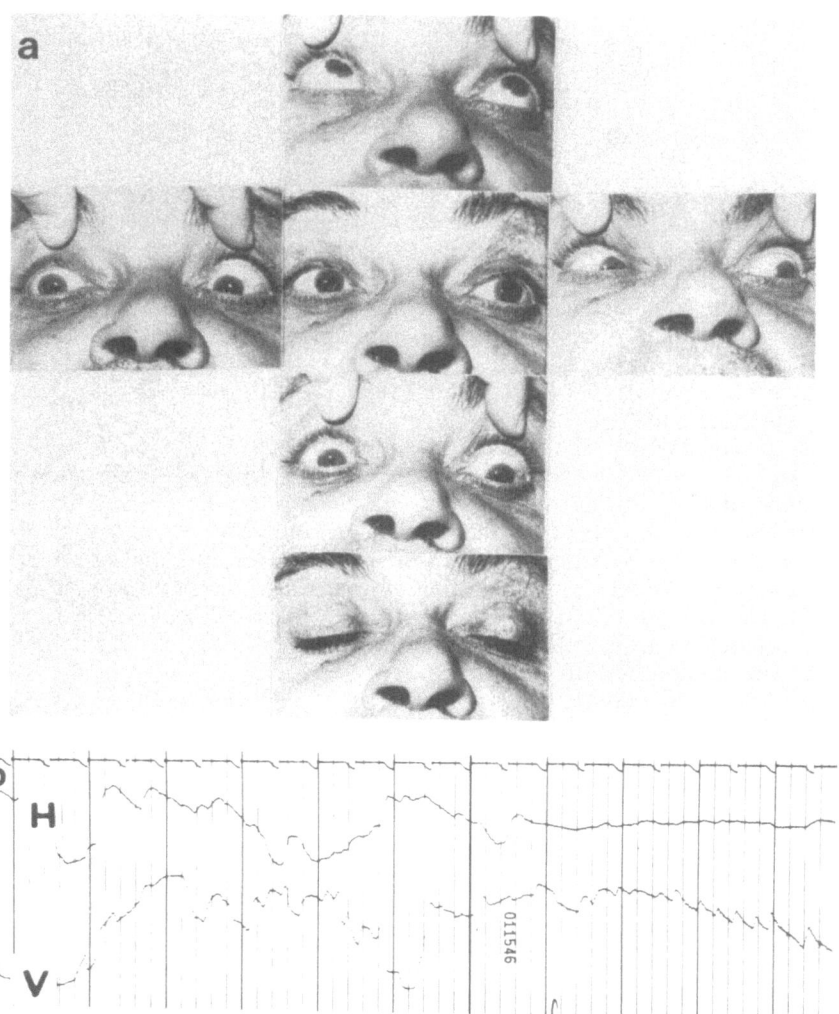

Abb. 5. a. Déviation conjuguée nach links, horizontale Blicklähmung nach rechts, vertikale nach unten. b. Li. Hälfte: Spontane Déviation in der Horizontalen und Vertikalen. Re. Hälfte: Nystagmischer Anteil der Vertikalparese (bei Blickhebung).

ein locked-in-Syndrom: alle Gliedmaßen waren gelähmt, Blickhebung und —senkung völlig ausgefallen, nur noch gewisse Horizontalbewegungen möglich. Am. 10.8. exitus letalis.

HORIZONTAL-VERTIKALE KOMPENSATIONSPHÄNOMENE

Wir kennen frühkindlich erworbene Nystagmen, die pathogenetisch in Beziehung zu Fehlbildungen in der Medianebene des Cerebrum, z.B. zur Platybasia (Cogan 1974) oder zum Fehlen des Septum pellucidum (Piper 1979) zu bringen sind. Der Nystagmus dieser Fälle schlägt vielfach in mehreren Ebenen und bietet Kompensationsmechanismen, die zur Auffindung der nystagmusarmen Zone dienen, wobei auch die Stellreflexe des Halses und Kopfes genutzt werden.

Fall 6. Matthias G., geb. 24.5.66; Untersuchung am 26.4.76 (Abb. 6).

Das Kind war unmittelbar nach der Geburt wegen einer Myelomeningozele operiert. Damals wurde augenärztlicherseits ein Sonnenuntergangsphänomen bei Hydrocephalus festgestellt. Das Kind ist seitdem mit einem Pudensventil versorgt. Jetzt ist neben einem Hydrocephalus noch eine totale Querschnittslähmung der unteren Extremitäten (Blase funktionstüchtig) vorhanden.

Sehschärfe: binokular 0,4–0,5 und N1/15 cm.

Gesichtsfelder intakt.

Fundus: Tortuositas.

Oculomotorisch ist eine Déviation und ein Nystagmus alternans zu beobachten, d.h. die Augen werden bei Gegendrehung des Kopfes mal extrem nach rechts (in der Phase des Linksnystagmus) und dann nach links (in der Phase des Rechtsnystagmus) gewendet; dementsprechend schlägt in der Mittellinie der Nystagmus in etwa 3 Min. Abstand nach links bzw. umgekehrt. Außerdem sieht man einen Vertikalnystagmus, der nach oben schlägt, aber auch optoklonusartige Ausbrüche erkennen läßt; er wird durch Kopfneigung nach hinten und Blicksenkung ausgeglichen.

Gewohnheitsmäßig hält das Kind den Kopf in Extremstellungen, wenn es in der Ferne genau beobachten will und fixiert — bei operativ vorbehandeltem Strabimus convergens mit Restwinkel — jeweils mit dem abduzierten

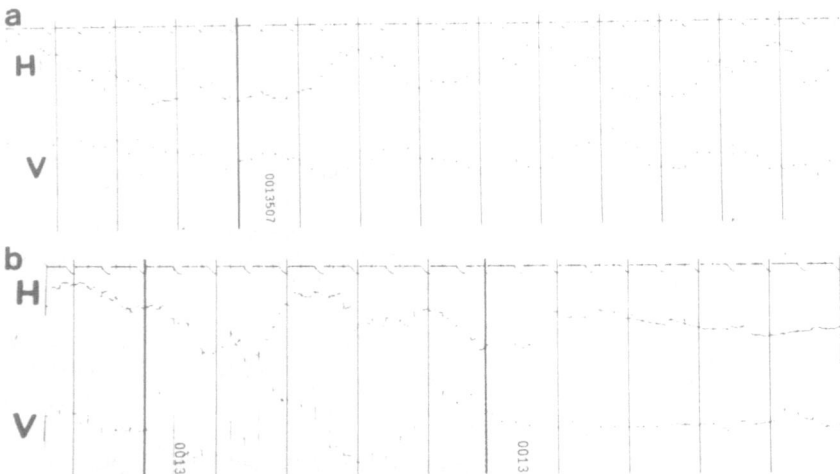

Abb. 6. a. Rechts-Phase in der horizontalen, Aufwärts-Phase in der vertikalen Ableitung. b. Kreisförmige Bewegungsführung. Linksphase. Opsoklonusartiger Charakter auch vertikal. Stop durch Fixation.

Auge. Im Leseabstand konvergieren die Augen um die Mittellinie, wobei der Kopf in den Nacken genommen wird.

Das Kind reduziert also den Horizontal- und Vertikalnystagmus durch extreme Seitwendung der Augen bis in die Endstellungen, und den Vertikalnystagmus beim Lesen durch Blicksenkung, wobei der Horizontalnystagmus alternans offenbar weniger stört.

DISKUSSION

In keinem der vorgestellten Fälle ließ das klinische Gesamtbild erkennen, daß die für Auslösung von Vertikalbewegungen besonders relevante mesencephale Substantia reticularis im mesodiencephalen Übergang elektiv betroffen worden war, ehestens noch in Fall 3. Die vertikale Symptomatik war meist mit Doppelseitigkeit bzw. medianer Lokalisation der Störung zu erklären. Im Fall 1 dürfte die Läsion in der parapontinen Substantia reticularis, also kaudal, im Fall 2 weit rostral in den Parietallappen des Großhirns gelegen sein. In den Fällen 4 und 5 handelt es sich um diffuse Störungen, die Schwerpunkte bilden (Fall 4) oder sich aus solchen aufbauen (Fall 5). Der Fall 6 weist trotz Hirnstamm- und Kleinhirnmechanismen wie Nystagmus alternans und Opsoklonus Kompensationskomplexe auf. Prognostisch kennzeichnet der begleitende Vertikalnystagmus zunächst eine akute Ödemphase; seine rasche Rückbildung ist damit ein günstiges Zeichen. Beteiligt sich über den Nystagmus hinaus noch die Grobmotorik in der Vertikalen, so ist die Prognose schlecht. Ist die Zusammenarbeit von Blickzentrierung, tonischen und sakkadischen Bewegungsintentionen in horizontalen und vertikalen Richtungen schon in früher Kindheit gestört, so bilden sich Kompensationsmechanismen heraus, die denen entsprechen, die beim idiopathischen Nystagmus mit Zwangsblickhaltungen zu beobachten sind.

LITERATUR

Bender, M.B. Brain control of conjugate horizontal and vertical eye movements, Brain 103, 23–69 (1980).

Bernsmeier, H. & F. Friedburg. Horizontale Blickparese, wo liegt die Läsion? Klin. Mbl. Augenheilk. 117, 650 (1980).

Cogan, D.G. Down-beat Nystagmus. Arch. Ophthal. 80, 757–768 (1968).

Cogan, D.G. Paralysis of down gaze. Arch. Ophthal. 91, 192–199 (1974).

Fisher, C.M. Some neuro-ophthalmologic observations. J. Neurol. neurosurg. psychiat. 30, 383–392 (1967).

Kömpf, D. Vertikale Augenbewegungen, Nervenarzt 49, 377–384 (1978).

Kornhuber, H.H. Physiologie und Klinik des zentral-vestibulären Systems in: Berendes, J. Link, R. Zöllner, F. (Herausgeber) HNO-Handbuch Vol. III, Band 3, Part 3 S. 2150–2351, Stuttgart, Thieme 1966.

Mehdorn, E., G. Kommerell & O. Meyenberg. Primary position vertical nystagmus: directional preponderance of the pursuite system? Albrecht v. Graefes Arch. Klin. Exp. Ophthal. 209, 209–217 (1979).

Pasik, P & C. Pasik. Oculomorph function in monkeys with lesions of the cerebrum and the superior colliculi in: Bender, M.B. (Herausgeber) The oculomotor system, New York, Harper and Row, 1964.

Piper, H.F. Das Elektrookulogramm als Spiegel der supranukleären Organisation und ihrer Störungen: Beobachtungen an Blicklähmungen in: Augenbewegungsstörungen Neurophysiologie u. Klinik, G. Kommerell (Herausgeber), J.F. Bergmann Verlag, München, 189–197 (1978).

Author's address:
Klinik für Augenheilkunde der Medizinischen Hochschule
Lübeck, F.R.G.

PRENUCLEAR SLOWLY PROGRESSIVE BILATERAL ABDUCENS PALSY IN MARIE'S CEREBELLAR ATAXIA

Divergence paralysis in cerebellar ataxia

T.W. VAN WEERDEN & W.A. HOUTMAN

(Groningen, The Netherlands)

SUMMARY

Uncrossed diplopia at distance fixation and not at near ('divergence paralysis') may be an early or even first complaint in patients with cerebellar ataxia. The esotropia progresses slowly, running parallel to the increasing severity of the ataxia. The ocular motor disturbance was interpreted as a prenuclear bilateral sixth nerve paresis caused by degeneration of pontine interneurons which mediate eye position signals to the abducens nuclei. The saccadic velocities as judged from the E.N.G. registration were normal.

INTRODUCTION

Cerebellar ataxia (Marie's disease) is now generally considered to consist of a number of different degenerative diseases which are characterized by a late onset slowly progressive cerebellar ataxia (Greenfield 1954; Eadie 1975, a, b, c). The most widely accepted classification is the one of Greenfield, who distinguishes on the ground of pathological changes: 1. Holmes type, or cerebello-olival atrophia, which shows an autosomal dominant mode of inheritance in most cases. 2. The olivo-ponto-cerebellar degenerations, a. the disease of Dejerine Thomas, which occurs sporadically; b. Menzel's type, which transmits by autosomal dominant inheritance, and shows mostly more widespread neurological disturbances, such as extrapyramidal, brainstem and spinal symptoms.

Paralysis of divergence is defined as the unability to exert the divergence necessary to bring the eyes into proper alignment at distance fixation (Burian 1971). The diagnosis is essentially based on the presence of uncrossed double vision at distance viewing, while binocular single vision is present up to a viewing distance of about 50 to 60 centimeters.

The angle of deviation is the same in primary position, as well as in lateral gaze. According to Bielschowsky (1935) the deviation will increase in upward, and decrease in downward gaze. Parinaud (1883) probably first mentioned the occurrence of divergence paralysis. He thought that the lesion might be located in the cerebellum. Jampolsky (1970) refuted the existence of divergence paralysis, and concluded that it was a manifestation of incipient bilateral sixth nerve palsy.

Docum. Ophthal. Proc. Series, Vol. 32, ed. by A.Th.M. van Balen & W.A. Houtman 263
© *1982, Dr W. Junk Publishers, The Hague. ISBN 90 6193 728 0*

We present six patients with cerebellar ataxia in which cases diplopia at distance was the first or an early manifestation of the disease or in which similar ocular motor disturbances were noticed.

CASE REPORTS

The clinical diagnosis and age of onset are summarized in Table 1. All patients had the clinical features of Marie's cerebellar ataxia. Onset was at middle age and the disease slowly progressed with increasing cerebellar ataxia especially of walking and standing. There were no spinal cord disturbances, except for case 1, who showed progressive pyramidal tract disturbances during the last two years of the disease. Clinical classification of the disease is not always possible, and cannot be conclusive in the absence of pathological data of family members (Eadie 1975, a, b, c). Pneumoencephalography and CT scanning may be helpful, (Le May & Abromoviez 1965; Aita 1978; Bories et al. 1972) but are not decisive.

Classification of the cases of this study was the most reasonable with regard to the data available.

All patients had normal visual acuity of both eyes, none of them showed optic disc pallor or pupil abnormalities, and except for the motor disturbances no eye signs were noted.

Case 1 and case 2 are described more fully in detail, because they are illustrative.

Case 1 (Table 2) male, 52 years old now, for the first time complained of double vision in 1969, especially during car driving. He was seen in 1971 at the out-patient clinic of neurology. At that time no ataxia was noticed. He was seen at the department of ophthalmology in 1974 and 1975. The diagnosis divergence paralysis or bilateral abducens palsy was made.

Prism glasses relieved his complaints temporary, but prescription had to be revised repeatedly because of increase of the angle of deviation. In the period 1975–1977 eye muscle surgery was performed elsewhere (bilateral recession of the medial rectus muscles up to 7.5 mm each, in two stages, and bilateral resection of the lateral rectus muscles at a third operation). Binocular single

Table 1.

Pat.	Sex	Age	Age of onset	Mode of inheritance	Type	PEG CT scan	Diplopia (at distance)
I	m	52	41	dom.	Menzel	+	++
II	f	58	47	spor.	Dejerine Thomas	+	++
III₁	f	65	50	dom.	Holmes	+	+
III₂	f	61	46	dom.	Holmes		±*
III₃	f	67	45	dom.	Holmes		–**
IV	m	70	55	dom.	Menzel		–**

*Intermittent.
** Esophoria in right and left gaze.

264

Table 2.

Pat.		Uncrossed diplopia at distance	Deviation – 2,5 m					Maddox wing	Fusional range
			P.P.	Re	Le	Up	Down		
I	1969	intermittent							
	1971	+ (70 cm.)	+2	+7	+4	+0	+4		
	1974	+	+9	+11	+11	+2	+11	−1	+14 – +4
	1975	+	+12	+12	+15	+9	+10	−2	
	1975–1977	surgical correction							
	1981	+ (40 cm.) cross dipl. 30 cm.	+5	+5	+6	+2	+6		+6 – +4
II	1971	onset							
	1975	+ (60 cm.)	+4	+2	+8	+3	+4	−1	+14 – +4
	1981	+ (30 cm.)	+12	+12	+15	+9	+10	+3,5	+15 – +9
III₁	1975	intermittent	+2	+3	+5	+2	+1	−3	+9 – −3
	1981	+	+4	+5	+7	+5	+5	−4	+7 – −1
III₂	1976	−	+1	+7	+7	+0	+4		+20 – +1
III₃	1976	−	+2	+6	+6			−3	
IV	1976	−	+3	+5	+6	+7	+7		+16 – −2

Deviations in prim. position, and 25 dg. eccentric gaze to the right (Re), to the left (Le), and in upward (Up) and downward (Do) gaze. Maddox wing and horizontal range in dg. arc. Esodeviations (+) and exodeviations (−).

265

vision at distance was retained until 1980. Then double vision reoccurred and the patient started to wear again his former prism glasses at increasing power. The patient complained now also of crossed diplopia at near vision because of marked convergence insufficiency.

The vertical fusional range was normal. Electronystagmography showed dysmetric saccades with normal velocities, and horizontal left and right gaze nystagmus. The CT scan demonstrated a moderate atrophia of the cerebellar cortex, with enlargement of the fourth ventricle and the cisterna magna.

During the last years of observation the neurological state deteriorated. At the end of observation time, there was a moderate dysarthria and an ataxia of fine hand movements and pyramidal disturbances of his legs developed. The last two years the patient was unable to stand and walk alone. Patients mother and one brother suffered also from the disease. In the brother double vision was a prominent complaint too.

Case 2, a 58 year old female, was first seen in 1975 because of double vision during the last four years. The double vision was of the divergence paralysis type. The angle of the deviation increased during the years of observation (Table 2). ENG showed horizontal gaze nystagmus in right and left lateral gaze, and dysmetric saccades. The saccadic velocity was normal.

During the first visit in 1975 the patient complained of some unsteadiness of walking during the last four years. There was some ataxia of the trunk, but the patient was able to walk and stand without support. The severity of the symptoms worsened during the years of observation. In 1981 there was a moderate dysarthria, an ataxia of the hand, and the patient was only able to walk with a stick. Affected family members were not known.

Case 3.1, female, born in 1917, is one out of three sisters who suffered from the disease. She was first seen in 1975, at the age of 58, because of double vision during the last 15 years. Both the ophthalmological and neurological state did not change remarkably (Table 2) up to 1981. One of the sisters did not complain of double vision. The other sister occasionally noticed diplopia at distance. Both showed an esodeviation in left and right gaze. ENG showed horizontal rebound nystagmus in left and right gaze, and some dysmetric saccades, but normal saccadic velocities in all of them. They complained of unsteadiness during walking. A moderate ataxia of the trunk was present.

Case 3.2, had a slight cerebellar tremor of the hands. In case 3.1 pneumo-encephalography revealed local atrophia of the vermal part of the cerebellum.

Case 4, was seen in 1976 at the age of 66 years. His grandfather, his mother and his three brothers were known to suffer from Marie's disease. Orthoptic examination revealed an esophoria with increasing deviation in right and left lateral gaze (Table 2). The patient did not complain of double vision, and can be considered to be a subclinical case.

DISCUSSION

The six cases which were diagnosed as Marie's cerebellar ataxia showed the typical features of the disease with late onset, slowly progressive ataxia of predominantly walking and standing. The ENG findings: dysmetric saccades, and gaze or rebound nystagmus are known features of cerebellar disease (Dichgans 1968).

The patients were presented because double vision at distance viewing was an early and prominent sign, or because similar ocular motor disturbances were found.

The angle of the deviation increased in some, running parallel with the neurological state of the patients, in others the double vision at distance and the neurological signs remained relatively unchanged. The findings in some cases were in accordance with the diagnosis of divergence paralysis, but in others a slight incomitance was noticed, though without restriction of abduction. Saccadic velocities were normal in all cases as judged by the ENG registrations. This is contrary to Kirkham et al. (1972) who found slowing down of the saccadic velocities in cases of 'divergence paralysis' caused by raised intracranial pressure.

Yet it is unlikely that we deal in our cases with a true divergence paralysis. It would be an attractive idea to find support to Parinaud's original thought for a location of vergence functions in the cerebellum, because cerebellar influence on the vergence system as on other ocular motor systems is hitherto unknown.

The normal vertical fusional range found in our patients does not argue for this idea. A more plausible explanation is a bilateral sixth nerve palsy. The subclinical cases and cases of intermittent double vision can then be explained by an intact (di)vergence function.

Because saccadic velocities were normal, and abduction was not restricted in our patients, the palsies can be presumed to be especially confined to the tonic innervation system which mediates the position of the eyes. Position signals are generated in pontine interneurons and from there mediated to the sixth nerve nuclei. Loss of these interneurons will cause a lower tonic innervation of the abducens nuclei and by this way a lower tonus in the lateral rectus muscles. Slowly degenerative changes in the pons are known amongst other sites in cerebellar ataxia.

Paralysis of divergence was recently reported in spinocerebellar degenerations by Itago (1981).

Divergence paralysis is mostly reported as an acute or subacute acquired syndrome in diseases which may be accompanied with small lesions in the brainstem (as multiple sclerosis, Wernicke encephalopathy, encephalitis, vascular disease of the brainstem, and head injuries) or in raised intracranial pressure (Lippmann 1944, Hogg & Schoenberg 1979). It is known, that raised intracranial pressure may cause functional disturbance in the paraventricular region of the brainstem. So it seems plausible that at least part of these so called divergence paralysis can be explained in the same way by a prenuclear pontine lesion causing loss of tonic position to the sixth nerve nuclei.

ACKNOWLEDGEMENT

We thank the neurologists E.J. Blokzijl and A.E.J. de Jager, the ophthalmologist W.A.D. Ham and the neuroradiologist W.J. Overbeek for the clinical and radiological information about the patients.

REFERENCES

Aita, J.F. Cranial computerized tomography and Marie's ataxia. Arch. Neurol., 35, 55–56 (1978).

Bielschowsky, A. Lectures on motor anomalies of the eyes. III. Paralysis of the conjugate movements of the eyes. Arch. Ophthalmol. 13, 569–583 (1935).

Bories, J., D. Fredy & J. Rosier. Etude tomo-encephalographique des atrophies cérébelleuses. Acta Radiologica Diagnosis, 13, 353–368 (1972).

Burian, H.M. Anomalies of the convergence and divergence functions and their treatment. Symposium on Strabismus. The C.V. Mosby Company, St. Louis (1971).

Dichgans, J. Okulomotorische Störungen bei Kleinhirnerkrankungen. In: Neurophysiologie und Klinik der Augenbewegungsstörungen. S. 235–248. Ed.: G. Kommerell. Bergmann Verlag, München (1978).

Eadie, M.J. Cerebello-olivary atrophy (Holmes type). In: Handbook of clinical neurology, 21, 403–415. Ed.: P.J. Vinken and G.W. Bruyn. North Holland Publ. Comp., Amsterdam (1975).

Eadie, M.J. Olivo-ponto-cerebellar atrophy (Déjérine-Thomas type). In: Handbook of clinical neurology, 21, 415–432. Ed.: P.J. Vinken and G.W. Bruyn. North Holland Publ. Comp., Amsterdam (1975).

Eadie, M.J. Olivo-ponto-cerebellar atrophy (Menzel type). In: Handbook of clinical neurology, 21, 433–450. Ed.: P.J. Vinken and G.W. Bruyn. North Holland Publ. Comp. Amsterdam (1975).

Greenfield, J.G. The spino-cerebellar degenerations. Oxford Blackwell Scient. Publ. (1954).

Hogg, J.E. & B.S. Schoenberg. Paralysis of divergence in an adult with aqueductal stenosis. Arch. Neurol. 36, 511–512 (1979).

Itoga, E. Spino-cerebellar degeneration with divergence paralysis as the earliest sign. Hiroshima Journal of Med. Science, 29, 1055–1061 (1980).

Jampolsky, A. Ocular divergence mechanisms. Trans. Am. Ophthalmol. Soc. 68, 730–822 (1970).

Kirkham, T.H., A.C. Bird & M.D. Sanders. Divergence paralysis with raised intracranial pressure. Brit. J. Ophthalmol., 56, 776–782 (1972).

Le May, M. & Abromoviez. The pneumoencephalographic findings in various forms of cerebellar degeneration. Radiology, 85, 284–290 (1965).

Lippmann, O. Paralysis of divergence due to cerebellar tumor. Arch. of Ophthalmol. 31, 299–301 (1944).

Parinaud, M.H. Paralysie des mouvements associés des yeux. Arch. Neurol., 5, 145–172 (1883).

Authors' address:
T.W. van Weerden
Department of Neurology
University Hospital
Oostersingel 59
9713 EZ Groningen, The Netherlands

ABSENCE OR HYPOPLASIA OF EXTRAOCULAR EYE MUSCLES

Clinical findings and surgical management

W. KONEN & W. RÜSSMANN

(Cologne, F.R.G.)

ABSTRACT

In one patient there was no insertion of the tendon of obliquus superior in sclera but in the Tenon's capsule. The clinical findings and the surgical management are demonstrated. In two patients we found a congenital dysplasie of the right rectus inferior. By looking for the embryological development of the orbit, the eye and the eye muscles we believe, that a deficient insertion of the recti muscles is probably the result of a disturbance in development of the orbit. The normal embryological development of the Tenon's capsule and the muscle sheaths is not influenced by an improper development of the muscles themselves. The long ciliar vessels also develop independently of the extrinsic eye muscles. No complication in form of a anterior necrosis are to be expected, if two additional recti muscles are removed during operation, even if a third recti muscle is missing, because of a congenital defect.

Hypoplasia of extrinsic eye muscle is extremely rare. It has been described by Casten (1940), Pietrowa (1958) and Giller (1962) for the rectus inferior. Combined hypoplasia of the rectus inferior and the rectus lateralis has also been indentified (Posey 1921–23). In 1959 Sousa identified a more extensive malformation, which included the obliquus superior, the rectus superior and the rectus inferior. Absence of eye muscles have also been diagnosed in combination with extensive malformations such as Moebius-syndrom.

The insertion of the rectus muscles is subject to considerable variation. Most of the variation is seen on the tendon of the obliquus superior muscle (De Decker 1977; Kaufmann 1972). We treated two patients, who had had a rectus inferior dysplasia of the right eye, and a third who had had an incorrect insertion of the obliquus superior on Tenon's capsule.

One of the patients, a five year old girl, came to us with classic symptoms of a right-sided obliquus superior parese combined with accommodative esotropia. There was an abnormal retinal correspondence, with correction of +2,0 dpt the visual acuity was 0,7.

Since no insertion of the obliquus superior on the sclera was found during the operation, the rectus superior was removed and the tendon of the obliquus superior was searched for on the medial side of the rectus superior

(Fig. 1). The tendon of the obliquus superior was isolated at last in the Tenon's capsule (Fig. 2). It had only about one fourth of the normal thickness. A histological examination identified the tissue as tendon. This remnant of a tendon was split into two strips, sparing the part next to the trochlear end. The split ends were attached to the sclera respectively 14 and 18 millimeters from the limbus on the temporal side of the rectus superior.

After the operation the function of the obliquus superior was decidedly improved. In a second operation a recession of both interni was performed. Now with bifocal correction there is microtropia.

In two patients we found the symptoms of a rectus inferior parese on the right eye. Both patients demonstrated an exotropia in the prism cover test. The head tilt test showed an increase in right hypertropia, if the head was tilted to the left shoulder. The patient carried his head tilted to the right shoulder in accordance with an incyclotorsion of 14 degrees. Because of a pronounced diplopia in the right field of vision, the patient turned his head 20 degrees to the right.

The third patient depressed his chin only slightly. A torsion was not observed. There was no diplopia. In the lower field of vision the right eye was suppressed.

In analogy to Hummelsheim we transposed one third of the internus muscle to the bottom of the right eye. In this case the operations reduced the incyclotorsion and the exotropia decidedly and the vertical deviation to a lesser degree. The results of the synoptometer measurement are still not satisfactory. But the patient refuses to allow another operation, because he considers his improved field of single binocular vision adequate.

The other patients demonstrated an encouraging improvement of motility

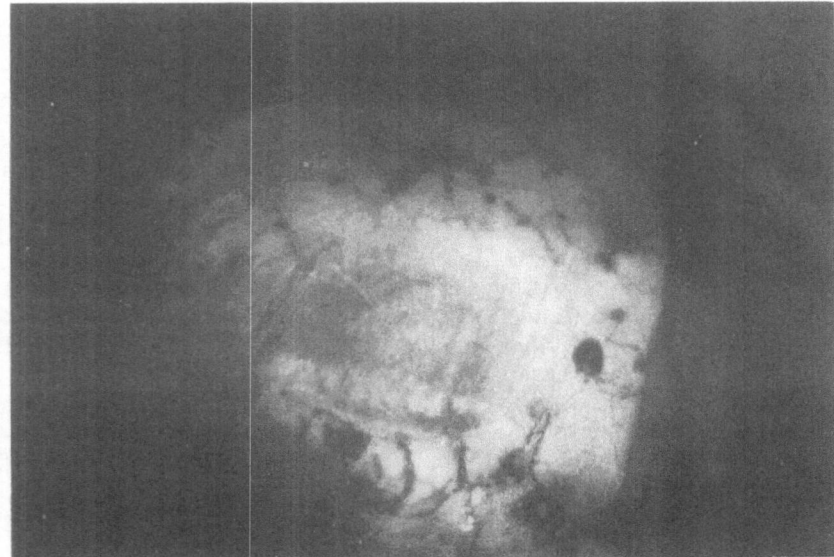

Fig. 1. Sclera after resection of rectus superior. There is no tendon of obliquus superior.

270

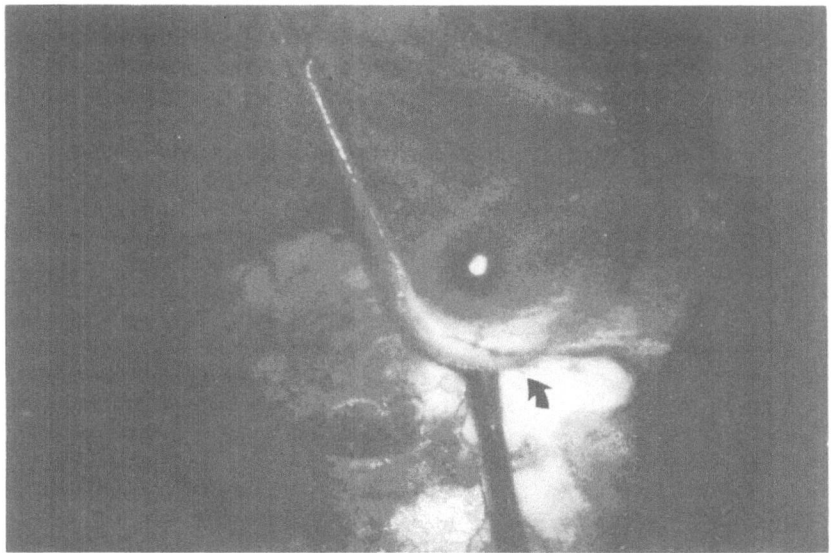

Fig. 2. The tendon of obliquus superior is isolated in the Tenon's capsule (arrow).

after a recession of the right superior rectus, a one third transposition of the internus muscle as above, and a new connection of the inferior muscle sheath to the sclera 6 millimeters from limbus.

The findings made during the operation were the same for both patients. The long ciliary vessels perforated the sclera 6 to 7 millimeters from the limbus (Fig. 3). From the point of perforation the ciliary vessels, lying directly on the sclera, going to the posterior pole of the eye. The vortex veins showed a unusually long intrascleral course. A membrane like a rudimentary muscle sheath could be isolated from Tenon's capsule (Fig. 4). When drawn, it demonstrated an elasticity greater than that of the rest of Tenon's capsule. It lay between the eye and the inferior oblique muscle. A detailed exploration as far as 20 millimeters behind the limbus revealed no muscle tissue. This muscle sheath was attached by the operation to the sclera 6 millimeters from the limbus.

The computer tomography in coronary projection directly behind the equator showed the inferior rectus muscle in the left orbit and in the right orbit an oedema after operation but no trace of an inferior rectus muscle (Fig. 5). Tomographs taken at a deeper level display a smaller orbit on the right and a small (white spot), which probably is the small underdeveloped inferior rectus muscle (Fig. 6).

Congenital paresis may be caused by an anomaly of oculomotor nuclei, or the nerves radiating from them, or by anomalies of the extrinsic eye muscles, their tendons and/or their fascia.

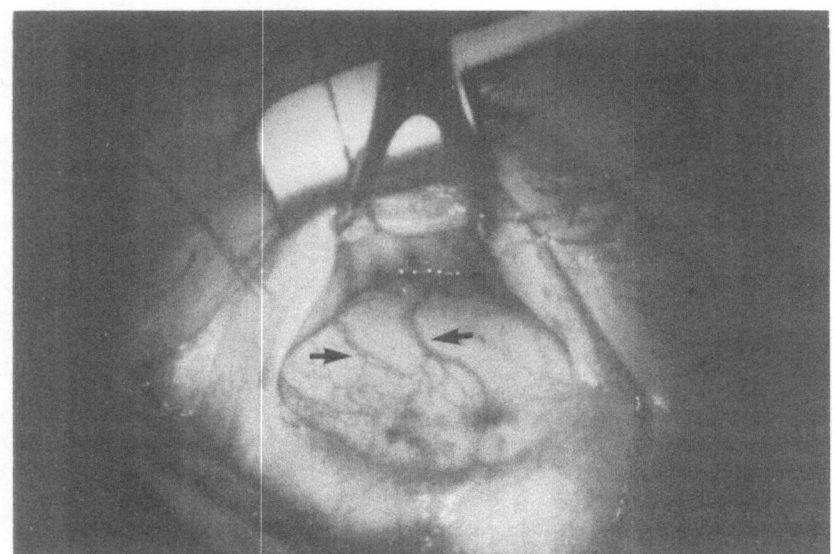

Fig. 3. Sclera after resection of rectus inferior. The long ciliary vessels can be seen (arrows).

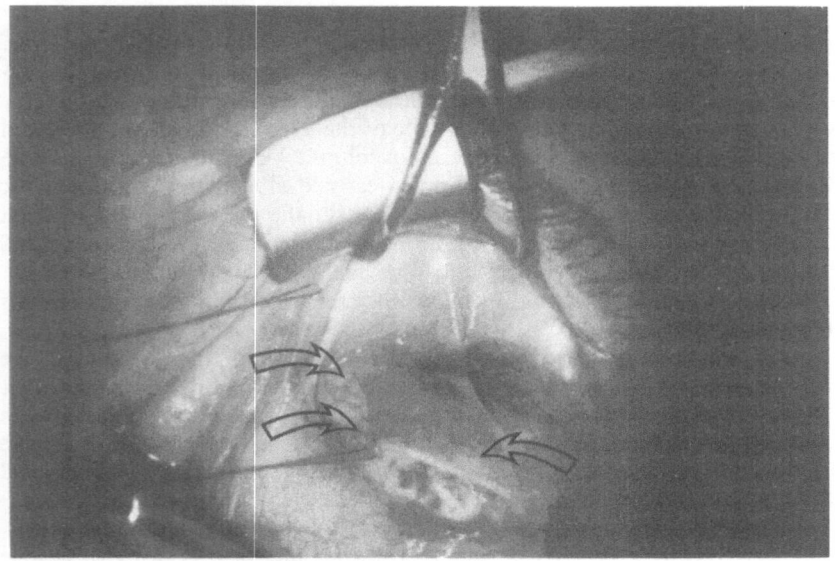

Fig. 4. The arrows shows a membrane like a rudimentary muscle sheath.

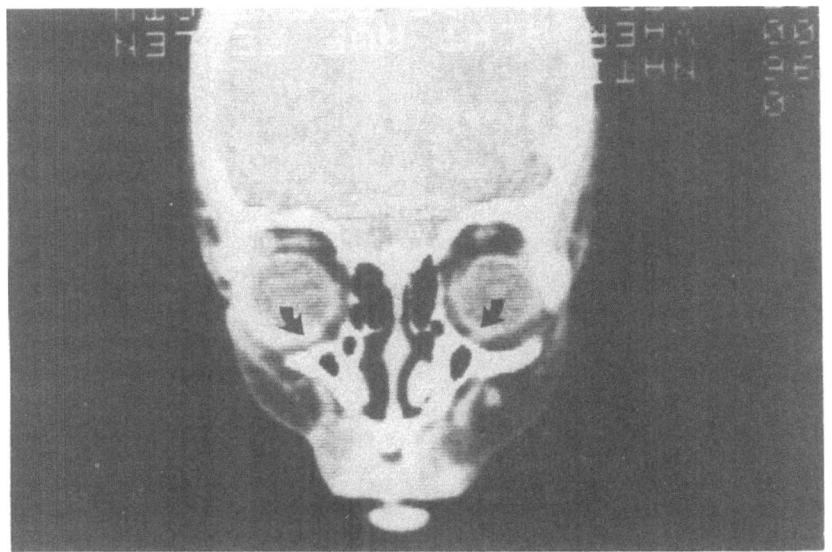

Fig. 5. There is oedema in the right orbit. Only on the left side the rectus inferior is present.

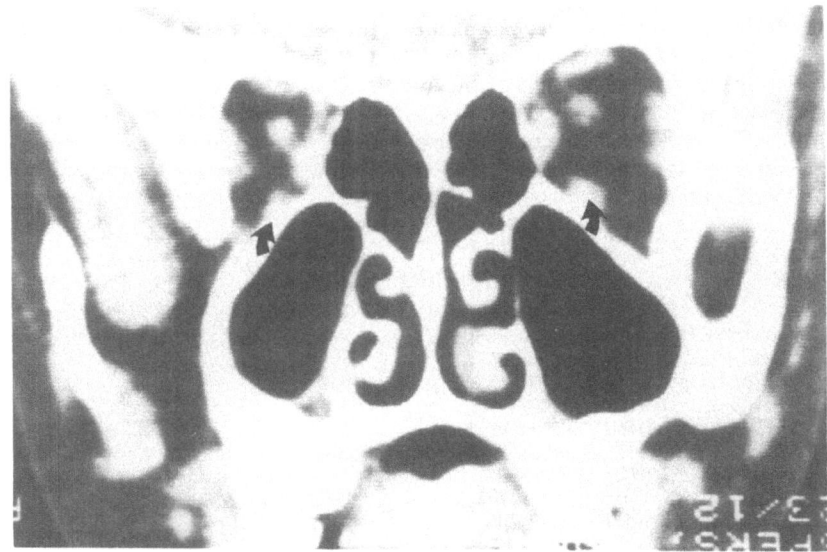

Fig. 6. The right orbit is smaller than the left orbit. There is a rudimentary rectus inferior in the right orbit (arrows).

273

How can these anomalies be explained?

The extrinsic eye muscle, the fascia, the ciliar vessels and the sclera develop from the paraxial mesodermal cells. The development of the extrinsic eye muscles is not caused by induction of the optic vesical. In the fifth to sixth week the paraxial mesodermal cells connect with the cells of the third, fourth, and sixth cerebral nerves and conically surround the optic nerve. The sclera grows from the limbus towards the optic cup. It connects to the mesoderm cells at the later point of muscle insertion. This connection in our cases has been hindered. I believe, that this is due to an incomplete development of the bony orbit by the visceral mesodermal cells, because the development of the bony orbit induces the development of the extrinsic ocular muscles primarily (Duke-Elder 1963).

This connection of the sclera and the mesodermal cells is critical, as the great number of anatomical variations by the muscle insertion shows.

The development of the muscle sheaths and Tenon's capsule takes place in the third month, also beginning at the limbus and going back to the orbit. The presence of the eyemuscle for the development of the muscle sheaths is not absolutely necessary. In our case there is a normal Tenon's capsule and a rudimentary muscle sheath.

The development of the long ciliar vessels depends on the presence of sclera. They develop independently of the recti muscles, under which they normally lie.

CONCLUSION

That means that a deficient insertion of the recti muscles is probably the result of a disturbance in development of the orbit. The normal embryological development of the Tenon's capsule and the muscle sheaths is not influenced by an improper development of the muscles themselves. The long ciliar vessels also develop independently of the extrinsic eye muscles. No complication in form of an anterior necrosis are to be expected, if two additional recti muscles are removed during operation, even if a third recti muscle is missing, because of a congenital defect.

REFERENCES

Casten. Arch. Ophthal. (Chicago)., 24, 55 (1940).
Pietrowa. Klin. oczna., 28, 209 (1958).
Giller. Arch. Ophthal., 68, 182 (1962).
Posey. Amer. J. Ophthal., 4, 524 (1921).
Sousa. Arch. port. Oftal., 11, 61 (1959).
De Decker, W. & H. Conrad. In: Augenbewegungstörungen: Symposion der DOG. p. 111—116 (1977).
Kaufman, H. & M. Kluxen. Klin. Mbl. Augenheilk., 160, 710 (1972).
Duke-Elder. System of Ophthalmology Volume III Part 1: p. 211—231 (1963).

Authors' address:
University Eye Hospital
Cologne, F.R.G.

POSTERIOR FIXATION SUTURE IN NONCOMITANT SQUINT

Round Table Discussion

PARTICIPANTS: CRONE (CHAIRMAN), DE DECKER, DELLER, FELLS, FROSINI, KAUFMANN, KOORNNEEF, PECHEREAU

Crone: We'll start this round table conference on the myopexy, the Faden operation. Well, I hope you will understand me, my mastery of the English is not so very great. I would have liked to ask an Englishman, a real Englishman, but the Faden operation is a very continental affair. Nevertheless, I am glad the invited speaker of this morning, Mr. Fells, is with us.

It is ten years ago that Cüppers first proposed this type of operation. I think he did not start with the Faden operation, but with a similar procedure. He pointed out with much emphasis that what were usually called weakening operations, recessions, were actual not weakening operations. In the same way strengthening operations were actual not strengthening operations, but adjustments to reposition the globe in another position.

If you really want to weaken a muscle, you have to do something more. I think, if my memory does not leave me in the lurch, that he started by proposing recession and resection in the same muscle to lessen the arc of contact.

In any case that type of operation was the first real weakening operation. Afterwards Cüppers changed his procedure into the myopexy, because in his view this procedure could be undone more easily. Of course this whole idea of the Faden operation, of weakening certain muscles, is an extremely logical idea. Because the basis is, that they could create an artificial paresis, just as Mr. Deller has formulated so well. With this method you do not only perform a surgery of the angle of deviation, but you really do a surgery of the direction of gaze.

Now, the reason for this round table discussion is this. While ten years have passed there are still very few quantitative data available about the efficacy of this operation, of this principle. What happened is that thousands of Faden operations have been done, and it became a very popular operation in several countries, but not in incomitant squint for which it was originally used and designed, on the contrary for concomitant squint. The operation was performed with the magic formula that it helped against variable angles, and that it helped against presumed blocking of nystagmus. It was supposed to work against what was called innervational factors. In the meanwhile, the original aim of the operation, to combat incomitance by creating another balancing incomitance, was more or less forgotten. This means that, from thousands of operations, there are many reports about the effect on

Docum. Ophthal. Proc. Series, Vol. 32, ed. by A.Th.M. van Balen & W.A. Houtman 275
© *1982, Dr W. Junk Publishers, The Hague. ISBN 90 6193 728 0*

convergence and so on, but very few about the effect on lateral gaze. I think that it is quite another topic than we are going to discuss here.

We have had the paper of Dr. Deller, which was quite straight forward in this point. We had two in itself very interesting papers, one of Frosini and one of Pechereau, who talked about Faden in comitant squint. Both were interesting. Frosini offered a surgical alternative to the Faden operation, and that means that he was not completely happy, evidently, with the result of the Faden operations, the technical results. The paper of Pechereau, who also spoke about Faden operations in concomitant squint was very interesting because he discussed possible failures, possible causes of failure of this myopexy. The paper of Mühlendyck, read by Kaufmann (we are very sorry that Mühlendyck is not here), and of De Decker dealt with paretic squint. That is also true for Koornneef's paper – perhaps not on paretic squint, but in any case on strongly incomitant squint. Well, there are many questions about these Faden operations. There is one to Dr. De Decker, and I suppose Dr. De Decker will also be able to answer the second.

This is to Dr. De Decker: 'Would you elaborate on the fact that you put your Faden or your posterior fixation suture on the lateral rectus muscle as far back as 19 mm. from the insertion?'. The other question is: 'How do you perform your Faden on the lateral rectus? There is the inferior oblique muscle. So it is difficult to put in place the suture without damaging the inferior oblique'.

De Decker: The second question is the easier one. The inferior oblique indeed is in the most cases in our way, so we cut it and refix it again. Do not try to compromise with that muscle staying there, but cut it away, and refix it when the attachment of lateral rectus is done.

The other question deals with the enormous amount of 19 mm on the lateral rectus. The length of the medial rectus within the orbit is much shorter than the length and the arc of contact of the lateral rectus (Fig. 1). Comparing it with 13 to 14 mm on a medial rectus, we can achieve an equal amount of artificial palsy by attaching the lateral rectus 17 to 19 mm behind its insertion. The measurement depends also on the size of the globe, but unless you reach an amount like this, you will achieve no effect. Does this answer the question?.

Crone: Yes, I fully agree that the arc of contact is about 6 to 7 mm longer. There is the other question – how do you attach the muscle so far backward without interfering with the insertion of the inferior oblique?

De Decker: I answered that first. We cut the muscle off its insertion and refix it later. I should add that it is surprisingly easy to go on with the posterior fixation itself, as there is a lot of space. My coworker, Dr. Krarup, has demonstrated here on Monday at the orbital part of the meeting that almost all muscular traumas enter the orbit from temporal, as there is space. As we can enter the orbit here without difficulties, it is easier to perform 19 mm on the lateral rectus than 14 mm on the medial rectus. It sounds very difficult, only, as many surgeons have never done it in practice.

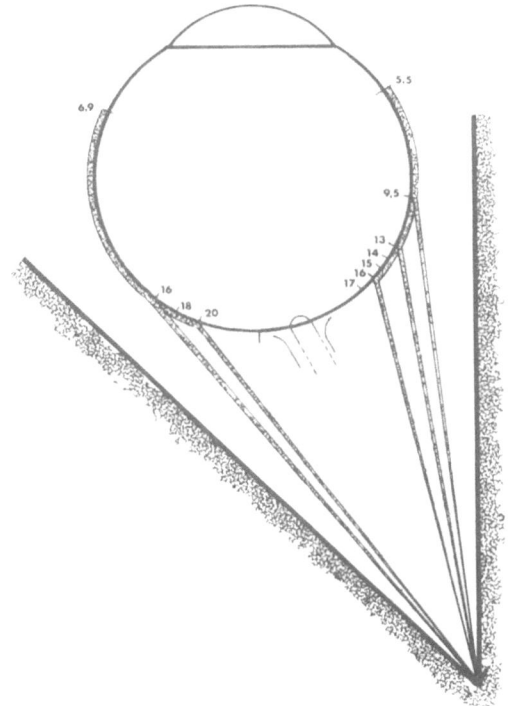

Fig. 1.

Crone: I agree with that. But I have the experience that even if you go as far back as possible, still the limitation of abduction is not as large as you would have expected. I tried to do it in a case of unilateral internuclear ophthalmoplegia, in a unilateral case. But the results were very unsatisfactory, yes, very poor.

Crone: Then we have a question to Dr. Deller. 'In case of superior oblique muscle palsy, you suggest Cüppers' Faden operation on the contralateral inferior rectus. What would you do in isolated inferior or superior rectus palsy?'. That is the first question. Then a second also addressed to you: 'I do not agree with your statement that the Faden operation creates a restitutio ad integrum'.

Deller: In order not to give too simple a reply, and to avoid the trend towards using one single language, I should prefer to answer in French.

It is evident that in cases of isolated palsies of the superior and inferior rectus muscles, which are very rare, for anatomical reasons the principle of compensatory surgery cannot be obeyed. This principle was formulated for the most frequently occurring palsies, those of the superior oblique and

277

lateral rectus muscles. I think that at least the majority of surgeons who use the retroequatorial myopexy will agree that this aspect of surgery cannot be usefully applied to the oblique muscles.

In the case of a superior rectus muscle palsy, a weakening procedure of the opposite inferior oblique muscle as proposed by Von Graefe — a recession, myotomy or myectomy — is appropriate as a first operation. In cases of isolated inferior rectus palsy I prefer a resection of this same muscle to a weakening procedure of the superior oblique muscle in order to avoid disturbing the binocular vision in downward gaze.

As to the second question, I would say that it is a problem of nomenclature. There is not an anatomical restitutio ad integrum, but rather a clinical restitutio. I mean by this a clinical recovery, in that double vision is removed in a particular direction of gaze. It is evident that in certain cases, where there is a complete lack of muscle action, one will reduce the excursions of both eyes in the direction of the underlying muscle paralysis. This is however of minor importance. We know that the eye movements do not usually exceed an amplitude of 15 degrees. After surgery, it is rare that the excursion be less than 15 degrees.

Crone: Thank you very much. A question to Mr. Kaufmann. Dr. Kaufmann demonstrated selected cases. Do you have data about the relation between the place of the Faden and its effect.

Kaufmann: It is exactly, what I said yesterday. I specified, how large the angle-reduction is following various amounts of the Cüppers-procedure. This study referred to a patient collective with non accommodative convergence-excess. The results showed a good correlation between the amount of posterior fixation suture and the reduction of the angle at distance and near-fixation.

Crone: Yes, thank you. I do not think perhaps that is the meaning of the question, because we are now talking on incomitant squint and the question can also be interpreted otherwise. Do you have data on the effect on the incomitant squint? How much artificial paresis can you create in degrees with a Faden of so many millimeters?

Kaufmann: Well, I have tried to apply the already mentioned results to cases of incomitant squint, that is, to compare the duction-excess of the sound eye with the convergence excess of comitant squint. Naturally, paretic cases are more inhomogeneous than comitant cases and therefore until now I have no definite statistical data. I am certain, that there is a correlation between amount and effect of posterior fixation suture also in paretic strabismus.

Crone: We all postulate that there is a relation between the distance of the Faden and the effect on incomitance. You don't have data because the number of patients is not large enough. Dr. Koornneef has no data because the number of cases is not large enough. Do you, Dr. De Decker, have data about that?

De Decker: I think so, but it is hidden in the information of my paper, in which the amount of Fadenoperation compared with the stabilization of changing angles has been shown. To answer your question it may be better to review 2 slides which we have seen before. Fig. 2 shows the increasing effect of a Fadenoperation (averaged from 6 patients by my coworker Dr. Conrad). Fig. 3 has been demonstrated by Prof. Kaufmann who has read Prof. Mühlendyck's paper. Mühlendyck's slide shows, following an idea, Cüppers has presented recently, that the degree of underaction of a paretic muscle can be plotted easily by recording the increasing overaction of the contra-

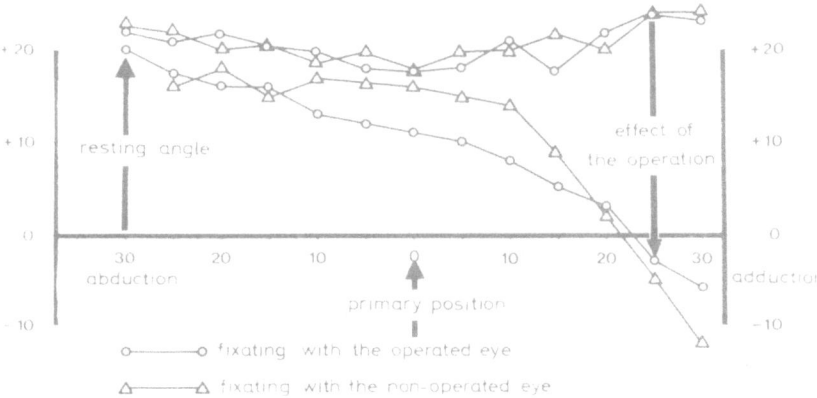

Fig. 2.

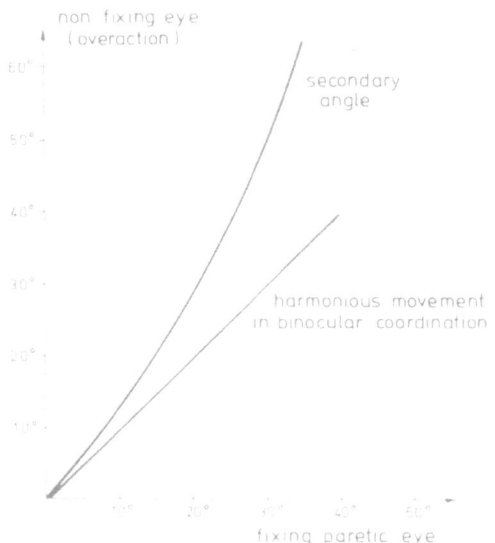

Fig. 3.

lateral synergistic muscle. Dr. Conrad's profile of action of a Fadenoperation shows the same type of exponential curve.

If we would be able to perform the Fadenoperation on the yoke muscle to an amount, which would create an artificial palsy of the yoke muscle with a slope that exactly compensates for the overactions of this muscle, then this would solve the problem. In my opinion it should be possible to collect the average effects of Fadenoperations on normal muscles, from 11 to 16 mm, and to compare the shape of these curves with the profile of the overaction (increasing secondary angle). This is a useful work, which should be done in the next years.

Crone: We continue with some other interesting things. Here is a question to Dr. Koornneef: 'How far does the superior oblique muscle interfere with a Faden operation on the superior rectus muscle?'. This is a question for an anatomist, I think.

Koornneef: I think it is dependent on how far you put your sutures and how the tendon of the superior oblique is actually moving back on the eye. As you know from the work of Fink, there is a considerable variation in the direction of the tendon of the superior oblique muscle. So I believe, while you are doing a Faden operation on the superior rectus muscle, you should always locate the superior oblique tendon, and try to avoid it. On the other hand, in our material we found that, doing Faden operations on the superior rectus muscle, it might even influence the action of the superior oblique.

If the superior oblique muscle tendon is not properly dissected out a Faden operation of the superior rectus might interfere with this insertion and consequently with its action.

Kaufmann: I propose in such cases to alter the position of the tendon of the superior oblique muscle and rectus muscle, that is, that after the procedure the rectus muscle rests upon the eye ball and the oblique muscle lies upon the rectus muscle. This technique guarantees after a large recession or a posterior fixation suture of the rectus muscle the unhampered mobility of the oblique muscle.

Crone: I am sure the myopexy does interfere with the superior oblique, so it is not a bad idea.

Crone: I have a question to Frosini. 'Why do you use fascia lata — an organic substance — and why don't you use plastic substance for their minor tissue reactions for the procedure of muscle lengthening?'. It is not a question exactly on the Faden operation, but it is about an alternative operation.

Frosini: I have some difficulty to choice the language, now. I should like to answer in French, for not letting alone my colleague Dr. Pechereau.

The use of fascia lata to lengthen a muscle was suggested by Professor Focosi, who used it first. The use of this organic material may be justified by the manner in which it is received by the host. In the beginning some cases

280

were reoperated because of over and undercorrections. It could be demonstrated by histological examination that nearly all the material was replaced by collagen that strongly resembled that of the host. It was also found in our cases that the muscle tissue and the fascia lata grow together perfectly. The fascia lata was fixed to the sklera very well on the place of needling, but there were no adhesions between the new tendon and the sklera. That's why we continued to use the material. The procedure allows to keep up the arc of contact. That is the aim of the procedure, that is different from that of the posterior fixation suture. I'll hope that at the next meeting in Florence, we will have the opportunity to discuss the results of this procedure and to compare them with those of others who used this type of operation. Perhaps data of electrophysiological methods will be presented and be available to compare the results.

Crone: Thank you very much. Now there is a question to Mr. Fells. Is there still place for a Hummelsheim operation in an abducens paralysis, since the Faden operation has been introduced?

Fells: I think that there are alternative methods for producing abduction besides the Hummelsheim procedure. I have tried to show that this morning and the reasons for them. The two operations that I have used so far are temporal transfer of the whole of the vertical recti in younger patients, and the Jensen procedure in older ones. With the Carlson-Jampolsky method we use half of the superior and half of the inferior rectus so that we are being as safe as we can with the blood supply and combine this with the advantages of the adjustable suture. It is in this modified form only that I think the Hummelsheim procedure may still have a place.

Crone: I thank you very much. I may say that my orthoptist Mrs. Everhard, has reviewed 20 cases of abducens paralysis. With Faden operation of the internal rectus muscle of averagely, I think, 12 or 13 mm, we found a decrease of incomitance at the 25 degree excursion of eleven degrees. But as in almost all our cases, there is a large spread, there is very little predictability of the effect in relation to the place of the suture.

Crone: I have a question to Mr. Pechereau. Dr. Koornneef reported about overcorrections and he wonders why you found only undercorrections. Please, can you explain that?

Pechereau: Only in cases of undercorrection we reoperated on the muscles which underwent a posterior fixation suture. And not in cases of overcorrection.

Crone: I am the only one who did not answer any question. I'll take the two easiest questions. 'Has any study been performed to determine if the stretching of a muscle due to the suture has any effect on the angle of deviation? That is to say that, if you stretch too much, you will get an adverse effect?' The answer is no, but in principle you would add a kind of resection to the myopexy.

The other question is: 'I would expect that every posterior fixation suture would require a recession of the same muscle, to avoid increase of tension in the rest position, because you elongate the way between the origin and the insertion of the muscle'.

Well, if that were true, then of course, you would always have to do a recession. But I think both effects, the one described in the first question and the other described in the second question, will more or less cancel out each other. The general idea is, and it is true in all of my cases, that the effect of the posterior fixation suture in the primary position is more or less negligible.

Well, those were the questions. I intended a kind of peroration, and to summarize the problem, but time does not permit that. Thousands of Faden operations have been performed in cases of comitant squint. I do not know whether future ophthalmologists will believe in the 'blocking syndrome' and its panacea, the Faden. The principal aim of this discussion was to emphasize the value of retroequatorial myopexy in the disorder for which it was originally designed: incomitant strabismus.

AUTHOR INDEX